# Cajal's Butterflies of the Soul

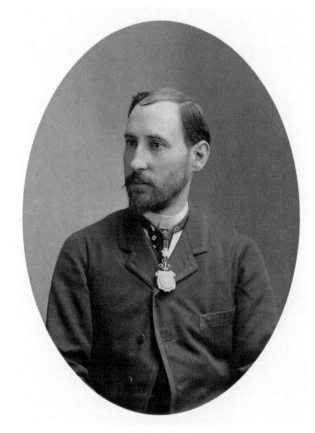

There can be no doubt, only artists are attracted to science [. . .]. I owe what I am today to my boyhood artistic hobbies, which my father opposed fiercely. To date, I must have done over 12,000 drawings. For a profane man they are strange drawings, the details of which are measured in thousandths of a millimetre although they reveal mysterious worlds emanating from the architecture of the brain. . .

*Santiago Ramón y Cajal, 1900*[*]

[*] Cajal at the age of 42 years. This paragraph was taken from an interview given by Cajal to a journalist in 1900 (María de los Ángeles Ramón y Cajal Junquera; *Cajal, Artista*, in *Paisajes Neuronales. Homenaje a Santiago Ramón y Cajal*. Madrid: CSIC, 2007).

# Cajal's Butterflies of the Soul

## SCIENCE AND ART

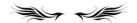

JAVIER DEFELIPE, PhD

INSTITUTO CAJAL (CSIC)
MADRID, SPAIN

OXFORD
UNIVERSITY PRESS
2010

**OXFORD**
UNIVERSITY PRESS

Oxford University Press, Inc., publishes works that further
Oxford University's objective of excellence
in research, scholarship, and education.

Oxford  New York
Auckland  Cape Town  Dar es Salaam  Hong Kong  Karachi
Kuala Lumpur  Madrid  Melbourne  Mexico City  Nairobi
New Delhi  Shanghai  Taipei  Toronto

With offices in
Argentina  Austria  Brazil  Chile  Czech Republic  France  Greece
Guatemala  Hungary  Italy  Japan  Poland  Portugal  Singapore
South Korea  Switzerland  Thailand  Turkey  Ukraine  Vietnam

Published by Oxford University Press, Inc.
198 Madison Avenue, New York, New York 10016
www.oup.com

Oxford is a registered trademark of Oxford University Press

Library of Congress Cataloging-in-Publication Data
DeFelipe, Javier.
Cajal's butterflies of the soul : science and art / Javier DeFelipe.
p. ; cm.
Includes bibliographical references and index.
ISBN 978-0-19-539270-8
1. Nervous system—Histology—History.   2. Neuroanatomy—History.   3. Neurosciences in art—History.
4. Medical illustration—History.   I. Ramón y Cajal, Santiago, 1852-1934.   II. Title.   III. Title: Butterflies of the soul.
[DNLM: 1. Nervous System—Pictorial Works. 2. Medical Illustration—Pictorial Works.
3. Neurology—history. WL 17 D313c 2010]
QM451.D34 2010
611'.01898—dc22
2009015442

The copyright for the Cajal's drawings and photographs is held by the Herederos de Santiago Ramón y Cajal. The copyright for the
drawings and photographs of Fernado de Castro pertains to the Archive Fernando de Castro. The images obtained from Cajal's
preparations and some figures from old illustrations, pictures, and documents were obtained from the Cajal Museum (Cajal Institute,
CSIC, Madrid). Some of the remaining figures were kindly supplied by the authors, or they were obtained from private collections as
indicated in the figure legends. The editors and the author have done everything possible to identify the owners of the copyrights of
the original illustrations reproduced in this book. We apologize for any possible error or omission in this sense and where such cases
come to light, these errors or omissions will be rectified immediately in subsequent editions.

9 8 7 6 5 4 3 2
Printed in the United States of America
on acid-free paper

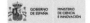

For my wife Alicia and my daughter Alicia

To know the brain—we said to ourselves in our idealistic enthusiasm—is equivalent to discover the material course of thought and will. [...] Like the entomologist hunting for brightly coloured butterflies, my attention was drawn to the flower garden of the grey matter, which contained cells with delicate and elegant forms, the mysterious *butterflies of the soul*, the beating of whose wings may some day (who knows?) clarify the secret of mental life. [...] Even from the aesthetic point of view, the nervous tissue contains the most charming attractions. In our parks are there any trees more elegant and luxurious than the Purkinje cells from the cerebellum or the *psychic cell*, that is the famous cerebral pyramid?

Santiago Ramón y Cajal,
*Recuerdos de Mi Vida*

On January 11, 1907, Amalio Gimeno (Minister for Public Instruction and Fine Arts) created the Council for Extension of Studies and Scientific Research by ministerial decree ("Junta para Ampliación de Estudios e Investigaciones Científicas," or JAE). This institution was created to end Spain's cultural and educational isolation and in an attempt to bring Spain up to the level of the most advanced European countries at the time. For this ambitious project to succeed, it was felt that the JAE must be presided over by the most relevant scientists. Hence, it was evident that Santiago Ramón y Cajal should be appointed as the first president of the JAE, with the collaboration of José Castillejo as its Secretary. The scientific and cultural program implemented by the JAE represented the most innovative project in Spain between 1907 and 1939, involving the creation of laboratories and research centers, awarding scholarships to study abroad, etc. In addition, it also brought leading Spanish thinkers and scientists into contact with those in other countries and continents, thereby opening up a new way of bringing people together through science and culture. The JAE pursued various goals, such as enabling students to undertake their higher studies in Spain and abroad, sending delegations to scientific conferences, establishing an overseas information and international relations service on issues concerning teaching, promoting scientific research, and protecting educational establishments involved in secondary and higher education. However, in the midst of the Spanish Civil War, on May 19, 1938, the JAE was shut down, its laboratories and centers were closed, and many of its scientists fled to exile. In 1939,

Franco's newly installed regime created the Spanish National Research Council ("Consejo Superior de Investigaciones Científicas," or CSIC) in the JAE's laboratories, premises, and centers. The CSIC was presided over by the Minister for Education, José Ibáñez Martín, with the close collaboration of José María Albareda, who was appointed Secretary General of the CSIC. The law passed on November 24, 1939 to create the CSIC established that "all the centres belonging to the dissolved Council for the Extension of Studies and Scientific Research (JAE), the Foundation for Scientific Research and Reform Trials, and those created by the Spanish Institute, would become part of the Spanish National Research Council."

We are very proud that Cajal, whom we truly consider to be our first President, is now considered the father of modern neuroscience and that he serves as an example for young scientists through his many teachings and scholarly approach to the study of the most enigmatic and attractive organ in the human being, the brain. Thus, it is with great pleasure that we participate in the production of this marvellous book, not only because it represents an excellent opportunity to commemorate the figure of Cajal but also because this book contains a fantastic collection of old illustrations. We are confident that these amazing drawings will serve as both an inexhaustible source for artistic inspiration in general and as a way to divulge and increase the interest in research into the nervous system.

Rafael Rodrigo
*President of the CSIC*
*Madrid, May 2009*

The Universidad Politécnica de Madrid (UPM; Technical University of Madrid) is the oldest and largest of the Spanish technical universities, covering most of engineering and architecture disciplines. Most of its schools are over 100 years old, dating back to the eighteenth and nineteenth centuries, and they existed independently until they were grouped together as the UPM in 1971. Hence, it is no exaggeration that much of the history of Spanish technology for over 150 years has been written by the Schools of Architecture and Engineering of this university, as for many years some of them were the only technical schools in existence in their fields in Spain. Indeed, many of the leading Spanish educators and researchers have been involved with the UPM either as students, teachers, or both.

Recently, the UPM has opened new avenues for research, which include expanding our particular interest in neuroscience, since unravelling the complexity of the brain from all possible scientific angles (morphological, genetic, molecular, physiological, and computational) represents the most ambitious and major challenge in science for many years. We think that an important starting point has been the implication of the UPM in the Blue Brain Project, which represents the first comprehensive, worldwide effort to reverse engineer the structure and function of the brain's components. The main aim of this project is to better understand the normal function and dysfunction of the brain through detailed simulations. The participation of Spain in this project constitutes the so-called Cajal Blue Brain, which involves several research groups belonging to various public research institutions.

The Cajal Blue Brain project was born with the idea of combining our expertise, long tradition, and resources in informatics and computational sciences with the excellent Spanish tradition in the field of the neuroanatomy that dates from Santiago Ramón y Cajal. Indeed, thanks to the school and the pioneering work of Cajal, renowned scientists and professionals have travelled worldwide and contributed to the remarkable advances in neurobiology. Thus, we would not only like to promote this research but to go a step further, embarking on the first large-scale attempt to unravel the complexity of the cerebral cortex at nanometer resolution through a multidisciplinary approach and employing new techniques. The development of these methods will open up new horizons and opportunities to examine the nervous system in general, both in health and disease, at a level of detail never reached before. Therefore, we are very pleased to participate in the production of this gorgeous book, not only as a tribute to Cajal but also as a further expression of our interest in developing new perspectives and tools to bridge neurobiology and computational neuroscience.

Javier Uceda
*President of the Universidad Politécnica of Madrid*
*Madrid, May 2009*

The *Fundación Centro de Investigación de Enfermedades Neurológicas* (*Fundación CIEN*; "Neurological Diseases Research Center Foundation") is a public institution in Spain supervised and coordinated by the *Instituto de Salud Carlos III*, a public research institution that pertains to the Ministry of Science and Innovation. The *Fundación CIEN* was created to endorse and organize a research network that supports, promotes, and coordinates research in all fields of neuroscience, including basic, clinical, and epidemiological issues, paying special attention to problems related to diseases of the nervous system. It is organized in such a way that research teams distributed across Spain are coordinated into scientific groups working on different areas of the neurosciences in order to not only share ideas and techniques but also the facilities provided by the *Fundación CIEN*. The foundation also manages the Center for Neurodegenerative Diseases within the Biomedical Research Network, which includes 63 research groups in Spain and around 800 investigators. In addition, it manages the Alzheimer's Project Research Unit, which is part of a new hospital dedicated primarily to the care of patients with Alzheimer disease.

Diseases of the brain affect the whole spectrum of society, with potentially devastating psychiatric and neurological consequences. The increase in age of our society is accompanied by an increase in the risk of developing brain diseases such as Alzheimer disease. Indeed, this disease is close to being considered a true worldwide pandemic problem. Vast resources have been invested around the world to fight this condition, such as the creation of the *Fundación CIEN*, although this still appears to be insufficient given the magnitude of the problem. Unfortunately, our society is not fully aware of the importance of studying the brain, perhaps due to the small amount of scientific information that reaches the general public in an effective manner. Thus, another important objective of the foundation is related to teaching and informing the public on issues related to neurological sciences. This wonderful book, where neuroscience and art are fused, represents a magnificent opportunity to bring the mysterious world of the brain to the general public. The work not only contains a beautiful collection of old drawings, but it also includes introductory information that will give readers unfamiliar with the nervous system a better understanding of the importance of the scientific illustrations produced in the early days of research into the nervous system. As a consequence, we decided to collaborate and to help make this project a reality from the very moment we became aware of the book. Furthermore, the book represents another good excuse to pay tribute to the father of modern neuroscience, Santiago Ramón y Cajal. Indeed, one of Cajal's masterpieces, his book *Estudios Sobre la Degeneración y Regeneración del sistema nervioso* (1913–1914), represented a major starting point in the battle against brain diseases. Thus, the *Fundacion CIEN* enthusiastically supports this book, since it represents an excellent tool to draw society's attention to the problems of the nervous system. We are confident that readers will be captivated by the beautiful illustrations in the book and that this will aid their introduction to the brain's complex neuronal jungle. No doubt, our society, and the scientific community in particular, must make an effort to better understand the brain in health and disease. Such efforts are not only motivated by the fact that the brain represents the essence of our humanity but also because it is the root of many frightful diseases for which we presently do not have a satisfactory solution. We hope that this book may serve to strengthen our resolve in the fight against brain diseases.

Julián Pérez
*Managing Director of the Fundación CIEN*
*(Instituto Salud Carlos III)*
*Madrid, May 2009*

ONCE UPON A TIME, the scientists who studied the microscopic world of the nervous system had to be true artists in order to communicate their observations. Indeed, if we go back to the nineteenth century, when the detailed analysis of the nervous system began, microphotography was not a well-developed technique. As a consequence, most scientific figures presented by the early neuroanatomists were their own drawings, providing a valuable "pretext" for those scientists to express and develop their artistic talent. Of course, the scientists did not reproduce the entire field of the histological preparations they observed through the microscope, but rather, they only illustrated those elements they thought were important for what they wanted to describe. As such, these illustrations were not necessarily free of technical errors and they may have been subject to the scientists' own interpretations, at times hindering their acceptance by their fellow scientists. Nevertheless, this interpretation of the image also represented an interesting source of artistic creativity. During this period the exchange of information between scientists was difficult, not least because some of these drawings were considered to be essentially artistic interpretations rather than accurate copies of the histological preparations. Indeed, this issue also makes it difficult for us to interpret some of these figures today. As a result, this period of scientific "art" and skepticism constitutes a fascinating page in the history of neuroscience. In the present book, we have included a total of 339 figures, most of which date from 1859 to 1932 and represent some characteristic examples of this golden era for artistic creativity in neuroscience.

It should be noted that the illustrations included in this book represent only a small sample of the thousands of figures that were produced during this period. Indeed, each time I discovered a beautiful figure, as if unearthing a hidden treasure, the feeling of joy that came over me was mixed with a sense of frustration…how many beautiful pictures had I still yet to see! Of course, I have not been able to go through all the articles and books of the time, yet perhaps this book will encourage other scientists to continue this quest for the hidden beauty in the neural forests once created by our old masters, many of which have been lost in our memory with the passing of time. In addition, only selected figures have been included due to space limitations and this selection reflects my own interests, which may not be fully shared by other readers. Nevertheless, I think this book will be of general interest, not only due to the captivating aesthetic appeal of the illustrations but also because they represent the bases of our current understanding of the nervous system. Indeed, in the words of Santiago Ramón y Cajal (1852–1934, **Fig. P-1**), in most cases they are "pieces of reality":

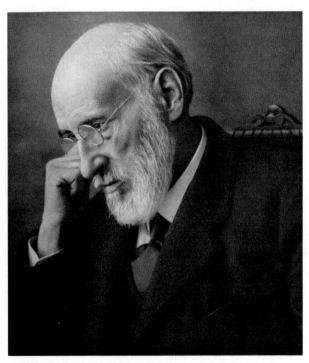

**FIGURE P-1.** Santiago Ramón y Cajal (1852–1934), 1920. Taken from Santarén JF (2006) Cronología 1852–1934. In *Santiago Ramón y Cajal. Premio Nobel 1906*, ed. J. F. Santarén. Madrid: Sociedad Estatal de Conmemoraciones Culturales.

A good drawing, like a good microscope preparation, is a fragment of reality, scientific documents that indefinitely maintain their value and whose study will always be useful, whatever interpretation they might inspire.

*Santiago Ramón y Cajal, 1899*

Fernando de Castro (1896–1967) (**Fig. P-2**), one of the most prominent disciples of Cajal, commented: "Science becomes art through the drawings of Cajal." Looking at the illustrations in this book, the readers will not only marvel at Cajal's drawings but will also find that many of the other early researchers that studied the nervous system were also true artists, of considerable talent and aesthetic sensibility.

These artistic skills were also shared by de Castro and Pío del Río-Hortega (1882–1945, **Fig. P-2**), as well as by other famous disciples of Cajal and many other important pioneers in neuroscience, including Deiters, Kölliker, Meynert, Ranvier, Golgi,

Retzius, Dogiel, and Alzheimer (**Fig. P-3**). Indeed, I was impressed by the wonderful, mostly unknown drawings of de Castro and del Río-Hortega. It is for this reason that I have included numerous drawings by these two great scientists and artists. The reader will find that many of the illustrations can be considered to belong to different artistic movements, such as modernism, surrealism, cubism, abstraction, or impressionism. Indeed, these illustrations may also provide artists with a source of inspiration since they reveal a fantastic and virtually unknown world of forms, a microuniverse with an aura of mystery. The coming together of the fields of art and science was beautifully explained by Cajal in an interview given by him to a journalist in 1900 (María de los Ángeles Ramón y Cajal Junquera; *Cajal, Artista*, in *Paisajes Neuronales. Homenaje a Santiago Ramón y Cajal*, Madrid: CSIC, 2007):

There can be no doubt, only artists are attracted to science [...]. For a profane man they are strange drawings, the details of which are measured in thousandths of a millimetre although they reveal mysterious worlds emanating from the architecture of the brain...

Another interesting aspect of the book is that many of the illustrations are virtually unknown to both young neuroscientists and to the general public alike. Indeed, the books and journals where these figures were originally published are frequently very hard to find or of limited access, making the present book all the more attractive. I would like to caution the reader that I have restrained from attempting to explain these figures in detail (with a few exceptions), as they cover many diverse fields of neuroscience. Instead, each image is accompanied with a title based on the description given by the original author, and I have identified its source to enable the readers interested in a particular figure to satisfy their curiosity regarding the significance of these early figures. The original labeling used to describe the illustrations has been preserved and, where possible, so have the original descriptions. Many of these figures have been retouched and restored in order to remove stains, wrinkles, or

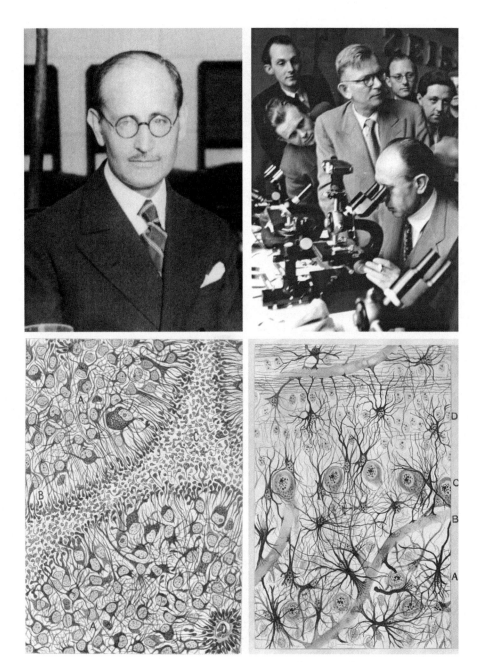

FIGURE P-2. (*Left*) Pío del Río-Hortega (1882–1945). (*Right*) Fernando de Castro (1896–1967), looking through the microscope at the Congress of Wiesbaden held in 1950 (Archivo Fernando de Castro). *Drawings*: *(left)* Del Río-Hortega (1922), (*right*) de Castro (1920). Del Río-Hortega P (1922) Constitución histológica de la glándula pineal. I. Células Parenquimatosas. In *Libro en honor de D. Santiago Ramón y Cajal*, Vol 1. Madrid: Jiménez y Molina, pp 315–359; de Castro F (1920) Estudios sobre la neuroglia de la corteza cerebral del hombre y de los animales. I. La arquitectonia neuróglica y vascular del bulbo olfativo. *Trab. Lab. Invest. Biol. Univ. Madrid* 18, 1–35.

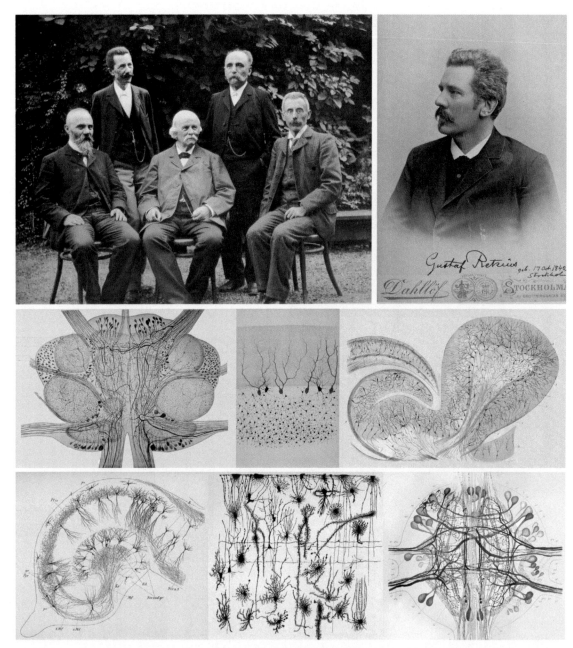

**FIGURE P-3.** (*Top left*) From left to right, first row: Giulio Bizzozero (1846–1901) and Camillo Golgi (1843–1926); second row, Edoardo Perroncito (1847–1936), Rudolf Albert von Kölliker (1817–1905), and Romeo Fusari (1857–1919). Courtesy of Paolo Mazzarello, University Pavia. (*Top right*) Magnus Gustaf Retzius (1842–1919) (Legado Cajal). *Drawings* (from left to right and up to down): Taken from Retzius G (1891) Zur Kenntniss des centralen Nervensystems der Crustaceen. *Biol. Untersuch. Neue Folge* 1, 1–50; Golgi C (1882–1883) Sulla fina anatomia degli organi centrali del sistema nervoso. *Riv. Sper. Freniat. Med. Leg.* Reprinted in *Opera Omnia*, Vol I. *Istologia Normale*, Chapter 16. Milano: Ulrico Hoepli, 1903; Fusari R (1887) Untersuchungen über die feinere Anatomie des Gehirnes des Teleostier. *Internat. Mschr. Anat. Physiol.* 4, 275–300; Kölliker A von (1893) *Handbuch der Gewebelehre des Menschen*, Vol II. *Nervensystem des Menschen und der Thiere*. Leipzig: Engelmann; Retzius G (1894) Die Neuroglia des Gehirns beim Menschen und bei Säugethieren. *Biol. Untersuch. Neue Folge* 6, 1–28; Retzius G (1891) Zur Kenntniss des centralen Nervensystems der Würmer. *Biol. Untersuch. Neue Folge* 2, 1–28.

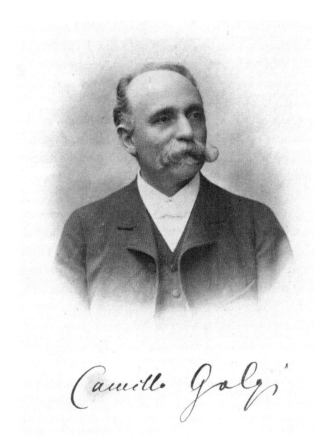

**FIGURE P-4.** Camillo Golgi (1843–1926). Taken from Golgi, C. *Opera Omnia*. Milano: Ulrico Hoepli, 1903.

other artifacts, and some of them are reproduced from original drawings.

The book has been divided into two Parts, Part I and II, the latter containing the main body of the work. Part I contains introductory information, including a general description of neurons and glia that will give readers unfamiliar with the nervous system a better understanding of the importance of the scientific illustrations produced in those days. This part also contains a section that refers to the methods used and the issues surrounding the interpretation of microscopic images through drawings in that period. However, the main section in Part I is titled "A Sketch History of the Microscopic Anatomy of the Nervous System," and this chapter has been divided into three sections that serve as an introduction to the three subdivisions established in Part II.

The second part of the book, Part II, contains the collection of 288 figures with the intention of transforming the reader into an observer. These illustrations have been divided into three main categories: Section 1, The Benedictine Period: The Early Days; Section 2, The Black Period: Neurons, Glia, and the Organization of the Nervous System; and Section 3, The Colorful Period: Internal Structure and Chemistry of the Cells. These titles are explained in Part I. Section 1 includes early figures of the nervous system before the discovery of the "*reazione nera*" (black reaction) by Camillo Golgi (1843–1926, **Fig. P-4**). In the hands of Cajal, this technique represented the principal tool that was to change the course of the history of neuroscience, signifying the birth of modern neuroscience. Section 2 is related to the Golgi method and other techniques used to analyze the morphology of neurons and glia, as well as the microanatomy, organization, and meaning of different regions of the nervous system (e.g., the pattern of connections between neurons, and the relationship between neurons and glia). The techniques to visualize the peripheral terminals of afferent and efferent nerve fibers are also included here. Indeed, some of these images show the structure and micro-organization of the nervous system as true maps, identifying the routes followed by nerve impulses through the intricate neural forest of the brain. Section 3 is mainly concerned with the internal structure of the cell body of neurons and glia revealed by a variety of staining procedures to visualize the nucleus and nucleolus, as well as the organelles present in the perikaryon. The first set of illustrations are not necessarily the oldest figures because, despite the years that passed since Golgi published this method in 1873, it was still not a commonly used technique when Cajal initiated his studies of Golgi-stained material in 1888. The second and the third sets of illustrations mostly coincide in time. Moreover, these illustrations not only deal with the normal nervous system but also with the alterations observed in the naturally diseased nervous system (e.g., Alzheimer disease), or after infection, trauma, and exposure to other external factors.

Many figures and particularly those dealing with the internal structure of the neuron also illustrate the response of neurons when experimental animals are manipulated in some way (e.g., their response to injury, electrical stimulation, or the toxic effects of chemical substances). The text included in Sections 1 and 2 of Part I are mainly based on articles on the history of the neuron, and they refer to the scientific atmosphere in Cajal's times. These articles were either published by myself (some of them in Spanish), or they were prepared in collaboration with Edward G. Jones. In addition, Section 3 not only deals with the early methods to selectively label the internal structure of the neurons or different histological aspects of the nervous system (in different colors), but it also contains a summary of how "multicolor microscopy" has evolved to date.

In producing this book, I am very grateful to the members of my laboratory: Lidia Alonso-Nanclares, Lidia Blázquez-Llorca, Ruth Benavides-Piccione, Isabel Fernaud, Ana García, Virginia García-Marín, Juncal González, Asta Kastanauskaite, Shira Knafo, Ángel Merchán, Paula Merino, Miguel Miguens, Alberto Muñoz, and José Rodrigo-Rodríguez, for their comments on the structure of the book and the figures, for their support, and for maintaining the laboratory at work while I was occupied in the preparation of the book. I would like to especially thank Ruth Benavides-Piccione and Alberto Muñoz for their criticisms on the text, and Ana Garcia for helping me with the scanning of the original drawings and in preparing the figure legends. The retouching of the images was largely done by myself, with much assistance from Roberto Rives.

I am deeply indebted to the publishers and the other organizations that have offered their support in producing this book: Oxford University Press, CSIC, Universidad Politécnica of Madrid, and Fundación CIEN /Instituto de Salud Carlos III. I would also like to express my gratitude to Mark Sefton for his editorial assistance and to María de los Ángeles Langa, librarian at the Instituto Cajal, for her help in obtaining some of the very inaccessible books and articles from which I obtained many of the figures presented here. I am also grateful to the granddaughters of Cajal, María de los Ángeles Ramón y Cajal Junquera and Silvia Cañadas, and to the son and grandson of Fernando de Castro, Fernando-Guillermo de Castro Fernández and Fernando de Castro Soubriet, respectively, for allowing us to use some of Cajal's and de Castro's original drawings and pictures. I also wish to thank Inigo Azcoitia, Ruth Benavides-Piccione, Marina Bentivoglio, Miguel Freire, Pablo García, Virginia García-Marín, Laurence Garey, Asta Kastanauskaite, Antonio Martín-Araguz, Paolo Mazzarello, Alberto Muñoz, Jorge Larriva-Sahd, Jeff Lichtman, Constantino Sotelo, and Tamily Weissman for kindly supplying or preparing some of the figures included in the book. I would like to extend my gratitutde to Craig Allen Panner (Executive Editor, Neuroscience and Neurology of Oxford University Press), Rafael Rodrigo, Miguel Ángel Puig-Samper, and Jose Manuel Prieto (President, Chief Editor, and Director of the Department of Publications of the CSIC, respectively), Javier Uceda and Gonzalo León (President and Vice President for Research, of the Universidad Politécnica of Madrid, respectively), and Julián Pérez (Managing Director of the Fundación CIEN/Instituto Salud Carlos III) for their enthusiastic support and help of this project.

Javier DeFelipe
*Madrid, April 2009*

PART I

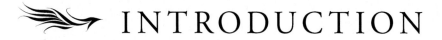 INTRODUCTION

My work began at nine o'clock in the morning and usually lasted until around midnight. Most curiously, my work caused me pleasure, a delightful intoxication, an irresistible enchantment. Indeed, leaving aside the egocentric flattery, the garden of neurology offers the investigator captivating spectacles and incomparable artistic emotions. In it, my aesthetic instincts were at last fully satisfied.

*Santiago Ramón y Cajal, Recuerdos de Mi Vida*

# Introductory Remarks

Santiago Ramón y Cajal (1852–1934) is considered the father of modern neuroscience for providing the first detailed analysis of the nervous system (DeFelipe, 2002a; **Fig. F-1**). Thus, we have honored his name in the title of this book, even though the figures contained in the main body of the text were composed by 95 different authors.

Cajal's studies and theories had a profound impact on the researchers of his era. He published almost 300 articles and several books of great importance, such as the classics *Textura del Sistema Nervioso del Hombre y de los Vertebrados* (Ramón y Cajal, 1899–1904) and *Estudios Sobre la Degeneración y Regeneración del Sistema Nervioso* (Ramón y Cajal, 1913–1914). He also received numerous awards and distinctions (**Fig. F-1 right and F-2, left**), including some of the most prestigious awards of his time: the Moscow Award (1900); the Helmholtz Gold Medal (1905); and the Nobel Prize for Physiology or Medicine (1906), which he shared with Camillo Golgi (1843–1926), the renowned Italian scientist who discovered the *reazione nera* (see "The Discovery of the *Reazione Nera*" in Section 2) and the organelle he defined as the "internal reticular apparatus" that was later called the Golgi apparatus (Bentivoglio, 1999). Over the years, Cajal has also received many tributes, such as the homage during the NASA Neurolab space flight mission in 1998 (**Fig. F-2, right**). The inclusion of "butterflies of the soul" in the title of this book refers

to one of Cajal's favorite topics: the human neocortex and the most common neuron in the cerebral cortex, the pyramidal cell that he sometimes poetically named butterflies of the soul. In his book *Recuerdos de Mi Vida*, he wrote the following paragraph when he started studying the cerebral cortex:

I felt at that time the most lively curiosity—somehow romantic—for the enigmatic organization of the organ of the soul. Humans—I said to myself—reign over Nature through the architectural perfection of their brains [...]. To know the brain—we said to ourselves in our idealistic enthusiasm—is equivalent to discovering the material course of thought and will. [...] Like the entomologist hunting for brightly coloured butterflies, my attention was drawn to the flower garden of the grey matter, which contained cells with delicate and elegant forms, the mysterious *butterflies of the soul*, the beating of whose wings may some day (who knows?) clarify the secret of mental life. [...] Even from the aesthetic point of view, the nervous tissue contains the most charming attractions. In our parks are there any trees more elegant and luxurious than the Purkinje cells from the cerebellum or the *psychic cell* that is the famous cerebral pyramid?

*Ramón y Cajal, 1917*

Throughout the nineteenth and early twentieth centuries, neuroscience is marked by two

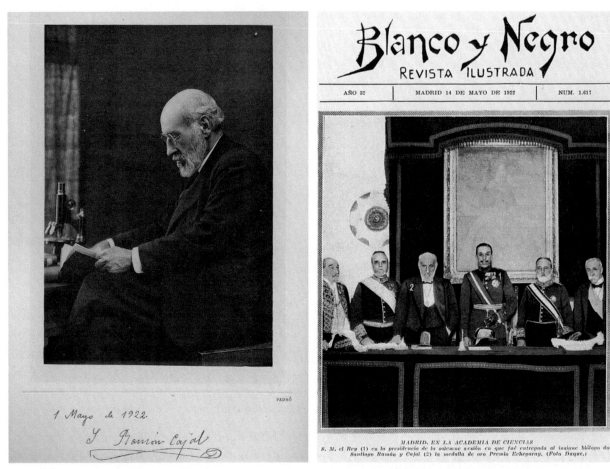

**FIGURE F-1.** (*Left*) Santiago Ramón y Cajal (1852–1934). (*Right*) Cover of the magazine *Blanco y Negro* (1922) to illustrate the award of the Echegaray Medal to Cajal at the Academia de Ciencias Exactas, Físicas y Naturales (Madrid), in the presence of His Majesty the King of Spain Alfonso XIII (1886–1941).

milestones: the developments in light microscopy and anatomical methods, and the progress made in localizing particular brain functions. Nevertheless, many of the ideas regarding functional localization, and in particular those related to mental attributes, have now been proven wrong. However, these studies were fundamental not only for the development of our present ideas on the function and physiology of the brain. From a structural point of view, anatomists began to consider that it might be possible to explain functional specialization through structural specialization (**Figs. F-3 and F-4**).

The nervous system is made up of two main classes of specialized cells: neurons and neuroglia (or simply glial cells as I shall refer to them in the remaining text). The function of the brain, and of the

nervous system in general, depends on the connections between neurons that are established through complex and specialized structures named synapses. These connections are organized into intricate networks or neuronal circuits, and they utilize electrochemical signals and neurotransmitters that are packed into small vesicles (synaptic vesicles) located in the presynaptic side of the synapse. In addition, close anatomical and functional coupling exists between neurons, glia, and blood vessels (see section, "The Beauty of the Nervous System: Neurons and Glia").

As the reader will see, neurons and glia are arranged so that they constitute a true forest. Indeed, some types of neurons, like the pyramidal cells of the cerebral cortex (**Fig. F-5a**) and the Purkinje cells of the cerebellar cortex (**Fig. F-5b**)—the most

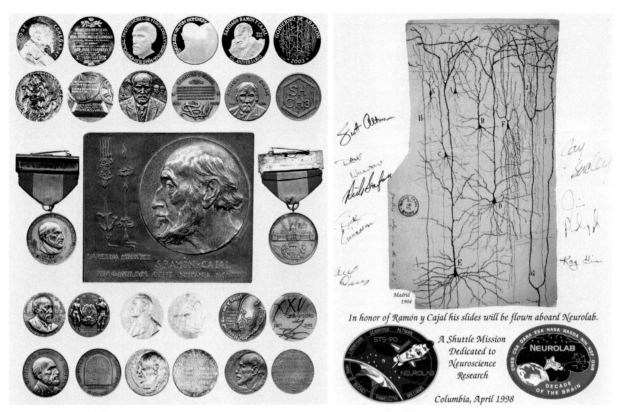

**FIGURE F-2.** (*Left*) Photograph showing a plaque and some medals that Cajal received in recognition of his studies. The images of the medals were kindly supplied by Pere Berbel (Instituto de Neurociencias, Alicante). (*Right*) Copy of one of the nine drawings of Cajal that traveled aboard the Space Shuttle Columbia as a tribute to him during NASA's Neurolab mission. The signatures are those of the crew members: Scott D. Altman, Jay C. Buckey, Richard M. Linnehan, Kathryn P. Hire, James A. Pawelczyk, Richard A. Searfoss, and Dafydd Rhys Williams. Neurolab was a NASA research mission to study how the nervous system responds in microgravity, a fundamental question for future long-duration space flights. Neurolab was born when the U.S. President declared the 1990s the Decade of the Brain, and NASA proposed the Neurolab mission as its contribution to this dictate. Other international space agencies also participated in the Neurolab mission. The seven-member crew were not only involved in various experiments with animals (rats, mice, fish, snails, and crickets) aboard the Space Shuttle Columbia, but they were also themselves subjected to a number of sophisticated biomedical studies. The Shuttle was launched on April 17, 1998 and landed on May 4, 1998 at the Kennedy Space Center in Cape Canaveral, Florida. The Shuttle reached an altitude of around 320 km above the planet's surface and traveled at a speed of approximately 7.5 km per second. Since the Shuttle orbited the earth every 92 minutes, during the 16-day spaceflight there were 16 sunsets and 16 sunrises every 24 hours. Accordingly, the Shuttle completed a total of 256 orbits around the earth.

characteristic neuronal type in the cerebellum—look like trees and due to their density and arrangement they constitute a thick forest (see the drawing in the center of **Fig. F-3**).

This is why Cajal and other scientists often referred to trees and forests in their descriptions of the brain and, in particular, of the cerebral cortex. Another beautiful example is the following comment from Cajal regarding cortical plasticity:

> The cerebral cortex is similar to a garden filled with innumerable trees, the pyramidal cells, which can multiply their branches thanks to intelligent cultivation, send their roots deeper and producing more exquisite flowers and fruits every day.
>
> *Ramón y Cajal, 1894*

These neuronal forests have served as an unlimited source of artistic and poetic inspiration to many scientists. Indeed, **Figure F-6** is an artistic illustration showing a mysterious object, the brain, arising through the mist and emerging from the entangled branches of the trees that are condensed into an enchanted neuronal forest.

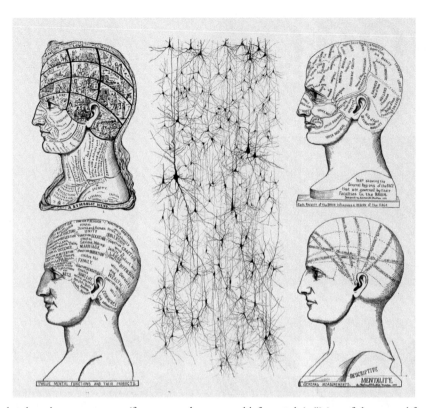

**FIGURE F-3.** Left and right columns represent (from top to bottom and left to right): "Map of the mental faculties"; "Twelve mental functions and their products"; "Each faculty of the brain influences a region of the face"; and "The measurements of the mentologist." Taken from Holmes W. Merton (Merton, H. W. *Descriptive Mentality from the Head, Face and Hand*. Philadelphia: MacKay, 1899). In the center is a drawing of the human cerebral cortex stained with the Golgi method and taken from Rudolf Albert von Kölliker (Kölliker, A. von. *Handbuch der Gewebelehre des Menschen*, 6th ed, vol II, first part. *Nervensystem des Menschen und der Thiere*. Leipzig: Engelmann, 1893). The ideas on the localization of brain functions inspired scientists to carry out comparative histology studies to investigate whether any structural peculiarities in the human cerebral cortex might explain specific human behaviors.

Pío del Río-Hortega (1882–1945; **Fig. F-7**), one of Cajal's outstanding disciples, wrote the following marvelous paragraph describing the relationships between neurons, glia, and blood vessels:

> In the landscape of the brain there are endless irrigation canals—blood vessels—and on their banks the bush-like cells—glia—collaborate in nerve function.

> *Del Río-Hortega, 1933*

It is interesting to note that trees have also served as artistic symbols to describe biblical texts, which on occasion mention cognitive alterations. In **Figure F-8**, King Nebuchadnezzar II of Babylon (sixth century BC) is shown with dementia and eating grass "like the beasts in the field"; his walking "on all fours" refers to the extreme bending of his trunk (camptocormia) due to his parkinsonism associated with Lewy body disease. As a main theme in the illustration, a tree is shown whose trunk represents the kingdom with its inhabitants, the birds in their branches (Martín-Araguz, 2006). Here, we can also imagine a charming bridge between literature, artistic drawings, and neuroscience (compare **Figs. F-5b** and **F-8**).

Another artistic example of these early scientists is again from Cajal himself. Indeed, he was a master of bringing together science and art not only through his drawings but also through his photography. In fact, he was a pioneer in the development of color photography (Ramón y Cajal, 1912; **Fig. F-9**).

In **Figure F-10** we can see two interesting photographs taken by Cajal himself. On the left of the

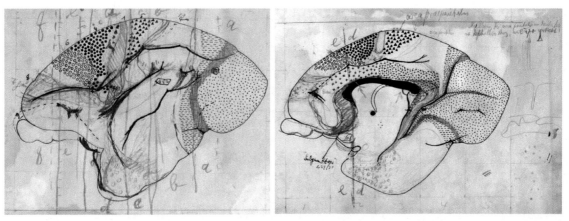

**FIGURE F-4.** Drawings by Korbinian Brodmann (1868–1918) showing the lateral (*left*) and medial (*right*) aspects of the brain of a prosimian lemur, with stippling of the various cortical areas. Brodmann was one of the great German neurologists in an exciting period at the turn of the twentieth century when the neuronal theory was only just coming to the fore. He is best known for his "maps" of the cerebral cortex, which are still commonly used today, and especially that of the human cortex first published in 1908 in the *Journal für Psychologie und Neurologie* as well as that from the following year in his famous monograph *Vergleichende Lokalisationslehre der Grosshirnride* (translated by Laurence Garey as *Localization in the Cerebral Cortex*, third edition. New York: Springer Science Business Media, Inc., 2006). Brodmann's printed black-and-white maps are reasonably well known, but it is rare to find copies of his original hand-drawn color figures. Brodmann undertook a study of the prosimian brain for his "Habilitation" thesis, which was surprisingly rejected by the Berlin Medical Faculty, although this drawing became Figure 98 in his 1909 monograph. The text and drawing are provided by Laurence Garey, with thanks to Marc Nagel (http://www.korbinian-brodmann.de/).

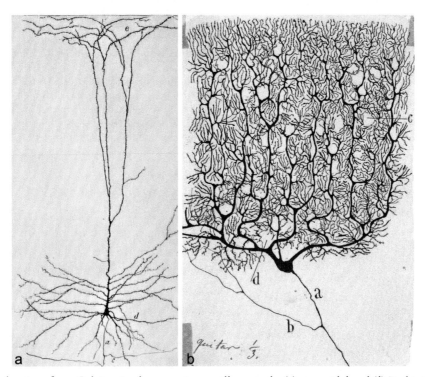

**FIGURE F-5.** Cajal's drawings from Golgi-stained preparations to illustrate the (*a*) pyramidal and (*b*) Purkinje cells in the human cerebral cortex and cerebellum, respectively. In (*a*), "a," "c," "d," and "e" indicate axon, collaterals, long basal dendrites, and terminal [dendritic] tuft, respectively. In (*b*), "a," "b," "c," and "d" indicate axon, recurrent collaterals, holes occupied by capillaries, and holes occupied by basket cells, respectively. These figures were reproduced in *Textura del Sistema Nervioso del Hombre y de los Vertebrados* (Cajal 1899–1904, figures 689 [*left*], and 10 and 365 [*right*]).

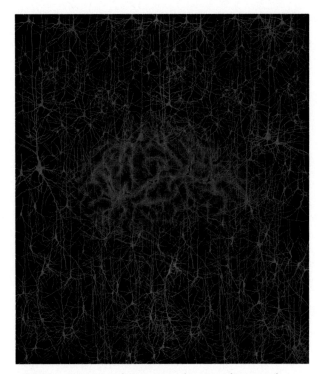

**FIGURE F-6.** Artistic composition showing a brain in the center that seems to be generated by the condensation of neurons (see text for further details).

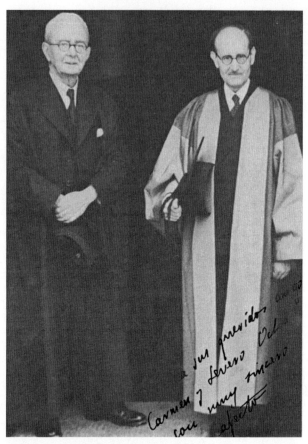

**FIGURE F-7.** Picture of Pío del Río-Hortega (1882–1945, *right*) when he received the honorary degree Doctor *Honoris Causa* from the University of Oxford. (*Left*) Charles Sherrington (1857–1952). This picture was dedicated to Severo Ochoa (1905–1993) and his wife Carmen García Cobián. Sherrington and Ochoa were awarded the Nobel Prize in Physiology or Medicine in 1932 and 1959, respectively.

figure Cajal is looking through a microscope, while on the right his daughter Paula is posing in a colorful dress with a basket of flowers. My interpretation of this photograph is that Cajal wants to tell us that science and art can coexist. The picture on the right seems to me as if Paula were like an angel or a muse of scientific inspiration.

Cajal also inspired poets like Juan Ramón Jiménez (1881–1958; Nobel Prize for Literature in 1956; **Fig. F-11**), who in his book *Españoles de Tres Mundos* wrote:

> I saw him once in a tram, a long afternoon that rained full and blind, putting on his reading glasses through his silver hair, forgotten, leaning against the glass window, and that was how he remained, staring leisurely, abandoned and melancholic, into the horizon.
>
> *Ramón-Jiménez, 1942*

In line with this poetic prose is the picture taken by Cajal himself in 1915 showing some trams in the Puerta del Sol, Madrid (**Fig. F-11**, *right*).

## THE BEAUTY OF THE NERVOUS SYSTEM: NEURONS AND GLIA

In the nervous system there are billions of neurons and even more glia (at least 10 times more). As the reader will see under the section "A Sketch History of the Microscopic Anatomy of the Nervous System," the discovery of the neuron has a long, fascinating history in which many researchers have participated up to the present day. Of course, glial cells are fundamental elements of the nervous system, and the history of these cells is tightly linked to that of the neuron. However, in the present book we shall only deal with these cells in a superficial manner. In general, neurons consist of a

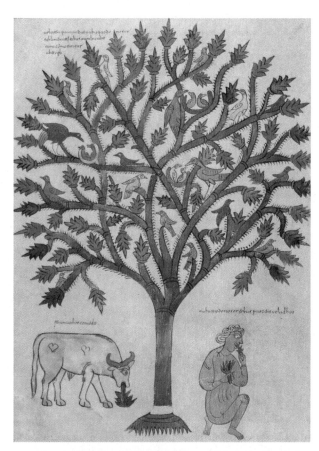

**FIGURE F-8.** This figure was taken from a Beato, a manuscript with miniatures from the tenth to thirteenth century, which contains comments by the Abbot Beato de Liébana (eighth century) on the Apocalypse and additions of various exegetic texts like the Commentary on the Book of Daniel of Saint Jerome. This miniature belongs to the Mozarabic Beato of San Miguel de Escalada (León, Spain), the work of the monk Maius in the tenth century. The tree is cut at its base showing the risk for the kingdom caused by the disease of King Nebuchadnezzar II (Martín-Araguz, 2006). King Nebuchadnezzar II, also called Nebuchadnezzar the Great, is mainly known for the conquest of Judah and Jerusalem, and for the construction of the Hanging Gardens of Babylon.

cell body or soma (usually 10–20 μm in diameter) that gives rise to several processes, of which only one forms the axon (0.5–2.0 μm thick) while the remainder form dendrites (1–5 μm thick). Neurons adopt a considerable variety of shapes and sizes, as well as many patterns of dendritic and axonal arborization (**Fig. F-12**). Glial cells are characterized by their relatively small soma (5–10 μm of diameter), which emit several thin (0.5–1.0 μm) and short processes that branch locally. There are two

major classes of glia: macroglia (astrocytes and oligodendrocytes) and microglia. The astrocytes are subdivided into protoplasmic and fibrous, while oligodendrocytes are subdivided into interfascicular and perineuronal satellites (**Fig. F-13**).

As for axons, they adopt one of two general designs: *(1)* axons that only branch near the cell body from which they originate, such that neurons with this kind of axon are named interneurons or short-axon cells (**Fig. F-12**, *right*); *(2)* axons that leave the region where the cell body of origin is located, and these cells are known as projection neurons (**Fig. F-12**, *left*). In this case, the axon can travel over enormous lengths, which can often be in the order of several millimeters or even meters (for example, pyramidal cells projecting to the spinal cord in large mammals like the giraffe). Furthermore, the axon of projection neurons frequently gives rise to collaterals along its trajectory and, in turn, these collaterals can give rise to local axonal arbors that may be located near to or a distance from the cell body of origin (**Fig. F-12**, *left*). As an example of the richness of dendritic and axonal arborization and of the complexity of the organization of the nervous system, it has been estimated that there are approximately 3 km and 400 m of axonal and dendritic length, respectively, and an average density of 90,000 neurons per mm$^3$ in the mouse cerebral cortex (Schüz and Palm, 1989). Furthermore, the brain is one of the organs of the body with the highest metabolic demands, and thus, there is a very dense network of blood vessels in association with the neurons and glia.

The exchange of information between neurons mainly takes place through two types of highly specialized structures: chemical synapses (the majority) and electrical synapses. The space between the cell bodies of the neurons, glia, and blood vessels—the neuropil—is occupied by a very dense network of axonal, dendritic, and glial processes. In the neuropil there is a high density of synapses, and, for example, there are approximately $1000 \times 10^6$ synapses per mm$^3$ of neuropil in the human temporal cortex. Indeed, the neuropil represents between 90% and 98% of the volume of the cerebral cortex (Alonso-Nanclares et al., 2008). Thus, the main problem when analyzing the

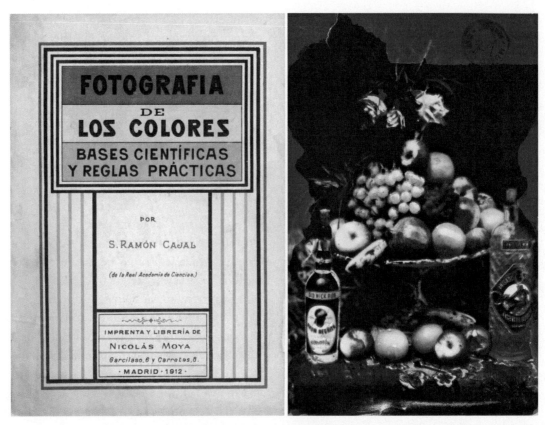

**FIGURE F-9.** (*Left*) Cover of Cajal's book *Fotografía de los Colores*, 1912. (*Right*) Cajal's photograph, a still life in color with flowers, fruit, and bottles (trichrome procedure on paper, 1907). Taken from María de los Ángeles Ramón y Cajal Junquera: *Cajal, Artista*, in *Paisajes Neuronales. Homenaje a Santiago Ramón y Cajal* (Madrid: CSIC, 2007).

nervous system is its extreme complexity, particularly in higher vertebrates (**Fig. F-14**).

Thus, throughout the history of neuroscience, scientists have sought to develop appropriate methods to analyze different aspects of the structure and function of the nervous system. Some of these methods were discovered at random, whereas others were designed to resolve a given problem. Nevertheless, the development of science not only depends on the methods available but also on the ways they are exploited. Thus, there are examples of methods that were available to scientists but that were not fully exploited until an individual made an important discovery or an astute interpretation that generated new concepts. This was the case of the Golgi method, which remained unexploited for many years before Cajal entered the scene to change the course of the history of neuroscience (DeFelipe, 2002a, 2006;

Jones, 2006; also see heading under Section 2 in this volume, "Cajal's First Study with the Golgi Method: Dendrites and Axons End Freely").

## A NOTE ON THE ILLUSTRATIONS

At the beginning of the nineteenth century and for several decades afterward, microphotography was not a well-established technique to study histology. Certainly, several types of microphotography accessories were available for light microscopy at that time, some of which were very sophisticated (**Fig. F-15**), but good techniques of microphotography had not yet been developed. Thus, obtaining high-quality microscopy images, particularly high-power microphotographs, was a difficult task. Moreover, the structure of the nervous system is very complex and the selective staining methods used, such as the Golgi method, do not define all

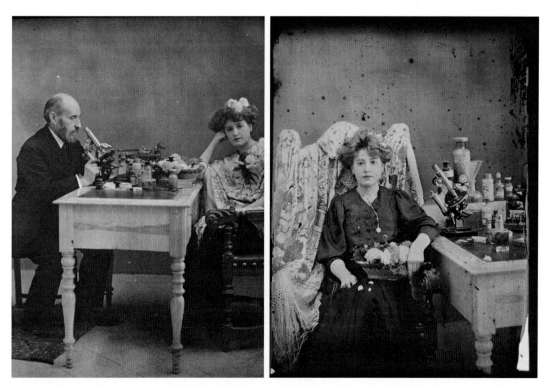

**FIGURE F-10.** Photographs taken by Cajal of himself and his daughter Paula. From the private collection of Silvia Cañadas, daughter of Paula Ramón y Cajal, and as also reproduced in the doctoral thesis of José María Martínez Murillo (2004).

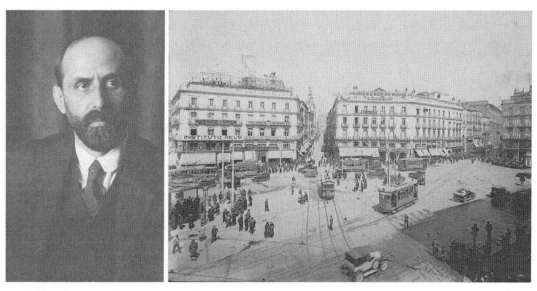

**FIGURE F-11.** (*Left*) Photograph of the poet Juan Ramón Jiménez (1881–1958). (*Right*) Photograph taken by Cajal of the Puerta del Sol, Madrid.

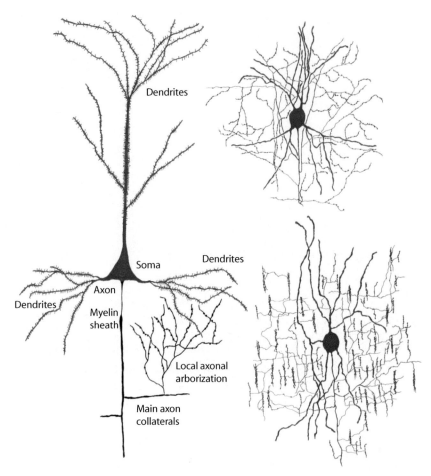

**FIGURE F-12.** Schematic drawings showing a typical pyramidal cell (*left*) and two interneurons (*right*: upper part, "common type," lower part, "chandelier cell") from the neocortex. The dendrites are shown in red.

the elements labeled in a given region in the same preparation or in the same focal plane. Therefore, the illustration of a given structure—with its possible connections—through microphotography was a difficult and often inefficient task. For these reasons, many of the drawings of the time were complex compositions, and the organization of a given region of the nervous system was shown synthetically. This is perhaps the most crucial aspect of these scientific drawings because it meant coupling artistic aptitudes with the interpretation of the microscopic images. In other words, the scientist had to discern between an artifact and a real element, and highlight the key features of the structure in an exact copy of the image obtained through the microscope. Thus, the illustration of histological

findings through drawings inevitably led to some skepticism (DeFelipe and Jones, 1992).

Readers interested in the various methods to reproduce microscopy images and the material used to produce these drawings can consult the work of Cajal itself. His book entitled *Manual de Histología Normal y de Técnica Micrográfica* (Handbook of Normal Histology and Micrography Techniques) is of particular interest, which was first published in 1889 (Ramón y Cajal, 1889a) and then re-edited over the years with additional and corrected content (e.g., Ramón y Cajal, 1893, 1914). An English version of this work was published with the help of his disciple Jorge Francisco Tello (1880–1958), considered to be Cajal's first disciple (Ramón y Cajal and Tello, 1933; see DeFelipe and Jones, 1992). In general, the

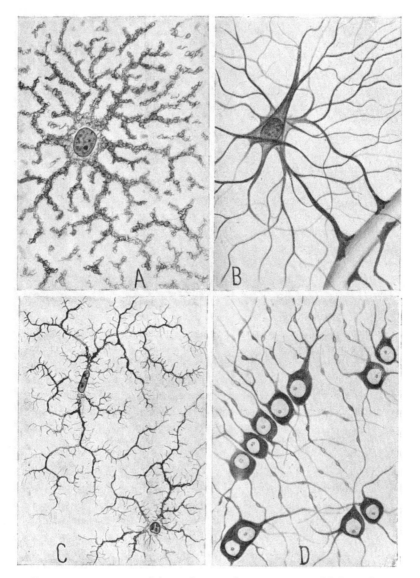

**FIGURE F-13.** Drawings to illustrate various types of glia in the central nervous system. (*A*) Protoplasmic astrocyte from the gray matter. (*B*) Fibrous astrocyte from the white matter. (*C*) Microglia. (*D*) Oligodendrocyte in the white matter (interfascicular form; taken from del Río Hortega, 1920). The discovery of glial cells is often attributed to Virchow, who in 1846 observed a nonneuronal connective or interstitial substance in the brain and spinal cord in which the elements of the nervous system were embedded (Virchow, 1846; quoted in Somjen, 1988). He referred to this using the term *Nervenkitt* (nerve-glue), later translated as "neuroglia" or simply "glia." However, these cells were mostly studied by Cajal and del Río-Hortega, using both the Golgi method and a variety of metallic impregnation techniques that they had developed, particularly Cajal's gold chloride sublimate method. One of Cajal's most important articles on neuroglia was published in 1913 (Ramón y Cajal, 1913), in which he described the detailed morphology of astrocytes and their relationship with neurons and blood vessels (see **Fig. F-33**). Furthermore, in this article Cajal described a *tercer elemento* (third element) that was different from neurons and astrocytes, and that he often described as "dwarf adendritic corpuscles." Some years later, two different types of these corpuscles were identified by del Río-Hortega in a detailed study using silver carbonate methods (del Río-Hortega, 1920, 1928): microglia and oligodendrocytes.

freehand drawings were made directly or with the aid of a camera lucida on different kinds of paper or cardboard, and using various types of pencils, pens, watercolor dyes, India ink, and other common drawing devices, either separately or in a variety of combinations. The camera lucida is a plotting device attached to the microscope that allows the observer to outline the optical microscope image that is projected upon a

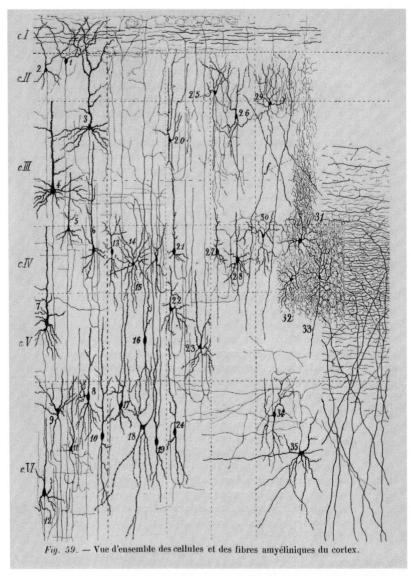

Fig. 59. — Vue d'ensemble des cellules et des fibres amyéliniques du cortex.

**FIGURE F-14.** Drawing made by Bonne (1906) showing the main types of cortical neurons and unmyelinated axons (*right*) based on the studies of Cajal. Numbers 1–12 stand for projection neurons, and 13–35 for short-axon cells.

drawing table (**Fig. F-16**). Thus, with this device the observer can visualize the paper, the pencil, and the histological preparation at the same time, allowing an accurate drawing of the objects to be produced.

However, I would caution the reader that the use of the camera lucida does not mean that the drawing was always an accurate observation, since it depended on the interpretation of the observer. Indeed, the scientist's drawings of the histological preparations only illustrated those elements thought to be important for what they wanted to describe. As such, these illustrations were not necessarily free of technical errors. Finally, unless otherwise specified, most of the images in the present work are digitalized reproductions from the figures that appear in the publications or, in some cases, of the original drawings. Many of these figures have been retouched and restored in order to remove stains, wrinkles, or other artifacts (**Fig. F-17**) using Adobe Photoshop CS3 software (Adobe Systems Inc., San Jose, CA).

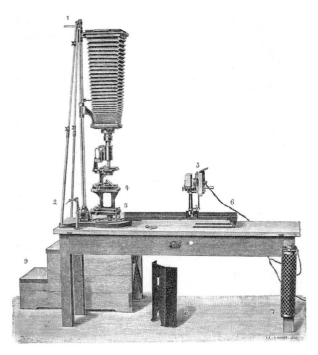

**FIGURE F-15.** Zeiss model for microphotography published by Cajal in his book *Manual de Histología Normal y de Técnica Micrográfica* (1914).

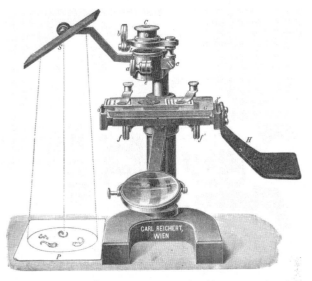

**FIGURE F-16.** Reichert microscope with Abbe camara lucida published by Cajal in his book *Manual de Histología Normal y de Técnica Micrográfica* (1914).

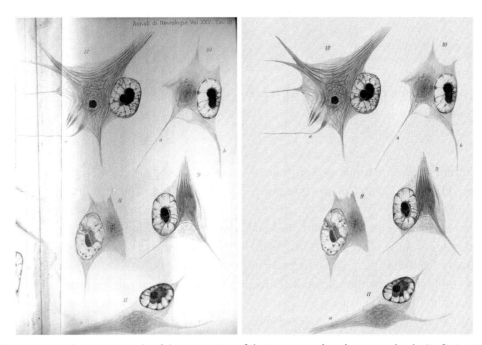

**FIGURE F-17.** Illustration to show an example of the restoration of the images used in the present book. (*Left*) Original image. (*Right*) After restoration. Taken from Fragnito, *Le Fibrille e la Sostanza Fibrillogena Nelle Cellule Ganglionari dei Vertebrati* (1907).

# A Sketch History of the Microscopic Anatomy of the Nervous System

The procedure of mechanical dissociation [...], applied to the analysis of the ganglia, of the retina, of the spinal cord or of the brain, the delicate operation of detaching the cells from their matrix of cement and of unravelling and extending their branched processes with needles, constituted a task for a Benedictine. What a delight it was when, by dint of much patience, we could completely isolate a neuroglial element, with its typical spider-like form, or a colossal motor neuron from the spinal cord, free and well separated with its robust axis cylinder and dendrites! What a triumph to capture the bifurcation of the single process [axon] from a dissociated spinal ganglia, or to clear a pyramidal cell from its neuroglial bramble thicket, that is, the noble and enigmatic cell of thought!

*Santiago Ramón y Cajal, Recuerdos de Mi Vida*

## SECTION 1

## THE BENEDICTINE PERIOD: THE EARLY DAYS

The first use of the word *cell* in histology is attributed to Robert Hooke (1635–1703), in his book *Micrographia* (1665, London; Turner, 1890). In the chapter "Of the schematisme or texture of cork and of the cells and pores of some other such frothy bodies," he employed the name "cells" in reference to the microscopic units that constitute the cork. Early microscopists had also described elements such as the cortical "glands" of Marcello Malpighi (1628–1694) and the "globules" of Antoni van Leeuwenhoek (1632–1723), while others proposed that all animal tissues are composed of tiny *globules* (globule theory). However, the detailed microscopic analysis of the nervous system did not begin until the early nineteenth century. At that time, using rudimentary optical microscopes, several researchers tried to apply the globule theory to the nervous system. One of the most notable researchers of that period was Everard Home (1756–1832), who argued that the abundance of globules and gelatinous substance in the cortex of the cerebrum and cerebellum, together with the large number of blood vessels in these structures, indicated that they were key elements

(Clarke and Jacyna, 1987): "the cortical substance is a very important part of [the brain]."

In the late 1820s and early 1830s, the introduction of achromatic lenses, coupled with other improvements in optical microscopy, led to the demonstration that the globules described by the earlier microscopists were artifacts produced by the chromatic and spherical aberrations of the optical lens used in old microscopes (Grainger, 1829). According to Hughes (1959), animal histology began after the classical publication of Thomas Hodgkin (1798–1866) and Joseph Jackson Lister (1786–1869) in 1827, who wrote the following on brain tissue (Hodgkin and Lister, 1827 quoted in Clarke and O'Malley, 1968):

> [...] one sees instead of globules a multitude of very small particles, which are most irregular in shape and size.

Studies on the cell in general led to the establishment of the cell theory toward the end of 1830, which is particularly associated to the botanist Matthias Jakob Schleiden (1804–1881) and the zoologist Theodor Schwann (1810–1882). This theory proposed that cells are the basic unit of animal and plant tissues, the seat of all vital processes (a "little organism"; Schleiden, 1838; Schwann, 1839). Rudolf Virchow (1821–1902) strongly supported the cell theory in his classic book *Die Cellularpathologie* (Virchow, 1858; **Fig. F-18**), writing the following interesting metaphor:

> whether vegetable or animal [...] cells are discovered to be the ultimate elements [...]. The structural composition of a body [...] always represents a kind of social arrangement of parts, an arrangement of a social kind, in which a number of individual existences are mutually dependent, but in such

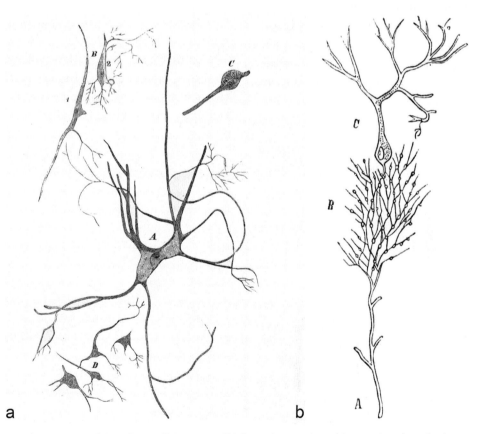

a                    b

FIGURE F-18. (*a*) Different types of "ganglion-cells" (nerve cells) from the spinal cord (A, B, C) and cerebral cortex (D). (*b*) Illustration of nerve cell connections ("...processes from ganglion-cells are connected with particularly complicated apparatuses") based on Gerlach. Virchow wrote in the legend to this figure: "Diagramatic representation of the disposition of the nerves in the cortex of the cerebellum, after Gerlach (Mikroscopische Studien/ plate I, fig. 3). *A*, white matter. *B, C*, grey matter, *B*, granular layer, *C*, cellular layer." Taken from Virchow (1858).

a way, that every element has its own special action, and, even though it derive[s] its stimulus to activity from other parts, yet alone effects the actual performance of its duties.

The application of the cell theory to the nervous system would logically lead to the formulation of the neuron doctrine (see Section 2, under "The Neuron Doctrine and the Law of Dynamic Polarization of Nerve Cells"). However, this was not a straightforward path due to the "special" characteristics of nerve cell connections (**Fig. F-18b**). In the words of Virchow:

> all nervous centres, the lowest as well as the most highly developed, are disposed upon an analogous plan; the only thing which, at least as yet, can be regarded as an especially characteristic peculiarity of the encephalon, is the circumstance [...] that in the cerebrum and cerebellum processes from ganglion-cells are connected with particularly complicated apparatuses (**Fig. F-18b**) [...] it is for the present uncertain whether they are to be regarded as the terminations of the nerves, or only structures placed in apposition to them.
>
> *Virchow, 1858*

Furthermore, given the absence of appropriate histological stains, many scientists and professors of anatomy at that time were sceptical about the usefulness of the microscopes. Indeed, it was believed that many of the images observed through these devices were artifacts, a source of errors and unsubstantiated assumptions. This situation was well expounded by Cajal himself:

> Many, perhaps most of the professors in those days underestimated the microscope, considering it even dangerous to the progress of Biology [...]! At that time, I remember a professor in Madrid who was never willing to look though the eyepiece of a magnifying instrument, and who referred to microscopic Anatomy as Celestial Anatomy [ironically useless anatomy]. This phrase, which became popular, is a good reflection of the attitude of that generation of professors.
>
> *Ramón y Cajal, 1917*

This scepticism was gradually overcome thanks to the technical advances in optical microscopy—especially with the introduction in the early 1860s of immersion objectives, which were subsequently improved from 1878 with the new models of transmitted light microscopes designed by the physicist Ernst Abbe (1840–1908) and manufactured in the factory of Carl Zeiss (1816–1888) in Jena (Álvarez-Leefmans, 1987; Merico, 1999)—and due to the introduction of new methods to analyze the nervous system.

## GLOBULES, GRANULES, CORPUSCLES (NERVE CELLS): KEY ELEMENTS OF THE NERVOUS SYSTEM

Gabriel Gustav Valentin (1810–1883) published an article in 1836 that according to Rudolf Albert von Kölliker (1817–1905), a prominent anatomist of that time, represented a milestone in the histology of the nervous system and the first good description of the elements of the nervous system (Kölliker, 1852, quoted in Shepherd, 1991).

**Figure F-19** is taken from Valentin (1836) and according to Clarke and O'Malley (1968), it represents the first microscopic image clearly showing a nerve cell (probably a Purkinje cell). In this figure the

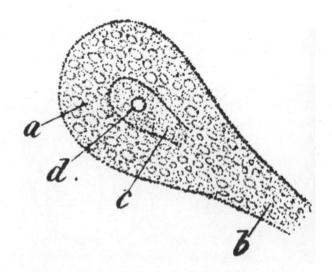

**FIGURE F-19.** Valentin's drawing of a globule (*Kugeln*) from the human cerebellar cortex (1836). This illustration represents the first microscopic image clearly showing a nerve cell. *a*, parenchyma (cell body); *b*, tail-like appendage (dendritic trunk); *c*, nucleus; *d*, small internal corpuscle (probably the nucleolus). The legend of the figure is based on that in Clarke and O'Malley (1968) and Shepherd (1991).

cell can be seen to have a well-defined contour (cell membrane) and substance in its interior (that he called *parenchyma*), a viscous fluid with numerous granules, containing a *nucleus* with an internal *corpuscle* (nucleolus). In describing this figure, Shepherd (1991) said: "Here, at a stroke, are the basic structures of the nerve cell body and the terminology that we recognize today." In the article by Valentin, the idea that globules (nerve cells), together with nerve fibers, were key elements in the central nervous system also emerged (Clarke and Jacyna, 1987).

The next important step in the development of our ideas on how the nervous system is organized was presented by Jan Evangelista Purkinje (1787–1869) at the Congress of Physicians and Researchers of Nature held in Prague on September 23, 1837. At this meeting, Purkinje described the first well-characterized nerve cell 1 year after the publication of Valentin's classic article (Purkinje, 1838). These cells were the large corpuscles of the cerebellum, later to be called Purkinje cells in honor of its discoverer (**Fig. F-20**). According to Clarke and Jacyna (1987), Purkinje gave Ehrenberg the credit for having first described the *ganglionic granules* in the ganglia. This finding prompted Purkinje to verify the existence of these elements in the central nervous system, and since he found that the granules of Ehrenberg were very similar to those found in the cortex of the cerebrum and cerebellum, it appeared that these corpuscles were very important in the functioning of the nervous system. The illustration of Purkinje is also of great significance, because it is the first description of the cytoarchitectonic layers in a region of the nervous system (Shepherd, 1991).

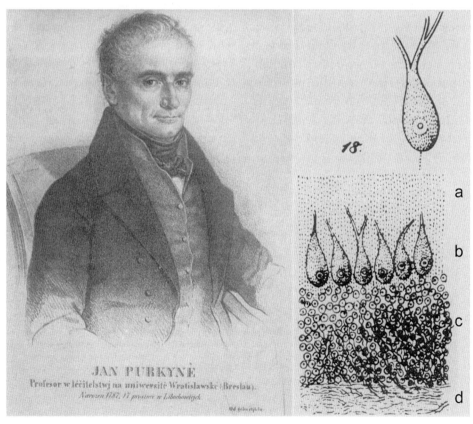

**FIGURE F-20.** Jan Evangelista Purkinje (1787–1869). On the right is the illustration of the first nerve cell identified (Purkinje, 1838), the large corpuscles of the cerebellum that were later called Purkinje cells. This illustration is also important because it is the first to show the cytoarchitecture of a region of the nervous system (Shepherd, 1991): *a*, molecular layer; *b*, large corpuscles; *c*, granules; *d*, fibers.

## RELATIONSHIP BETWEEN NERVE CELLS AND NERVE FIBERS: THE DEVELOPMENT OF MICROANATOMICAL METHODS

For a long time the relationship between nerve cells and nerve fibers remained unclear. Indeed, in the mid-nineteenth century there were two hypotheses: that a nerve fiber is an outgrowth from a single cell (e.g., Bidder and Kupffer, 1857; His, 1886), or, alternatively, nerve cells and fibers are two independent elements in the nervous system. In this latter case, it was proposed that the nerve fibers differentiate within a continuous protoplasmic meshwork during very early stages of development (Hensen, 1864: "protoplasmic bridge" theory). An essential step in the microanatomical analysis of the nervous system was the initial introduction of methods to mechanically dissociate this tissue manually with dissection needles, with or without the use of chemical agents to harden the tissue and facilitate the dissection of nerves, ganglia, and nerve cells. Using this method, in 1833 and 1836 Christian Gottfried Ehrenberg (1795–1876) described *granules* (nerve cells) in the gray matter of the brain and ganglia, noting that these elements were often multipolar with several processes. However, Ehremberg did not attribute any special significance to the granules; rather, these findings simply served to demonstrate that the gray matter of the nervous system was not a homogeneous amorphous mass, as assumed by several authors at that time (Clarke and Jacyna, 1987). These observations were confirmed by several researchers that initially proposed that all these processes were similar in nature. However, several authors soon indicated that only one of the processes had the characteristics of a nerve fiber (Barker, 1899).

Among these scientists Robert Remak (1815–1865) is considered to be the first to clearly illustrate the continuity between the axon and cell body, and to distinguish the two main types of fibers that we recognize today: myelinated and unmyelinated fibers, described in 1838 by Remak as a *primitive band within a very thin-walled tube* and an *organic fiber* (Van der Loos, 1967; Brazier, 1988). Otto Friedrich Karl Deiters (1834–1863) improved the dissociation method by introducing the treatment of the tissue with potassium dichromate. In 1865, he made the important generalization that all multipolar ganglion cells of vertebrates have two morphological and functional types of processes (Deiters, 1865): an axon continued with a fiber of myelin, then called a *Achsencylinderfortsatz* (prolongation of the cylinder-axis), a term introduced in 1839 by J. F. Rosenthal (a student of Purkinje: Shepherd, 1991); and several short, branching processes (dendrites) that he called *Protoplasmafortsätze* (protoplasmic prolongations; **Fig. F-21**).

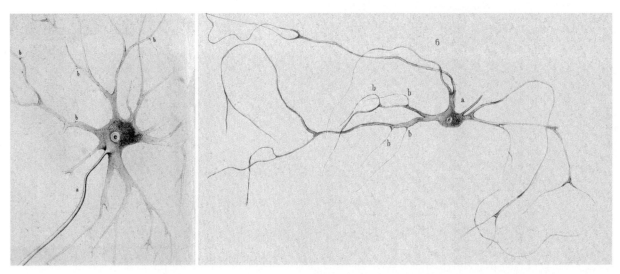

**FIGURE F-21.** Drawings made by Deiters (1865) to illustrate nerve cells (spinal cord of the ox). Method of mechanical dissociation. He distinguished a principal axon (*a*) originated from the soma and several thin axons that arise from the dendrites (*b*, "second axonic system"). According to Cajal, the erroneous interpretation of this second axonic plexus was the germ of the reticular theory.

The next truly relevant event was the development of methods to obtain *thin and transparent sections*, mainly introduced by Benedict Stilling (1810–1879) in 1842. This method consisted of obtaining serial thin sections after hardening the nervous tissue by freezing or using potassium dichromate. Stilling's method was improved by several scientists, who incorporated other techniques to harden and stain the tissue. Among which, the most important was the method of Joseph von Gerlach (1820–1896), who introduced ammoniated carmine and gold chloride, a method of staining that allowed him to formulate the famous reticular theory (see following section, "The Reticular Theory").

During the subsequent four decades, little progress was made in understanding the structure and function of the nervous system. For example, in the classic book of Kölliker published in 1852, the year Cajal was born, the structure of the nervous system was described in a very simple manner **(Fig. F-22)**.

The main reason for this lack of information was due to the fact that with the histological techniques available, the visualization of nerve cells was incomplete, since it was often only feasible to observe the cell body and the proximal portions of the dendrites and axon. Thus, it was not possible to follow the trajectory of the thin axons or to visualize the terminal axonal arbors. Hence, it was still not technically feasible to tackle one of the key needs to study the organization of the nervous system, the tracing of the connections between neurons, or in other words to outline neural circuits. In the words of Cajal:

> The great enigma in the organization of the brain revolves around our need to ascertain how the nervous ramifications end and how neurons are mutually connected. Referring to a simile already

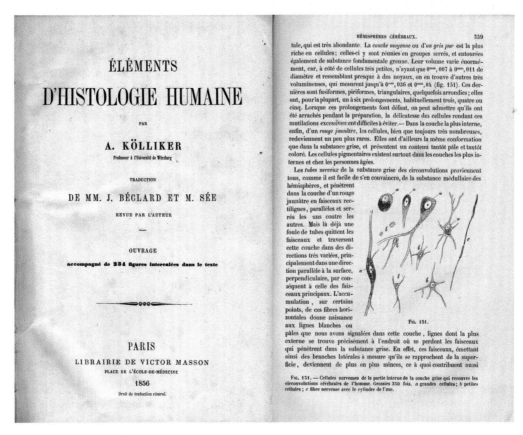

**FIGURE F-22.** French edition (1856) of Kölliker's classic book *Handbuch der Gewebelehre des Menschen* (1852). In Fig. 151 various morphological types of nerve cells in the human cerebral cortex are shown.

mentioned, the idea was to inquire how the roots and branches of the trees in the grey matter terminate, so that in such a dense jungle, in which there are no gaps thanks to its refined complexity, the trunks, branches and leaves touch everywhere.

*Ramón y Cajal, 1917*

As outlined in Section 2, this technical void was resolved primarily with the discovery of *reazione nera* (black reaction) by Camillo Golgi (1843–1926).

## THE RETICULAR THEORY

At that time, the prevailing hypothesis about the organization of the nervous system was the reticular theory, which proposed that the elements of the nervous system form a continuum. It was Joseph von Gerlach (1820–1896) who really developed the reticular theory (**Fig. F-23**), and thus he is considered the father of this theory (Gerlach, 1872).

Part of the success of this theory was due to the idea that if the nervous system consisted of a continuous network of processes, without interruptions, it could be relatively easy to explain how the nervous

currents in the brain could pass from one nerve cell to another. Hence, the passing of information from one nerve cell to another would be due to the continuity of their processes. **Figures F-23b and c** show drawings of Aleksander Dogiel (1852–1922), supporting the reticular theory. **Figure 23b** shows a drawing illustrating two neurons connected through a thick common dendrite ("interprotoplasmic bridges") rather than existing as independent elements. This is a particularly interesting figure since it was produced with the aid of a camera lucida, a good example for demonstrating that the use of this device did not preclude the observer from making incorrect observations. Indeed, there were two major opponents of the reticular theory, Wilhelm His (1831–1904) and August-Henri Forel (1848–1931), which according to Cajal (1909–1911):

> …they struggle against the doctrine of the networks, and they prepared our minds to accept the theory of contacts and of the free ending of the nervous processes.

Both these scientists reached the same conclusion separately, based on different observations. His found

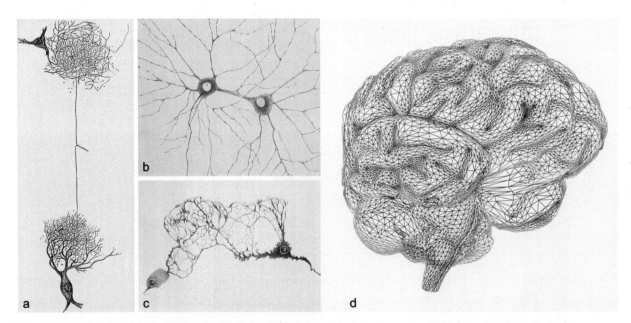

**FIGURE F-23.** Reticular theory. (*a*) Drawing made by Gerlach (1872) showing two nerve cells from the spinal cord of the ox (prepared with carmine and ammonia). According to this author, the conduction of nervous activity takes place through a network of neural elements formed by dendrites (dendritic network) and axons (axonal network). (*b* and *c*) Drawings of ganglion cells of the human retina and cells of the dog gallbladder ganglia made by Dogiel in 1893 and 1899, respectively. (*d*) Schematic illustration to show the brain as made up of a mesh of neuronal processes. This drawing of the brain was kindly provided by Juan Sanz (computer animation specialist).

that the surface of the nerve cells did not anastomose with other nerve cells and he proposed that the nerve cell was the embryological or genetic unit of the nervous system (His, 1886, 1889). Forel began to work in the laboratory of Bernard von Gudden (1824–1886), where he learned the experimental methods to study von Gudden degeneration and the connections in the nervous system. This method was devised by August Waller (1816–1870) to study spinal nerve degeneration, through which secondary degeneration was discovered (better known as Wallerian degeneration in honor of its discoverer). Waller (1850, 1852) found that when an axon is sectioned, the portion separated from the cell body (*trophic center*) degenerated and disappeared, whereas the portion joined to the cell of origin maintained its structure. The method of von Gudden consisted of inducing secondary atrophy in central structures of the nervous system after extirpating the sense organs or the cranial nerves of young animals. As a consequence, atrophy of the nerve cells from which the damaged axons originated would occur first, and later these cells would completely disappear (von Gudden, 1870). Forel (1887, 1890–1891) was opposed to the reticular theory based on the pathological and physiological evidence obtained with the method of von Gudden. Forel argued that after a lesion in a given region, cell atrophy was restricted to a particular group of cells, without extending to another group of cells, as would be expected if they formed a mesh.

According to Cajal (1899–1904), the ideas of His and Forel were not accepted by the reticularists for mainly methodological reasons, and also because their studies were performed in embryonic or young animals:

> It was necessary to demonstrate *de visu*, and in the adult, that nervous ramifications terminated freely, and in conditions in which it were not possible to question this fact, neither due to the embryonic nature of the material presented, nor because of the incomplete staining of the fibres.

For example, Hans Held (1866–1942) described a separation in the trapezoid nucleus of the embryo or in newborn animals, a line of demarcation (*Grenxline*) between the giant basket terminals (*Endkörb*)—later called chalices of Held—and the cell body of the neurons with which they contacted. However, he proposed that during development these terminal axons were fused to the cell bodies (**Fig. F-24:** Held, 1897a, 1897b). This idea was generalized to other parts of the nervous system (Held, 1902, 1904, 1905), indicating that axon terminals were not only fused with the cell bodies but also with the dendrites. As a result, the reticular theory represented the main concept regarding the organization of the nervous system.

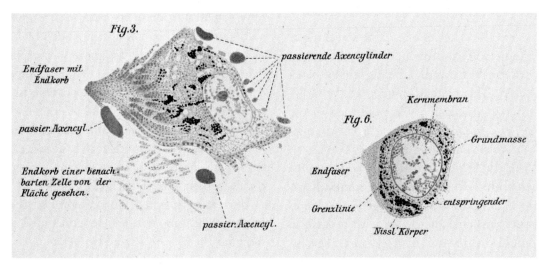

FIGURE F-24. Drawings made by Held (1897a) to show the development of the giant baskets terminals in the trapezoid nucleus stained with erythrosine/methylene blue. According to Held, in the newborn animal (*Fig. 6*; 9-day-old dog, paraffin section 3 μm thick) there is a demarcation line (*Grenxlinie*) between the terminal fiber (*Endfaser*) and the cell body. However, in the adult (*Fig. 3*; rabbit, paraffin section 1.5 μm thick) Held thought that the terminal axons were fused to the cell body.

SECTION 2

# THE BLACK PERIOD: NEURONS, GLIA, AND THE ORGANIZATION OF THE NERVOUS SYSTEM

## THE DISCOVERY OF THE *REAZIONE NERA*

On February 16, 1873, a revolution began in the world of neuroscience. On this date, Golgi sent the following letter to his friend Niccolò Manfredi (Mazzarello, 1999):

> I spend long hours at the microscope. I am delighted that I have found a new reaction to demonstrate even to the blind the structure of the interstitial stroma of the cerebral cortex. I let the silver nitrate react with pieces of brain hardened in potassium dichromate. I have obtained magnificent results and hope to do even better in the future.

Golgi referred in this letter to a new technique to stain the nervous system that allowed neurons and glia to be visualized, labeling them black (*reazione nera*). This method, named as the Golgi method after its discoverer, was published in the *Gazzeta Medica Italiani* on August 2, 1873 (Golgi, 1873): *Sulla Struttura della Sostanza Grigia del Cervello* (On the Structure of the Gray Substance of the Cerebrum). Thanks to a very simple staining protocol, requiring a "prolonged immersion of the tissue, previously hardened with potassium or ammonium dichromate, in a 0.50 or 1.0% solution of silver nitrate," for the first time it was possible to observe neurons and glia in a histological preparation (**Fig. F-25**) with all their parts—cell body, dendrites, and axon in the case of neurons

(**Fig. F-26**, *right*); cell body and processes in the case of glia (see below).

It is true that Deiters' old method of the mechanical dissociation (1865) enabled the morphology of a neuron to be completely visualized (**Fig. F-21**), although it was a technique that was very difficult to perform. Moreover, the Golgi method has the advantage that it allowed the cells to be observed "in their natural position and shape," as Cajal said, that is, in situ, without any possible artifacts that might be introduced by dissociation. Another important advantage of the Golgi method was that only a small portion of the neurons in a given preparation were stained, permitting individual neurons to be examined with the greatest morphological detail, for instance, allowing dendritic spines to be discovered. Thus, it was at last possible to characterize and classify neurons, and to potentially study their connections. These characteristics of the Golgi method gave rise to another great advance, namely that of tracing the first accurate circuit diagrams of the nervous system (DeFelipe, 2002b).

Interestingly, when Golgi examined the silver-impregnated preparations, he concluded that the reticular theory enunciated by Gerlach was wrong, since Golgi thought that dendrites ended freely and that only the axons and their collaterals were seen to anastomose. Therefore, he suggested that the nervous system consisted of a *rete nervosa*

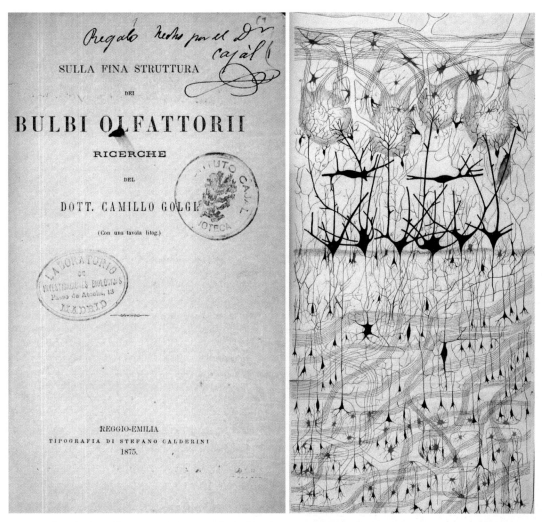

**FIGURE F-25.** (*Right*) The first illustration by Golgi of a Golgi-impregnated preparation of the nervous system. "Semi-schematic drawing of a fragment of a vertical section of the olfactory bulb of a dog," taken from Golgi (1875). Cajal said in *Recuerdos de Mi Vida*: "I expressed in former paragraphs the surprise which I experienced upon seeing with my own eyes the wonderful revelatory powers of the chrome-silver reaction and the absence of any excitement aroused in the scientific world by its discovery. How can one explain such strange indifference? Today, when I am better acquainted with the psychology of scientific men, I find it very natural.... Out of respect for the master, no pupil is wont to use methods of investigation which he has not learned from him. As for the great investigators, they would consider themselves dishonoured if they worked with the methods of others." (*Left*) Cover of the work *Sulla fina struttura del bulbi olfattorii*. Reggio-Emilia: Stefano Calderini, 1875.

*diffusa* (diffuse nervous network), an idea that he supported even during his Nobel Price lecture in 1906 (**Fig. F-26**).

## THE GOLGI METHOD, CAJAL, MAESTRE DE SAN JUAN, AND SIMARRO

For a long time after the discovery of the Golgi method, the vast majority of the scientific community failed to take advantage of it. Part of the reason for this can be seen in the very training that Cajal himself received at this time. When Cajal was studying for his doctorate and attended the doctoral course of normal and pathological histology, one of the principal texts used was the *Tratado de Histología Normal y Patológica* (1879, Madrid) by Aureliano Maestre de San Juan (1828–1890: **Fig. F-27**), professor of histology at the Faculty of Medicine in Madrid. Indeed, it was this professor who introduced

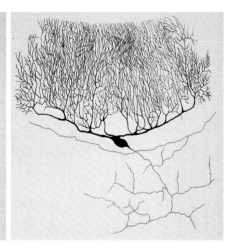

## LA DOTTRINA DEL NEURONE

### TEORIA E FATTI

(CON 19 FIGURE INTERCALATE NEL TESTO)

*Conferenza tenuta l' 11 Dicembre 1906 presso l' Accademia delle Scienze di Stoccolma in occasione del conferimento del Premio Nobel per la Medicina (\*)*

Può sembrare un fatto singolare che, mentre io sempre mi sono dichiarato decisamente contrario alla dottrina del neurone, pur riconoscendo che il punto di partenza di essa è da ricercarsi proprio nei miei studi, abbia scelto per tema di questa mia conferenza appunto la questione del neurone e che questo accada quando da molte parti si afferma che la dottrina già volge al tramonto.

**FIGURE F-26.** (*Left*) Introductory paragraph of the Nobel Prize lecture given by Golgi in 1906 (Golgi, 1929). (*Right*) Drawing made by Golgi to illustrate a Purkinje cell of the cerebellum (Fig. 4 of his lecture). The axon is shown in red. When they jointly received the Nobel Prize for Physiology or Medicine in 1906, the lectures of Cajal and Golgi provided a good reflection of the state of scientific thought at the time (DeFelipe, 2002a). Golgi started his lecture "The Neuron Doctrine" by saying (kindly translated by Fiorenzo Conti, University of Ancona, Italy): "It might appear odd that, having always opposed the neuron doctrine—though its point of departure is undoubtedly to be found in my own studies—I should choose this very problem as the subject of my lecture, particularly at a time when this doctrine is considered by many to be on the wane." By contrast, Cajal's Nobel lecture "The Structure and Connections of Neurons" expounded his most fundamental results and vigorously opposed Golgi's stance. Regarding Golgi's Nobel lecture, Cajal later said in his autobiography *Recuerdos de Mi Vida*: "Contrary to what we all expected, instead of pointing out the valuable facts which he [Golgi] had discovered, he tried to refloat his almost forgotten theory of the interstitial nervous nets."

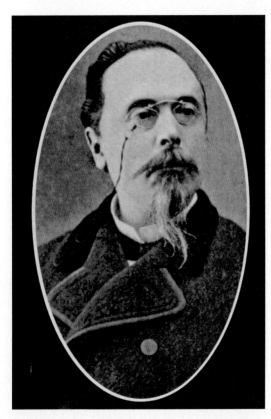

**FIGURE F-27.** Portrait of Aureliano Maestre de San Juan (1828–1890).

Cajal to the field of the microscopy. According to Cajal, he was so impressed by some of the beautiful histological preparations that Mastre de San Juan showed him that he decided to set up a laboratory of microscopy "as an indispensable complement of descriptive anatomy."

However, in Maestre de San Juan's book, published in 1879, and in the second edition of 1885 (**Fig. F-28**), there is no mention of the Golgi method. This was also true of another interesting book that Cajal used, *Tratado Elemental de Anatomía y Fisiología Normal y Patológica del Sistema Nervioso* (1878, Valencia) by José Crous (1846–1887), professor of medical pathology. In Crous's book, the rudimentary knowledge of the organization of the brain at that time is nicely reflected (**Fig. F-29**). However, despite the years that had passed since its publication, the Golgi method was not commonly referred to in most of the contemporary texts available at that time.

Nevertheless, Cajal was aware of the existence of the Golgi method, even though he had not tested it because he thought it was a useless method:

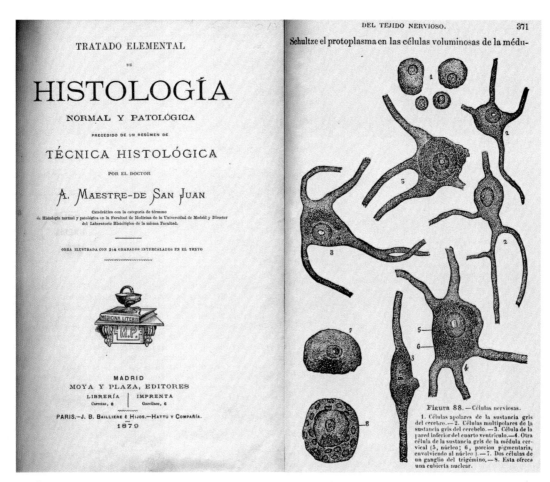

**FIGURE F-28.** (*Left*) Cover of the book of Maestre de San Juan *Tratado Elemental de Anatomía y Fisiología Normal y Patológica del Sistema Nervioso* (1879, Valencia). (*Right*) Morphological types of nerve cells taken from this book of Maestre de San Juan. Cajal would have read the following regarding the morphological types of nerve cells in this book: "The nerve cell may or may not present prolongations of its protoplasm, and from that come their division into: 1º., apolar, that is to say, without any protoplasmic prolongation…; and 2º., others [nerve cells] that show a variable number of prolongations."

But, as I mentioned, the admirable method of Golgi was then (1887–1888) unknown to the immense majority of neurologists or was underestimated by the few who had precise information about it. Ranvier's book, my technical bible of those days, devoted only a few descriptive lines of to it, written in an indifferent style. It was evident that the French savant had not tried it. Naturally, the readers of Ranvier, like myself, thought this method to be unworthy to be used.

*Ramón y Cajal, 1917*

If we compare **Figure F-22** of Kölliker (1852) with **Figure F-28** of Maestre de San Juan, we can see that although 27 years had elapsed since the publication of

Kölliker's book, both drawings are very similar. This represents a good example of the slow progress in microanatomy due to the lack of appropriate methods or to the incapacity to exploit the methods available.

It was in this scientific scenario that Luis Simarro (1851–1921), a psychiatrist and neurologist (**Fig. F-30**) who was also an enthusiast of histology, first showed Cajal a Golgi-impregnated preparation in 1887 (**Fig. F-31**).

I owe to Luis Simarro the unforgetable favour of having been shown the first good preparations made by the method of silver chromate which I ever saw, and of his having called my attention to the exceptional importance of the book of the Italian savant

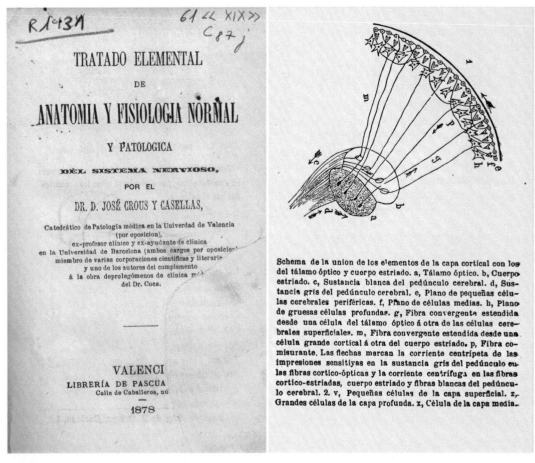

TRATADO ELEMENTAL

DE

ANATOMIA Y FISIOLOGIA NORMAL

Y PATOLOGICA

DEL SISTEMA NERVIOSO,

POR EL

DR. D. JOSÉ CROUS Y CASELLAS,

Catedrático de Patología médica en la Univerdad de Valencia
(por oposicion),
ex-profesor clínico y ex-ayudante de clínica
en la Universidad de Barcelona (ambos cargos por oposicion)
miembro de varias corporaciones científicas y literaris
y uno de los autores del complemento
á la obra deprolegómenos de clínica m
del Dr. Coca.

VALENCI
LIBRERÍA DE PASCUA
Calle de Caballeros, nú

1878

Schema de la union de los elementos de la capa cortical con los
del tálamo óptico y cuerpo estriado. a, Tálamo óptico. b, Cuerpo
estriado. c, Sustancia blanca del pedúnculo cerebral. d, Sustancia gris del pedúnculo cerebral. e, Plano de pequeñas células cerebrales periféricas. f, Plano de células medias. h, Plano
de gruesas células profundas. g, Fibra convergente estendida
desde una célula del tálamo óptico á otra de las células cerebrales superficiales. m, Fibra convergente estendida desde una
célula grande cortical á otra del cuerpo estriado. p, Fibra co-
misurante. Las flechas marcan la corriente centrípeta de las
impresiones sensitivas en la sustancia gris del pedúnculo eu-
las fibras cortico-ópticas y la corriente centrífuga en las fibras
cortico-estriadas, cuerpo estriado y fibras blancas del pedúnculo cerebral. 2. v, Pequeñas células de la capa superficial. z,
Grandes células de la capa profunda. x, Célula de la capa media.

**FIGURE F-29.** Taken from Crous (1878): "Scheme of the union of the elements of the cortical layer with those of the optic thalamus and corpus striatum. a, optic thalamus. b, corpus striatum. c, white substance of the cerebral peduncle [ . . . ] Arrows indicate the centripetal and centrifugal currents [ . . . ]."

devoted to the examination of the fine structure of the gray matter.

*Ramón y Cajal, 1917*

## CAJAL'S FIRST STUDY WITH THE GOLGI METHOD: DENDRITES AND AXONS END FREELY

Cajal was rapt by this marvelous staining method and he immediately started to use it to analyze practically the entire nervous system in several species. One year after his meeting with Simarro, Cajal had published his first important article based on results obtained with this method in the avian cerebellum (**Fig. F-32**). In this study entitled *Estructura de los Centros Nerviosos de las Aves* (Ramón y Cajal, 1888), Cajal made two great contributions. First, he

described the existence of dendritic spines (which he also named), structures that currently generate particular interest as they are highly plastic and they are the main postsynaptic site for excitatory synapses in the cerebral cortex. Second, Cajal confirmed Golgi's conclusion that dendrites end freely but in contrast to Golgi, Cajal added the decisive conclusion that this also applies to axons and their branches:

> We have carried out detailed studies to investigate the course and connections of the nerve fibres in the cerebral and cerebellar convolutions of the human, monkey, dog, etc. We have not been able to see an anastomosis between the ramifications of two different nervous prolongations, nor between the filaments emanating from the same expansion of Deiters [axons]. While the fibres are interlaced in

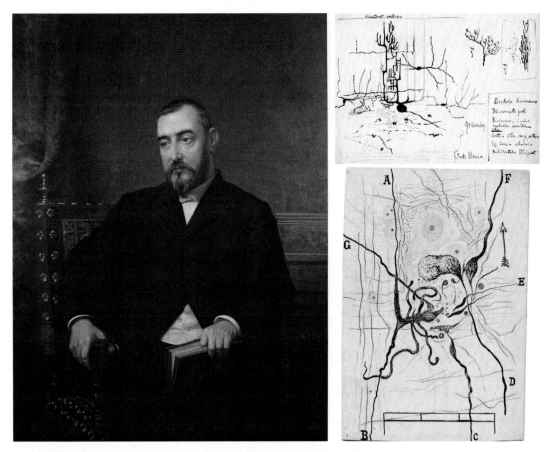

**FIGURE F-30.** (*Left*) Luis Simarro (1851–1921, Legado Cajal, Instituto Cajal). (*Right, top*) Drawing from Simarro showing cells of the human cerebellum stained with the Golgi method (Legado Simarro, Universidad Complutense, Madrid. See **Fig. F-31**: Courtesy of Iñigo Azcoitia, and Alberto Muñoz, Universidad Complutense). (*Right, bottom*) Simarro's drawing of a senile plaque ("plaque of Fischer") that was reproduced by Cajal in Fig. 310 of the book *Estudios Sobre la Degeneración y Regeneración del Sistema Nervioso* (Vol. 2, Madrid: Moya, 1913–1914): "Details of a plaque of Fischer in formation. *A*, hypertrophied projection axon, next to the plaque, to which it sends a thick collateral ending in a bulb and numerous terminal branches; *D, G, F*, fibres ending in buds or balls in the region of the plaque. (From a drawing of Simarro.) [...] It appears as if the sprouts had been attracted towards the region of the plaque under the influence of some special neurotropic substance" (see DeFelipe and Jones, 1991). The original drawing is held in the Archivo Fernando de Castro.

a very complicated manner, engendering an intricate and dense plexus, they never form a net [...] it could be said that each [nerve cell] is an absolutely autonomous physiological canton [unit].

*Ramón y Cajal, 1888*

The historical moment when Cajal discovered the properties of the Golgi method is beautifully described in several of his writings, especially in the French translation of *Textura*, which represents an excellent example of his typical vivid writing style and enthusiasm:

In summary, a method was necessary to selectively stain an element, or at most a small number of elements, that would appear to be isolated among the remaining invisible elements. Could the dream of such a technique truly become reality, in which the microscope becomes a scalpel and histology a fine [tool for] anatomical dissection? A piece of nervous tissue was left hardening for several days in Müller's pure liquid [potassium dichromate] or in a mixture of this [fixative] with osmic acid. Whether it was the distraction of the histologist or the curiosity of the scientist, the tissue was then immersed in a bath of

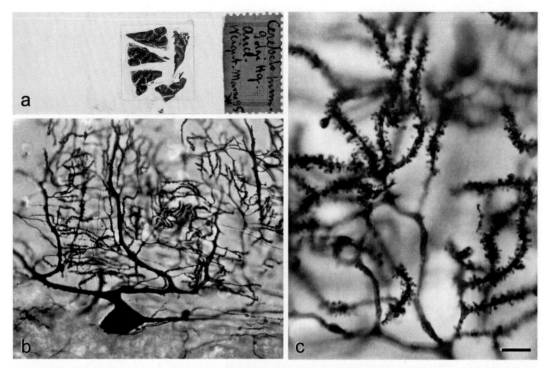

**FIGURE F-31.** (*a*) Photograph of a preparation from Simarro of the human cerebellum stained with the Golgi method in combination with the Weigert method. (*b*) Low-power photomicrograph showing a typical Purkinje cell. (*c*) Higher magnification of (*b*) showing dendritic spines. Scale bar: 30 μm in (*b*); 4.5 μm in (*c*). The histological images (Legado Simarro, Universidad Complutense, Madrid) were taken by Iñigo Azcoitia and Alberto Muñoz (Universidad Complutense). Dendritic spines were discovered by Cajal in 1888 (see **Fig. F-32** and text for further details).

silver nitrate. The appearance of gleaming needles with shimmering gold reflections soon attracted the attention. The tissue was cut, and the sections were dehydrated, cleared, and then examined [with the microscope]. What an unexpected spectacle! On the perfectly translucent yellow background sparse black filaments appeared that were smooth and thin or thorny and thick, as well as black triangular, stellate or fusiform bodies! One would have thought that they were designs in Chinese ink on transparent Japanese paper. The eye was disconcerted, accustomed as it was to the inextricable network [observed] in the sections stained with carmine and hematoxylin where the indecision of the mind

has to be reinforced by its capacity to criticize and interpret. Here everything was simple, clear and unconfused. It was no longer necessary to interpret [microscopically] the findings to verify that the cell has multiple branches covered with 'frost,' embracing an amazingly large space with their undulations. A slender fibre that originated from the cell elongated over enormous distances and suddenly opened out in a spray of innumerable sprouting fibres. A corpuscle confined to the surface of a ventricle where it sends out a shaft, which is branched at the surface of the [brain], and other cells [appeared] like comatulids or phalangidas.* The amazed eye could not be torn away from this contemplation. The technique

---

* Comatulids are marine crinoid invertebrates like sea lilies and feather stars. Phalangidas (or opiliones), also known as water harvestmen, are arachnids that superficially resemble true spiders, but they have small, oval-shaped bodies and long legs. Cajal is probably referring to some neuroglial cells that, when stained with the Golgi method, have a morphology that resembles these invertebrates (see **Fig. F-33**).

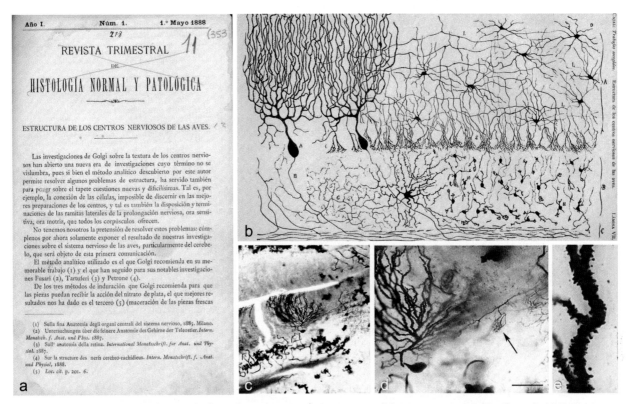

**FIGURE F-32.** First illustration by Cajal of a Golgi-impregnated preparation of the nervous system (Cajal, 1888). (*a*) First page of the article and (*b*) illustration whose legend states: "Vertical section of a cerebellar convolution of a hen. Impregnation by the Golgi method. A, represents the molecular zone, B, designates the granular layer and C the white matter." (*c*) Photomicrograph from one of Cajal's preparations of the cerebellum of an adult bird stained with the Golgi method. (*d*) Higher magnification of (*c*) to illustrate a Purkinje cell and a basket formation (*arrow*). (*e*) Dendrite of the Purkinje cell, which is covered by spines. In the text, Cajal said: "…the surface of [the dendrites of Purkinje cells] appears to be covered with thorns or short spines…(At the beginning, we thought that these eminences were the result of a tumultuous precipitation of the silver but the constancy of its existence and its presence, even in preparations in which the reaction appears to be very delicate in the remaining elements, incline us to believe this to be a normal condition)." Scale bar: 200 μm in (*c*); 60 μm in (*d*); 8,4 μm in (*e*). The histological images were obtained by Pablo García-López, Virginia García-Marín, and Miguel Freire (Legado Cajal, Instituto Cajal).

that had been dreamed of is a reality! The metallic impregnation has unexpectedly achieved this fine dissection. This is the Golgi method! […] whose clear and decisive images enables us to cast off the famous net of Gerlach, [as well as] of the [dendritic] arms of Valentin and Wagner, and of so many other fanciful hypothesis.

## THE NEURON DOCTRINE AND THE LAW OF DYNAMIC POLARIZATION OF NERVE CELLS

From the outset of Cajal's studies with the Golgi method in 1887, he provided many examples from throughout the nervous system to support his observation that dendrites and axons end freely. For example, he considered that the free arborization of neurons would more easily explain plastic changes in the brain through the formation of new connections:

As opposed to the reticular theory, the theory that cellular processes could develop free arborizations seems not only the most likely, but also the most encouraging. A continuous pre-established net—like a lattice of telegraphic wires in which no new stations or new lines can be created—somehow rigid, immutable, incapable of being modified, goes against the concept that all we hold of the organ of thought, which within certain limits, is malleable

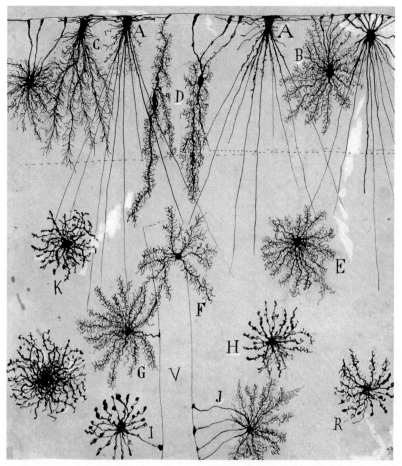

**FIGURE F-33.** Cajal's drawing of Golgi-impregnated neuroglia. The figure legend states: "Neuroglia of the superficial layers of the cerebrum: child of two months. Golgi Method. A, B, [C], D, neuroglial cells of the plexiform layer; E, F, [G, H, K], R, neuroglial cells of the second and third layers; V, blood vessel; I, J, neuroglial cells with vascular [pedicles]." The astrocyte vascular end-feet on blood vessels confirmed the observation made by Golgi in 1885, who often noticed that Golgi-impregnated processes from neuroglial cells were frequently in contact with both blood vessels (vascular end-feet or "sucker processes") and neurons. This finding prompted Golgi to suggest that the main function of glial cells was to supply nutrients to the nerve cells.

and capable of being perfected by means of well-directed mental gymnastics.

*Ramón y Cajal, 1894*

Therefore, how the connections between neurons were established was another important issue that had to be addressed by scientists. This was summarized by Cajal in *Recuerdos de Mi Vida* in the following poetic and characteristic anthropomorphic prose that he often used to describe various aspects of the nervous system:

What mysterious forces preside the appearance of the processes [dendrites and axon], promoting their

growth and ramification, provoking the coherent migration of the cells and fibres in predetermined directions, as if obeying a wise architectonic plan, and finally establishing those protoplasmic kisses, the *intercellular articulations* [synapses] that appear to constitute the final ecstasy of an epic love story?

*Ramón y Cajal, 1917*

Obviously, it is not the same to think that nerve currents flow through a continuous rather than a discontinuous network of neuronal processes (**Fig. F-34**). Thus, the new ideas about the connections between neurons led to novel theories on the

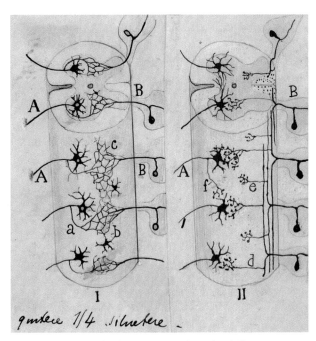

**FIGURE F-34.** Cajal's drawing to explain the differences between the neuron and the reticular theories. The figure legend states: "Scheme to compare the concept of Golgi regarding the sensory-motor connections of the spinal cord (I) with the results of my investigations (II). *A*, anterior roots; *B*, posterior roots; *a*, collateral of a motor root; *b*, cells with a short axon which, according to Golgi, would intervene in the formation of the network; *c*, diffuse interstitial network; *d*, our long collaterals in contact with the motor cells; *e*, short collaterals." This figure was reproduced as Figure 9 in *Recuerdos de Mi Vida*.

relationship between neuronal circuits and brain function. Cajal wrote:

> The cell bodies [dendrites and axons] terminate freely but nevertheless, the flow of currents is not impeded in such an infinitely interrupted, fragmented nervous system. How can such currents flow? There can be only one answer, by contact, in much the same way that electric current crosses a splice between two wires.
>
> *Ramón y Cajal, 1909–1911*

## ARROWS IN THE ILLUSTRATIONS: THE DIRECTION OF THE NERVOUS CURRENTS

The reader will note that some of Cajal's drawings and those of other scientists included arrows, which indicate the direction of the nervous currents. An important consequence of the neuron doctrine was Cajal's theory of the law of dynamic polarization of nerve cells (DeFelipe, 2009). At that time, the direction of impulse activity within the neurons remained a puzzling question to researchers, as nicely expounded by Cajal in *Recuerdos de Mi Vida*:

> In what direction does the nervous impulse travel within the neuron? Does it spread in all directions, like sound or light, or does it pass constantly in one direction like water in a watermill?
>
> *Ramón y Cajal, 1917*

It was commonly thought that dendrites played a nourishing role, while axons transmit nervous impulses in a cellulifugal direction (a generalization mostly based on the cellulifugal conduction in the axons of the spinal motor neurons). However, there was no general consensus or clear ideas about the role of dendrites in the processing of information. In 1889, Cajal thought it was clear that the dendrites play a role in receiving currents (Ramón y Cajal, 1889b), at least in certain cases, and 2 years later he tried to generalize this idea in the Law of Dynamic Polarization (Ramón y Cajal, 1891). This law was based on the direction followed by the impulses in regions of the nervous system, where, through their activity, it was apparently clear what anatomical routes the impulses followed, such as in the visual and olfactory systems (**Fig. F-35**):

> If in such inquiry, the [dendritic] arborization is always shown as a *receptor* apparatus and the [axonal arborization] as an apparatus for the *application* of the [impulses]. By analogy, we would have attained a rule to judge the direction of the currents in the [nerve cells within the central nervous system].

Cajal proposed that neurons could be divided into three functionally distinct regions: a receptor apparatus (formed by the dendrites and soma), an emission apparatus (the axon), and a distribution apparatus (terminal axonal arborization). He later realized that the soma does not always intervene in the conduction of the impulses and that sometimes impulse activity goes directly from the dendrites to the axon (Ramón y Cajal, 1897: **Fig. F-36**). Thus,

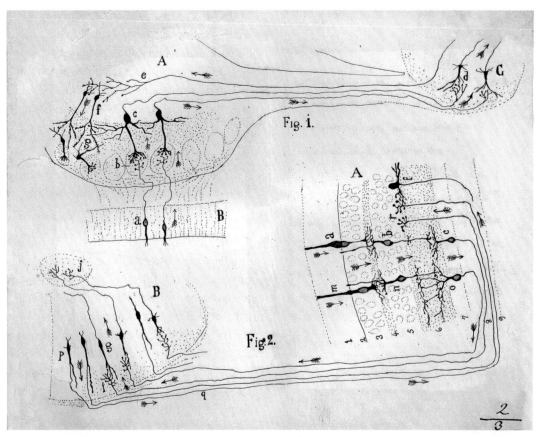

**FIGURE F-35.** Cajal's scheme showing the current flow in the visual and olfactory systems. This drawing was reproduced in his article "Significación fisiológica de las expansiones protoplásmicas y nerviosas de las células de la substancia gris" (*Rev. Ciencias Méd.* 22, 673–679; 715–723, 1891). The legend states: "*Fig. 1.* Scheme of cellular connections in the olfactory mucosa, olfactory bulb, tractus, and olfactory lobe of the cerebrum. The arrows indicate the direction of the currents. *A*, olfactory bulb; *B*, mucosa; *C*, olfactory lobe. *a, b, c, d.* One-way or centripetal pathway through which sensory or olfactory excitation passes. *e, f, g,* Centrifugal pathway through which the [nervous] centres can act on the elements of the bulb, granules and nerve cells, whose protoplasmic processes penetrate the glomeruli." "*Fig. 2.* Scheme of the visual excitation pathway through the retina, optic nerve and optic lobe of the birds. *A*, retina; *B*, optic lobe. *a, b, c,* represent a cone, a bipolar cell and a ganglion cell of the retina, respectively, the order through which visual excitation travels. *m, n, o,* parallel current emanating from the rod also involves bipolar and ganglion cells. *g,* cells of the optic lobe that receive the visual excitation and transfer it to *j,* the central ganglion. *p, q, r,* centrifugal currents that start in certain fusiform cells of the optic lobe and terminate in *r,* in the retina at the level of the spongioblasts; *f,* a spongioblast." Arrows indicate the direction of current flow.

the Law of Dynamic Polarization was changed to the Theory of Axipetal Polarization:

> The soma and dendrites display axipetal conduction, whereby they transmit the nervous waves towards the axon. Conversely, the axon or cylinder-axis has somatofugal or dendrifugal conduction, propagating the impulses received by the soma or dendrites towards the terminal axonal arborizations. [...]. This formula can be applied universally without exception, both in vertebrates and invertebrates.

Cajal's early studies with the Golgi method were so decisive that they represented the main core of the review published by Wilhelm von Waldeyer-Hartz (1836–1921) in the journal *Deutsche Medizinische Wochenschrift* in 1891 (**Fig. F-37**, *left*). In this article, the term *neuron* was introduced to denominate the nerve cells and the so-called neuron doctrine become popular. By the end of the nineteenth century this theory was the most accepted theory to explain the organization of the nervous system, in which the neuron was considered as the anatomical,

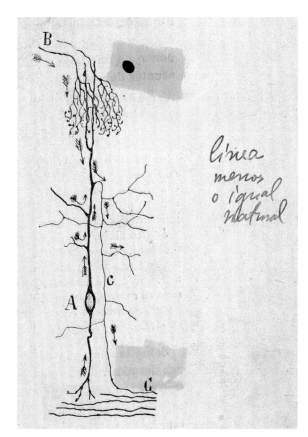

*línea menos o igual normal*

**FIGURE F-36.** Cajal's drawing reproduced in his article "Leyes de la morfología y dinamismo de las células nerviosas" (*Rev. Trimest. Micrográf.* 2, 1–28, 1987). The legend states: "Crosier cell of the optic lobe of the sparrow. *A*, soma; *B*, fibres arriving from the retina; *C*, central white matter; *c*, axon. Arrows indicate the direction of the current [flow]."

physiological, genetic, and metabolic unit of the nervous system (Shepherd, 1991; Jones, 1994, 2006). The many, fundamental contributions of Cajal to the neuron doctrine were summarized by himself in several articles and books, and especially in *Neuronismo o Reticularismo?* published in 1933 (**Fig. F-37**, *right*).

Nevertheless, despite the wealth of experimental data (from physiological and Wallerian secondary degeneration studies) and histological observations supporting the neuron doctrine, the crucial observation that there was a physical separation between the neurons took a long time to appear since the light microscope was not powerful enough to resolve this question. Thus, the neuron doctrine was generally accepted but with certain doubts, and exceptions were proposed up to the middle of the twentieth

century. This situation was beautifully summarized by Charles Sherrington (1857–1952) in his classic book *The Integrative Action of the Nervous System* (**Fig. F-38**). Sherrington, who in 1897 introduced the term *synapse* for the hypothetical one-way contact between axon terminals and somata or dendrites, wrote the following with regard to this subject:

> As to the existence or non-existence of a surface of separation or membrane between neurone and neurone, that is a structural question on which histology might be competent to give valuable information. In certain cases, especially in Invertebrata, observation (Apathy, Bethe, etc.) indicates that many nerve-cells are actually continuous one with another. It is noteworthy that in several of these cases the irreversibility of direction of conduction which is characteristic of spinal reflex-arcs is not demonstrable [...]. But in the neurone-chains on the gray-centred system of vertebrates, histology on the whole furnishes evidence that a surface of separation does exist between neurone and neurone. [...] It seems therefore likely that the nexus between neurone and neurone in the reflex-arc, at least in the spinal arc of the vertebrate, involves a surface of separation between neurone and neurone; and this as a transverse membrane across the conductor must be an important element in intercellular conduction. [...] In view, therefore, of the probable importance physiologically of this mode of nexus between neurone and neurone it is convenient to have a term for it. The term introduced has been *synapse* (Foster and Sherrington, 1897).
>
> *Sherrington, 1947*

It was not until the introduction of electron microscopy in the 1950s that the structural issues raised by Sherrington could be resolved. Along with the development of new methods to prepare nervous tissue for fine structural analysis (for example, fixation in osmium tetroxide and/or aldehydes, epoxy embedding, etc: Robertson, 1953; Palade and Palay, 1954; De Robertis and Bennett, 1955; Palay, 1956; De Robertis, 1959; Gray, 1959a, 1959b), this technique made it possible to examine the ultrastructure of the synapse. In this way one of the main tenets of the neural doctrine could be confirmed: presynaptic and

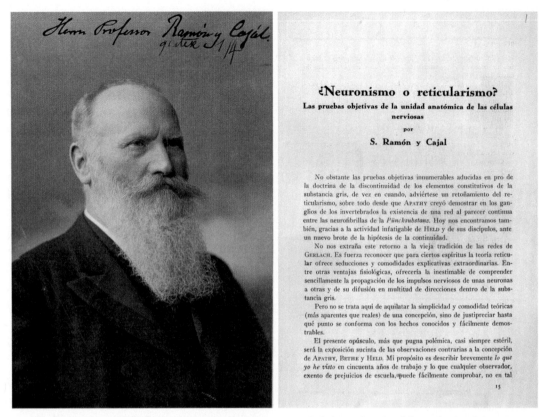

**FIGURE F-37.** (*Left*) Portrait of Wilhelm von Waldeyer-Hartz (1836–1921) dedicated to Cajal (Legado Cajal, Instituto Cajal). (*Right*) First page of the article of Cajal ¿Neuronismo o Reticularismo? (1933), where he summarized the main observations against the reticular theory.

postsynaptic elements are physically separated by a space about 10 to 20 nm wide (**Fig. F-39**), known as the synaptic cleft (reviewed in Peters et al., 1991).

Thus, the observations and theories of Cajal were essentially confirmed. However, the appearance of new techniques to study the nervous system at the anatomical, physiological, and molecular level has shown that there are many exceptions that challenge the neuron doctrine and the law of dynamic (or axipetal) polarization. For example, axons have been found to form synapses with other axons (axo-axonal synapses) and presynaptic elements are not necessarily axonal but they can be dendrites or somata. Thus, a variety of synaptic relationships have been observed, including dendro-dendritic, somato-somatic, somato-dendritic, dendro-somatic, dendro-axonic, and somato-axonic synapses (Peters et al., 1991). Furthermore, neurons are not only connected by point-to-point chemical synapses, but they may also be coupled electrically, while the direction of transmission may be bidirectional through gap junctions (Bennett, 2000). The plasma membranes of adjacent neurons are separated by a gap of about 2 nm, although they contain small channels (gap junctions) that connect the cytoplasm of the adjoining neurons, permitting the diffusion of small molecules and the flow of electric current (Bennett and Zukin, 2004; Hormuzdi et al., 2004). Moreover, the transmitter released at synaptic or nonsynaptic sites may diffuse and act on other synaptic contacts, or on extrasynaptic receptors (Fuxe et al., 2007). Finally, glial cells are not only key components of the nervous system because of their numerous structural, metabolic, and protective functions, but it has also been shown that astrocytes are involved in information processing

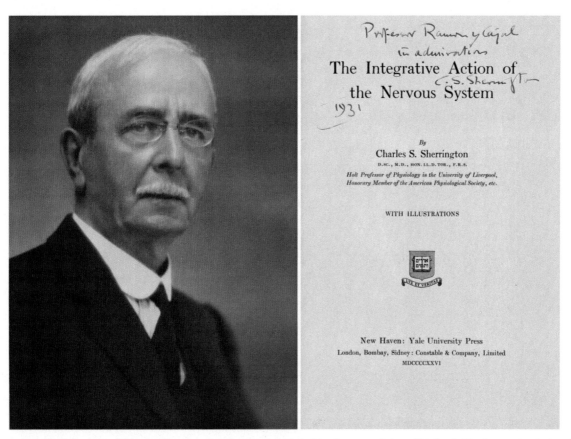

**FIGURE F-38.** (*Left*) Portrait of Charles Sherrington (1857–1952) included in the 1947 edition of his book *The Integrative Action of the Nervous System*. Reprinted with permission of The Royal Society. (*Right*) Cover of the book published in 1926 dedicated to Cajal.

through bidirectional signaling between these cells and neurons (Araque et al., 2001). These different features represent further complexity in the system, making it even more difficult to establish the information flow and wiring of neural circuits (DeFelipe, 2002b). Nevertheless, chemical axo-dendritic synapses are by far the most common type of synapse (followed by axo-somatic synapses), at least in mammals. Other types of synapses are not found in all regions of the nervous system and when they are present, they are usually only established between certain types of neurons. Therefore, we agree with the conclusion of Shepherd (2004) that the idea of the nerve cell as an independent cellular unit, with an overall polarization to mediate its input-output functions, continues to be one of the foundations on which our concepts of nervous activity are based (DeFelipe, 2009).

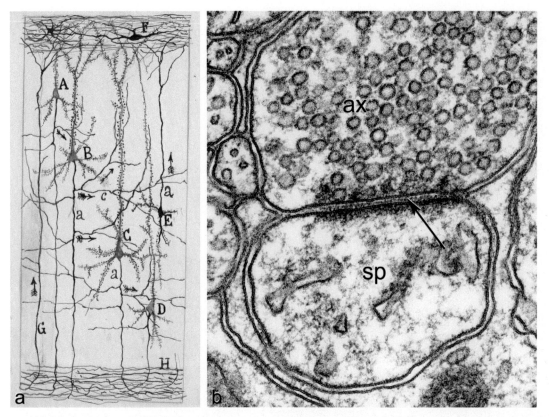

**FIGURE F-39.** (*a*) Schematic drawing by Cajal to show synaptic connections and the possible flow of information through neural circuits in the cerebral cortex. The legend states: "A, small pyramid; B and C, medium and giant pyramids respectively; a, axon; [c], nervous collaterals that appear to cross and touch the dendrites and the trunks [apical dendrites] of the pyramids; H, white matter; [E, Martinotti cell with ascending axon]; F, special cells of the first layer of cerebral cortex; G, fibre coming from the white matter. The arrows mark the supposed direction of the nervous current." Taken from *¿Neuronismo o Reticularismo?* (Ramón y Cajal, 1933, Figure 48). In the text, Cajal says, "Note how these collaterals cross and enter into transversal or oblique contact with a great number of the dendritic shafts. It is probable that collaterals rest on the spines which cover the protoplasmic surfaces [dendrites] like down." Thus, Cajal proposed that dendritic spines established synapses but, as shown in (*b*), it was necessary to wait several decades until the advent of electron microscopy to visualize the space that exists between the axon terminals and the dendrites. (*b*) Electron micrograph of a typical synapse. In this figure a synapse established between a parallel fiber varicosity (ax) and a spine of a Purkinje cell dendrite (sp) in the molecular layer of the rat cerebellum is shown. The presynaptic varicosity is filled with spherical synaptic vesicles that contain the neurotransmitter (glutamate). The synaptic cleft (between the pre- and postsynaptic membranes) is indicated by an arrow. (Courtesy of Constantino Sotelo, Instituto de Neurociencias, Alicante.)

[…] because of the different chemical composition of cells and intercellular substances, it is apparently a miracle that when exposed to a mixture of several dyes, each of them choose, fix and retain one of these colours and always the same one. As a result, polychromatic images can be obtained where the cellular nuclei, for example, display red colours with a smooth range of tones, the protoplasm, yellow and orange colours, and the [intercellular substance], green and blue colours […] through these tools, the histologist not only discerns the beauty of the forms and groups of cells, but also their chemical composition, enabling him to deduce the normal or altered functional properties of these cells.

*Del Río-Hortega, "Arte y Artificio de la Ciencia Histológica"*

SECTION 3

# THE COLORFUL PERIOD: INTERNAL STRUCTURE AND CHEMISTRY OF THE CELLS

## ON THE EARLY USE OF SELECTIVE COLORANTS TO STUDY THE NERVOUS SYSTEM

It is important to emphasize that different fixation and staining protocols are necessary to observe and analyze specific architectonic aspects of the nervous system, and the morphology and cytology of neurons or glia. These techniques have been developed over the years and rely on the use of a wide variety of chemicals (pyridine, methylene blue, mercuric chloride, osmic acid, silver solutions, etc). For instance, lipids and myelin are well preserved when the tissue is fixed in formol followed by mordanting in potassium dichromate, and this improves the visualization of myelin sheaths when stained with hematoxylin. The lipids of myelin are removed if the fixative includes solvents like alcohol, ether, or chloroform, whereas if these solvents are omitted the lipids of the myelin sheath can be stained with osmic acid. Thus, there are specific methods to visualize different types of glial cells and not neurons, or methods to label mainly neurons, with their dendritic and axonal processes, or techniques that stain the neurofibrils but not other cytoplasmic organelles. Selective staining procedures were discovered to examine the different types of organelles in the perikaryon (e.g., Nissl bodies, mitochondria, neurofibrils, Golgi apparatus, inclusions such as pigments, fat and lipids, etc). Indeed, as Alan Peters, Sanford Palay, and Henry Webster stated in their book *The Fine Structure of the Nervous System* (New York: Oxford University Press,

1991): "Our image of the nerve cell at the light microscope level is like a collage of many overlapping views, patiently accrued during a century of study."

Thanks to the extraordinary variety of techniques used to unravel the complex structure and organization of the nervous system, a beautiful microscopic world has been discovered with an almost infinite combination of forms and multiple colors. The coming together of art and science was nicely presented by Pío del Río-Hortega (1882–1945):

> After using a technical process of those that required the careful combination of several complementary colours: red and green, yellow and blue, the histologist finally got a true picture from which three sources of pure emotion could be derived: that which stems from the beauty of the landscape itself, with its polychromatic nature, its tones and [depth]; that which emanates from the observer himself, who feels the hidden satisfaction of achieving his purpose; and that which emerges from the novelty of the details resolved, [that is] the discovery of ignored truths.
>
> *Del Río-Hortega, 1933*

## THE FIRST EXPLOSION OF COLOR: THE NORMAL AND ALTERED CYTOLOGY OF NEURAL CELLS

The first explosion of color appeared in the field when scientists began to examine cytoplasmic organelles in detail to address the possible changes associated with the functional state of nerve cells. For this purpose, a variety of methods were developed that involved the use of different dyes. Through these colorants, they could analyze cytological characteristics and infer the chemical composition in both normal and altered states. One of the starting points was the study of nerve cells from a dynamic point of view that began in the 1880s and 1890s. Did all the nerve cell's connections with other neurons remain immutable, or are neurons dynamic elements capable of continuously altering their connections? Did the activity of neurons produce chemical or morphological changes in their constitution? What follows is a summary of some of the early studies on the internal structure of the neuron.

One of the most important pioneering studies of these issues was performed by Flesch in 1886. This author observed that there were two very well-differentiated types of neurons in the Gasser ganglion of the trigeminal nerve, distinguished by their affinity for the dyes: cromophilic and cromophobic cells. Flesch and his colleagues reached the conclusion that these differences were due to internal chemical modifications related to the functional state of the cells at the moment of tissue fixation (e.g., Flesch and Koneff, 1886). Later, several scientists, including Cajal (1896), studied this differential staining in several ganglia and regions of the central nervous system and, in general, it was concluded that the cromophilic nerve cells were possibly in a resting state, while the cromophobic cells correlated with a more active state.

At the end of the 1880s, the histological changes associated with the functional state of neurons began to be approached experimentally, mostly after electrical stimulation or by examining the tissue after normal neural activity. The pioneers in these studies included Hodge (1888, 1889, 1892) and Korybutt-Daszkiewicz (1889). The studies of Hodge were particularly influential since in addition to investigating the effects of electrical stimulation of the dorsal root ganglia of several species of vertebrates, he analyzed the phenomenon of their normal activity in invertebrates. For example, Hodge

examined the histological changes in the cerebral ganglia of bees that had been fixed in the morning, after resting overnight, and he compared the results with the changes observed in the cerebral ganglia fixed in the evening, after a day of normal activity. Hodge's studies were soon followed by those of others in several species (e.g., Vas, 1892; Lambert, 1893; Mann, 1894; Lugaro, 1895). The most frequent experimental procedure was to stimulate the sensory or sympathetic ganglia at one site and compare this with the intact contralateral side. The changes described varied, and they included changes in the size and position of the nucleus, vacuolization and modifications in the staining of the cytoplasm, and changes in the size of the cell body. However, the electrical stimulation used did not represent the normal physiological activity of neurons. Thus, Mann (1894) inspired by the research of Hodge, examined the histological modifications induced by physiological and regular activity in several regions of the brain. He compared the motor areas of the brain and spinal cord between two dogs, one of which had been resting while the other was active for 10 hours (**Fig. F-40**). He said:

> ...in the fresh brain the nerve cells appear as deep blue bodies on a light background, while in the worked brain they are very pale or quite colourless, and they appear as light figures on a darker background.

The changes found in the internal structure of the motor neurons motivated Mann to analyze whether similar changes occurred in sensory cells. He analyzed the effects of light on the retina and the optical centers in the brain, including the visual cortex, of dogs that were allowed to move freely for 12 hours with one eye covered up and the other exposed to light (**Fig. F-41**). The main conclusions reached by Mann were that activity was accompanied by an increase in the size of the cells, the nuclei, and the nucleoli of sympathetic, motor, and sensory ganglion cells. By contrast, the fatigue of neurons was associated with the shriveling of the nucleus and probably also of the cell, as well as with the formation of diffuse chromatic material in the nucleus.

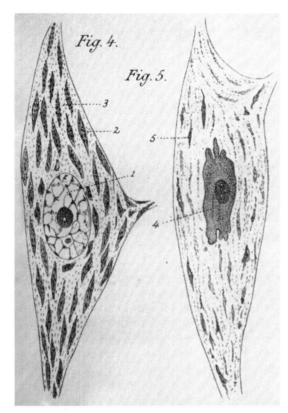

**FIGURE F-40.** Mann's drawings (1894) of motor cells from the lumbar region of the spinal cord of dog, fixed in HgCl₂ and stained in Toluidine-blue. (*Left*) "Fig. 4 from a fresh dog: (1) pale nucleus, (2) dark Nissl's spindles, (3) bundles of nerve-fibrils." (*Right*) "Fig. 5 from the fatigued dog, with (4) dark shrivelled nuclei and (5) pale spindles."

Following the ideas of Mann, Demoor (1896) and Pergens (1896) studied the effect of visual deprivation in several optic centers in the dog and in the retina of fish. Demoor examined the effect of closing one eye for a given time, while Pergens investigated the effect of the lack of light on retinal cells. They both identified cytological changes. However, since the observations in different studies were not uniform after electrical stimulation, or even when similar experiments were performed, and because the histological methods were often poor, Cajal (1899–1904) concluded that this type of research should be continued and that the stimulation of neurons in these experiments should be performed under physiological conditions.

Some years later, Cajal and his disciples used the reduced silver nitrate method, a new technique that Cajal had developed in 1903 (Ramón y Cajal, 1903a, 1903b), to study the neurofibrillar structure of the neurons. This method was based on that published by Simarro (1900) to study the neurofibrillar structure of the neuronal cytoplasm. According to Tello (1935), Cajal had observed variability in the staining that he was unable to interpret. At that time, Tello had begun to study neurofibrils in several animals (Tello, 1903, 1904) and he had observed that in reptiles, there were

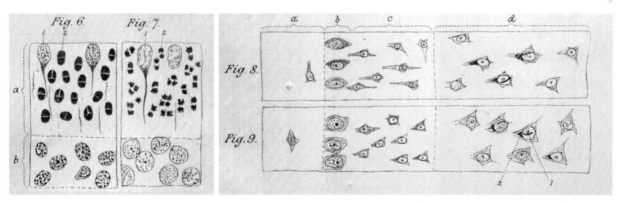

**FIGURE F-41.** Mann's drawings (1894) of the retina of a dog and the visual cortex of a rabbit. In the figure legend he states: "Figures 6 and 7 retinae of dogs fixed in corrosive sublimate, stained in Toluidine-blue. Fig. 6 from eye kept dark. Fig. 7 from eye exposed for twelve hours to ordinary daylight on a sunny day. (*a*) layer of nuclei of cones (1) and rods (2), (*b*), middle ganglionic layer. Figures 8 and 9 from lower aspect of occipital lobe of rabbit. Fixed in sublimate, stained in 1 per cent, watery solution of Eosin for 1 minute and Toulidine-blue ½ per cent for 15 minutes. Fig. 8 corresponds to eye kept dark. Fig. 9 corresponds to eye exposed for two hours of flashes of light. *a* = molecular layer; *b* = layer of cells, first described by Ramón y Cajal, for which I suggest the name "submolecular; *c* = layer of small pyramidal cells; *d* = layer of large pyramidal cells. 1. Intra-nuclear chromatic crescents (centrosomes?). 2. Chromatic material on apex of nucleus."

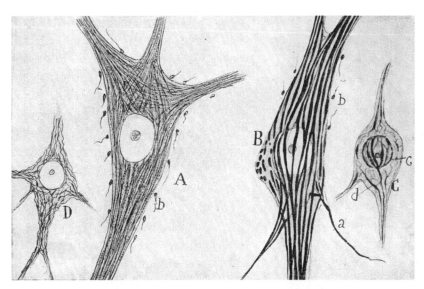

**FIGURE F-42.** Illustration used by Cajal to show the normal variations of the neurofibrillar plexus in cells of the lizard spinal cord. A and D, motor and funicular corpuscles in activity (30 hours of [incubation] at 30°C); B and C, motor and funicular cells of the lizard spinal cord maintained at normal temperature (12°C); *a*, axon; *b*, terminal club endings; *c*, perinuclear [neuro-fibrillar] net; *d*, thickened primary filament. Reduced silver nitrate method. This figure was reproduced as Figure 864 in *Textura* (Ramón y Cajal, 1899–1904).

fewer and much thicker neurofibrils than in other animals. Tello (1935) commented that he performed these studies in winter with lethargic lizards and snakes, but when carried out on lizards that were "excited" since their tail was pulled up when spring was approaching, there were many more neurofibrils and they were of a similar thickness to those in mammals. Hence, Cajal thought that the thickening of the neurofibrils could be due to the cooling during winter hibernation. This idea was verified after forcing the lizards to wake up by prolonged incubation in the oven, observing that the neurofibrils were thinner, as in amputated lizards (**Fig. F-42**). In volume 2 of *Textura* (Ramón y Cajal, 1889–1904), Cajal commented:

> [ . . . ] when spring arrives or the temperature rises where the reptile is resident, or it is excited by any procedure that activates the spinal cord, the thin neurofibrils reappear and are multiplied enormously [ . . . ] The recent studies of Tello in our laboratory have proved that changing the resting state to a state of [activity] [**Fig. F-42**] can be achieved by just warming up the reptile for half an hour [ . . . ]. Note [in **Fig. F-42**] the enormous difference in the

reticulum between the two states and bear in mind that we have used perfectly normal conditions for this experiment (whose results are absolutely consistent in all reptiles) [ . . . ] Regarding the mechanism by which the temperature or the state of activity produces such very interesting variations of the reticulum, our studies are still insufficient to formulate a solid explanation.

Cajal studied the variation in the number, shape, and thickness of the neurofibrils in several vertebrates (including mammals) and invertebrates, in both normal and pathological conditions (e.g., Ramón y Cajal, 1904a, 1904b). He reached the conclusion that there was a consistent relationship in some animals between the thickness of the neurofibrils and the state of activity or inactivity (normal or pathologically induced). According to Cajal (1909–1911), these studies were confirmed by many researchers (e.g., Marinesco, 1904, 1906; Dustin, 1905; Rebizzi, 1906), but the significance of these changes could not be explored and this line of research was practically abandoned.

During the first three decades of 1900, marvelous drawings were produced to illustrate different characteristics of the normal and altered cytology and histology of the nervous system in general. The staining procedures not only included a large number of reagents and methods, such as eosin, toulidine blue, reduced silver nitrate, silver carbonate, methylene blue, erythrosine, carmine, hematoxylin, etc., but also the numerous modifications introduced by different scientists, like Weigert's staining for glia, Cajal's gold chloride sublimate method, the method of Mann-Alzheimer, the method of Alzheimer-Mallory, the method of Bielschowsky, etc. For example, the drawings of Emil Holmgren (1866–1922) showing normal nerve cells of the leech, lamprey, crayfish, and spiny dogfish are particularly beautiful (**Fig. F-43**).

As shown in **Figure F-44**, the drawings of senile plaques made by Alois Alzheimer (1864–1915), Oskar Fischer (1876–1942), Georges Marinesco (1863–1938), and Walther Spielmeyer (1879–1935) have a great aesthetic appeal, as well as show changes in neurons in cases of dementia precox (Rezza, 1913: **Fig. F-45**).

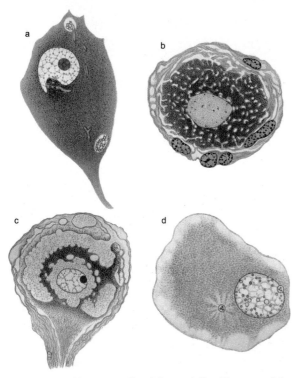

**FIGURE F-43.** (*a*) Nerve cells of the medulla oblongata of the lamprey (*Petromyzon*), (*b*) esophageal ganglion of the crayfish (*Astacus fluviatilis*), (*c*) of the esophageal ganglion of the leech (*Hirudo medicinalis*), (*d*) and of the spinal cord of spiny dogfish (*Acanthias*). Taken from Holmgren (1900).

Another example of the wonderful drawings produced at that time is shown in **Figure F-46,** where various aspects of the degeneration of the nervous system are shown by Fritz Lotmar (1878–1964) in a wealth of detail and color.

Finally, **Figure F-47** illustrates the correlation between a drawing of Cajal and a very nice preparation he made showing the violet impregnation of the neurofibrils obtained with his reduced silver nitrate/gold toning (treatment with gold chloride) technique.

I would like to warn the reader that in many cases the chemical reaction that labels the cellular and subcellular elements in the nervous system is unknown. Furthermore, in some cases the labeling has proved to be an artifact of the techniques or the authors' incorrect interpretation. However, in general these tools represent the roots of our knowledge of the cytology, histology, and anatomy of the nervous system. Indeed, these techniques and the methods derived from them continued to be used for decades. Ted Jones, one of the most distinguished modern neuroanatomists, states:

> It is salutary for us to recognize that the years subsequent to Cajal's last major papers in the early 1920s were years in which the techniques at the disposal of neuroanatomists remained those that Cajal himself had used or that had been in existence even before he commenced his research. Not that these were years of impoverished discovery [ . . . ] the post-Cajal years were those of active research on the long tract connections in the nervous system, an area in which the Golgi technique could yield little. But it is also true to say that these important investigations on the spinal, brainstem and thalamocortical pathways were conducted with techniques that predated Cajal's perfection of the Golgi technique.
>
> *Jones, 2007*

Over the years, neuroanatomy has evolved considerably thanks to the use of classical techniques and to the introduction of new procedures (Jones and Hartman, 1978), such as axonal transport methods to trace connections; electron microscopy to better understand synaptic connectivity; immunocytochemistry to map protein expression and the distribution of particular types of neurons; in situ

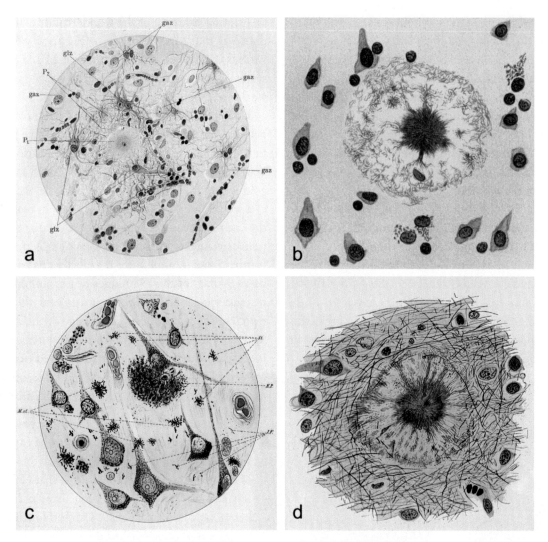

**FIGURE F-44.** Drawings of senile plaques from (*a*) Alzheimer (1911), (*b*) Fischer (1912), (*c*) Marinesco and Minea (1912), and (*d*) Spielmeyer (1922) using different techniques: Weigert method to stain glia, Carbol methylene blue/methylene violet, staining using a "Cajal's modified method," and Bielschowsky silver impregnation, respectively.

hybridization to map gene expression; intracellular labeling of physiologically characterized neurons to visualize their morphology; and other powerful techniques to examine the organization of the nervous system. For example, after the renaissance of the Golgi method in the 1960s and 1970s, mainly after the publication of several important contributions (e.g., Sholl, 1956; Colonnier, 1966; Marin-Padilla, 1969; Szentágothai, 1969; Scheibel and Scheibel, 1970; Valverde, 1970; Lund, 1973; Jones, 1975; reviewed in DeFelipe, 2002b), several methods appeared to intracellularly label individual neurons. One of these

methods consists of combining light and electron microscopy tracing of cells after intracellular application of horseradish peroxidase (HRP; Cullheim and Kellerth, 1976; Jankowska et al., 1976). The main advantages of this method were that it permitted a far more complete visualization of axon arbors than the Golgi method, as well as coupling the physiological characterization of the HRP-labeled neurons with an electron microscopy study of the synapses formed by these cells. Further combinations of different techniques (degeneration methods, immunocytochemistry, etc) for correlative light and electron microscopy

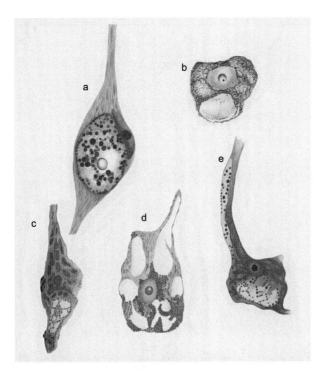

**FIGURE F-45.** Drawings showing the changes in neurons of the medulla oblongata associated with dementia precox, using different methods: (*a*) Mann-Alzheimer method; (*b*) Bielschowscky method; (*c*) Weigert method to stain neuroglia; (*d*) Daddi-Herxheimer method; and (*e*) Alzheimer-Mallory method. Taken from Rezza (1913).

soon followed. The application of these methods permitted the more detailed examination of the afferent and efferent connections and chemical characteristics of Golgi-impregnated neurons, of retrogradely HRP-labeled neurons, and of neurons physiologically characterized and intracellularly labeled to visualize their morphology with Lucifer Yellow, biocytin, neurobiotin, HRP, or other markers (for reviews, see White, 1989; Nieuwenhuys, 1994; Somogyi, 1990; DeFelipe, 2002b; Fairén, 2005). Finally, as we will see below, molecular/genetic approaches are now among the most appealing new tools to activate, inactivate, and label active neurons and synapses (Marek and Davis, 2003; Dymecki and Kim, 2007; Kuhlman and Huang, 2008), such as the generation of genetically modified mice that express fluorescent proteins in subsets of cells (e.g., the Brainbow mouse; Lichtman et al., 2008).

## THE SECOND EXPLOSION OF COLOR: FLUORESCENCE MICROSCOPY AND CONFOCAL LASER SCANNING MICROSCOPY

In the late 1970s, fluorescence microscopy and the use of fluorescent dyes or fluorochrome stains to visualize a molecule of interest in specimens became a commonly used technique in neuroscience. For instance, Kuypers and colleagues studied long-range connections using bisbenzimide and Nuclear Yellow to produce green and golden-yellow retrograde labeling of a neuron's nucleus, and True Blue and Fast Blue were used to produce blue retrograde labeling of the neuron's cytoplasm (Kuypers et al., 1980). At the same time, the availability of a variety of neural-specific antibodies and secondary antibodies conjugated to different fluorescent tags (e.g., rhodamine-conjugated [red] and fluorescein-conjugated [green] secondary antisera) facilitated colocalization studies to be performed in which two or more substances could be identified in a given neuron (e.g., Hendry et al., 1984). Combinations of various techniques served to examine other aspects of the organization of the nervous system. For example, combining retrograde tracing and fluorescent dye injection with indirect immunofluorescence histochemistry permitted the neurochemical characterization of neurons that could be identified by their projection site and their labeling in different colors (e.g., Skirboll et al., 1984). Thus, multicolor images using several fluorophores could be obtained by combining several single-color images. However, one of the limitations of fluorescent microscopy is that interference of the fluorescent emissions occurs above and below the focal plane; therefore, it is not possible to obtain high-resolution optical images of thick specimens. This problem was resolved with the introduction of confocal laser scanning microscopy, which became a standard technique toward the end of the 1980s. Since confocal microscopy images are acquired point by point (optical sectioning) and these images can be computer reconstructed in three dimensions, it is possible to analyze with relative ease complex spatial relationships between neural elements visualized with different colors in thick sections (**Fig. F-48**).

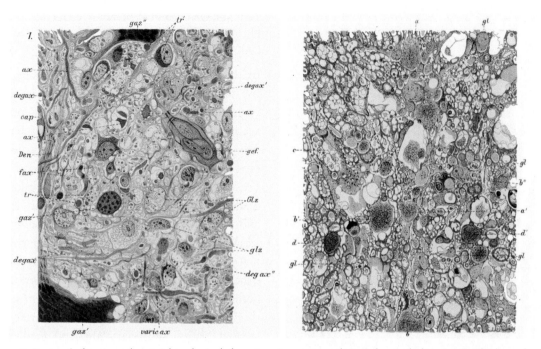

**FIGURE F-46.** Lotmar's drawings showing histological alterations in acute myelitis and encephalitis (1918). The legend states: (*Left*) "Degeneration of fine nervous structures 'axis cylinder, eventually thin dendrites' in the marginal region of the anterior horn. Method of Mann." (*Right*) "Axon swelling general view of a transversal section through the marginal region of a focus in the white matter of the spinal cord showing axon swelling. Fuchsin staining."

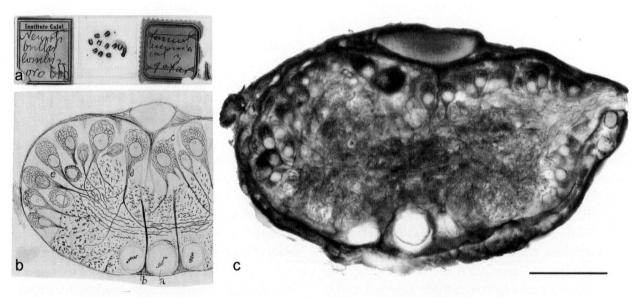

**FIGURE F-47.** (*a*) Photograph of Cajal's preparation of an earthworm stained with his reduced silver nitrate/gold toning method. (*b*) Cajal's drawing (1904c) of a transverse section of a ganglion of the earthworm's (*Lumbricus agricola*) ventral chain. The legend states: "*a*, colossal tube [axon]; *b*, neuroglial column; *c*, multipolar corpuscle [neuron]; *d*, commissural cell; *e*, unipolar elements [cells]." (*c*) Photomicrograph taken from a section in (*a*) to illustrate the same structures as observed in Cajal's drawing. Scale bar: 500 μm. The histological images were obtained by Virginia García-Marín, Pablo García-López, and Miguel Freire (Legado Cajal, Instituto Cajal).

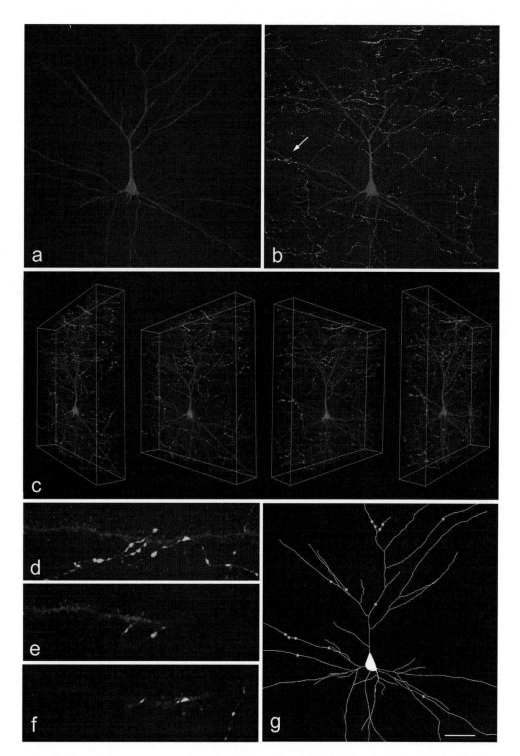

**FIGURE F-48.** (*a*) Confocal microscopy stack of 64 serial images showing a pyramidal neuron intracellularly injected with Lucifer Yellow in the human temporal cortex. (*b*) By combining the image in (*a*) with that obtained following immunocyto-chemistry for tyrosine hydroxylase (TH) in the same section, it is possible to establish the relative location of TH-labeled axons (green) with respect to the dendritic arbor of the pyramidal cell. (*c*) 3D visualization of the stack of serial images shown in (*b*) at different angles. (*d–f*) High-magnification images of the region indicated in *b* (arrow), showing an example of TH-labeled axonal appositions with the dendritic spines (*e*) and shafts (*f*) of the labeled pyramidal cell. (*g*) Map showing the distribution of putative TH-labeled inputs (green dots) along the length of the apical and basal dendrites of the 3D reconstructed pyramidal neuron. Sections were double-stained using a rabbit and a mouse antiserum against Lucifer Yellow and TH, respectively. Labeling was visualized with a biotinylated horse anti-mouse IgG and a mixture of Alexa fluor 594-conjugated goat anti-rabbit (red) and streptavidin-conjugated Alexa fluor 488 (green). Scale bar: 50 μm in *a, b, g*; 10 μm in *d, e, f*. See text for further details. The injections and figure were prepared by Ruth Benavides-Piccione (Instituto Cajal; see Benavides-Piccione et al., 2005).

For instance, to quantify the spatial relationship between catecholaminergic fibers and the dendritic arbor of pyramidal neurons in the human cerebral cortex, cells can be labeled by injecting them with Lucifer Yellow, and then immunocytochemistry can be performed for the rate-limiting catecholamine-synthesizing enzyme tyrosine hydroxylase to visualize catecholaminergic fibers in the same sections. In double-labeled sections (**Fig. F-48**), a three-dimensional reconstruction of pyramidal cells (red) can be performed with the Neurolucida software and the putative appositions of tyrosine hydroxylase-positive fibers (green) are marked in serial stacks of confocal microscopy images of each injected cell (Benavides-Piccione et al., 2005). In this way, a map of catecholaminergic appositions with the dendritic arbor of neurons can be obtained. At present, thanks to the widespread use of confocal microscopy and the availability of new fluorophores, fluorescent proteins, and immunofluorescence reagents, confocal microscopy has become an indispensable tool to analyze the nervous system, giving rise to a new colorful period in the neurosciences (**Fig. F-49**).

## THE THIRD EXPLOSION OF COLOR: THE GREEN FLUORESCENT PROTEIN AND THE BRAINBOW

Another major innovation in imaging has come in recent years from the identification of the green fluorescent protein (GFP), originally isolated from the jellyfish *Aequorea victoria*. The GFP gene can be introduced into intact cells and organisms in such a way that when the gene for GFP is fused to the gene encoding a given protein, the expressed protein preserves its normal activity while GFP maintains its fluorescence, providing us with a very useful marker for gene expression (Tsien, 1998). Engineering of GFP has permitted brighter and more stable variants to be generated, with various excitation and emission spectra, marking a new era for imaging in cell biology (Giepmans et al., 2006). The impact of GFP and its variants has been extraordinary. Indeed, Martin Chalfie, Osamu Shimomura, and Roger Y. Tsien were awarded the 2008 Nobel Prize in Chemistry "for their discovery and development of the green fluorescent protein." The application

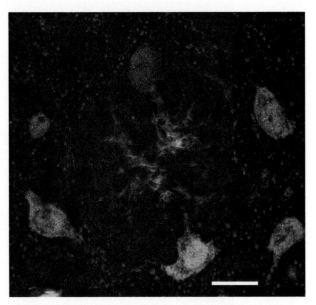

**FIGURE F-49.** Confocal microscopy analysis of GABAergic innervation of neurons near amyloid plaques in a mouse model of Alzheimer disease (APP/PS1 transgenic mouse). Triple fluorescence immunohistochemistry to examine neurons visualized with NeuN (green) in contact with plaques labeled with Thioflavine-S (blue) that were innervated by GABAergic terminals that were in turn visualized with an antibody against the GABA transporter 1 (GAT1, red). This figure represents a stack of three optical images each separated by 0.2 μm in the z-axis. Scale bar: 25 μm. From Virginia García-Marín, Lidia Blázquez-Llorca, and Javier DeFelipe (Instituto Cajal).

of this technology to study brain circuits now represents one of the most exciting, beautiful, and promising areas in neuroanatomy. For example, transgenic mice have been generated in which red, green, yellow, or cyan fluorescent proteins (called XFPs) are selectively expressed in neurons, such that the labeling is similar to the Golgi staining but in bright colors. Mice expressing spectrally distinct XFPs can be crossed to generate "bicolor" or "tricolor" animals in which the possible connections between the labeled neurons can be visualized (Feng et al., 2000).

One of the most fascinating new tools is the combinatorial color method, called Brainbow, in which rather than labeling neurons in one of two or three colors, they can be labeled in one of more than 100 colors (Livet et al., 2007). The combinatorial expression of red, green, and blue XFPs at

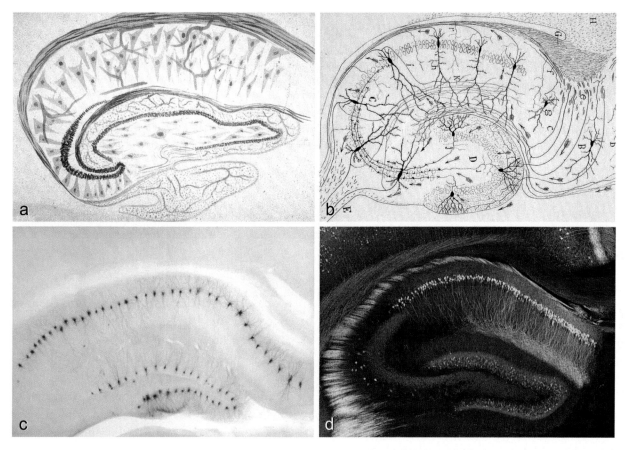

**FIGURE F-50.** Hippocampus visualized with different techniques from the nineteenth through the twenty-first centuries. (*a*) Drawing of the hippocampus dated in 1876—before the classic studies performed with the Golgi method—from Giulio Bizzozero (1846–1901) who introduced Golgi to experimental research and histological techniques (kindly provided by Marina Bentivoglio, University of Verona). (*b*) Drawing taken from Cajal (1901–1902) showing the structure and connections of the hippocampus from small mammals based on the Golgi method. (*c*) Photomicrograph of a section from the mouse hippocampus where neurons were injected with Lucifer Yellow and then processed with a light-stable diaminobenzidine reaction product (brown color). The injections and figure were prepared by Asta Kastanauskaite (Instituto Cajal). (*d*) An image taken from a mouse that was genetically modified to express fluorescent proteins in subsets of cells kindly provided by Tamily Weissman and Jeff Lichtman (Harvard University). Neurons are labeled in color because they express different combinations of yellow, blue (cyan), or red fluorescent proteins. The curved hippocampal formation is shown where the cells within the dentate gyrus and CA regions are labeled to different extents. Curving around the hippocampus, fibers can be seen coursing through both the corpus callosum (red, to the right), which carries information between the cerebral hemispheres and the alveus (green, to the left), which transmits information from the hippocampus to the entorhinal cortex. This picture represents a portion of an image that included the neocortex above the hippocampus and that was the winner of Neuroscapes 2006 award. This exhibition was inaugurated in Barcelona on April 6, 2006 before its international launch during the Cajal Centenary Conference on the Cerebral Cortex, held at the CosmoCaixa Science Museum (Barcelona), April 25–29 (*Paisajes Neuronales, Homenaje a Santiago Ramón y Cajal*, Madrid: CSIC, 2007). As an example of the interest of the general public on the beauty of the brain, since the inauguration of Neuroscapes in Barcelona, several cities in Spain (including Valladolid, Cuenca, Logroño, Murcia, Madrid, Cádiz, Almería, and Las Palmas) and around the world (New York, Chicago, Melbourne, Jerusalem, Ribeirao Preto, Sao Paolo, Rio de Janeiro, Salvador de Bahia, Belo Horizonte and Brasilia) have already hosted the exhibition. Moreover, several cities around the world have expressed an interest in hosting the exhibition.

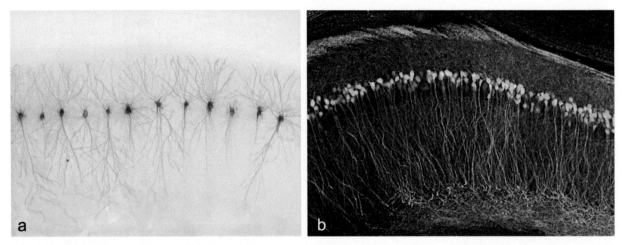

**FIGURE F-51.** Higher magnification of **Figure F-50c and d**, respectively.

various levels can generate a large spectrum of colors. Lichtman et al. (2008) drew the nice analogy between the Brainbow and an RGB video monitor "which combines different intensities of three channels (red, green, and blue) to generate almost the entire color spectrum that the human visual system can perceive." Since several Brainbow lines are available, it is expected that this "technicolor approach" will help us discover new aspects of neuronal circuits, enabling us to analyze them on a large scale. We have shown how the methods to analyze neuronal circuits have evolved dramatically over the years in **Figure F-50**, from the era of Cajal to the present day. In **Figure F-51**, a higher magnification of **Figure F-50c and d** is shown to demonstrate the neurons labeled with modern techniques in greater detail (intracellular injections and XPSs).

# Closing Comments on the Brain and Art

While reflecting on the Brainbow mouse, the comment of the Russian writer Vladimir Nabokov (1899–1977) comes to mind: "which is as if genes were painting in aquarelle." Nabokov, mainly known for his novel *Lolita* (1955), was a grapheme-color synesthete—synesthetes are individuals displaying synesthesia, a phenomenon in which stimulation of one sensory or cognitive pathway leads to associated experiences in a second, unstimulated stream (e.g., Hubbard, 2007 and references contained therein)—made this comment in a television interview in 1962 (published in *The Listener and BBC Television Review* 68, 856–858: "Vladimir Nabokov on His Life and Work"). Afterward, he said, "I have this rather freakish gift of seeing letters in color," and the interviewer asked him, "What colours are your own initials, VN?" Nabokov answered:

> V is a kind of pale, transparent pink [...]: this is one of the closest colours that I can connect with the V. And the N, on the other hand, is a grey-ish-yellowish oatmeal colour. But a funny thing happens: my wife has this gift of seeing letters in colour, too, but her colours are completely different. There are, perhaps, two or three letters where we coincide, but otherwise the colours are quite different. It turned out, we discovered one day, that my son [...] sees letters in colours, too. [...] Then we asked him to list his colours and we discovered that in one case, one letter which he sees as purple, or perhaps mauve, is pink to me and blue to my wife. This is the letter M. So the combination of pink

and blue makes lilac in his case. Which is as if his genes were painting in aquarelle.

It is amazing that this metaphor of Nabokov has become virtually real with the Brainbow mice, where rather than in aquarelle, genes are painted with fluorescent proteins, a great revelation for literary and artistic inspiration for a grapheme-color synesthete like Nabokov.

Certainly, artistic creativity is a product of the brain, which interprets the external world by processing the information it receives through its neuronal circuits. However, the similarities between scientific illustrations and some paintings created by artists make me wonder whether the artist was unconsciously painting not only what his brain was interpreting, but to some extent, what his own brain contains. Indeed, the photomicrography images of crystallized neurotransmitters, when visualized using polarized light microscopy, resemble the cubist paintings or abstract art of Franz Marc (1880–1916) or Juan Gris (1887–1927: **Fig. F-52**).

Finally, **Figure F-53** shows an artistic composite illustration comprising a collage of digital images of the major neurotransmitters in the brain (glutamate, GABA, norepinephrine, serotonin, acetylcholine, and dopamine) superimposed on a picture of a human brain.

This cocktail of "colorful" neurotransmitters is intended to show that the inexhaustible artistic creativity of the human mind seems to have a parallel multicolored world within the microscopic universe of the brain.

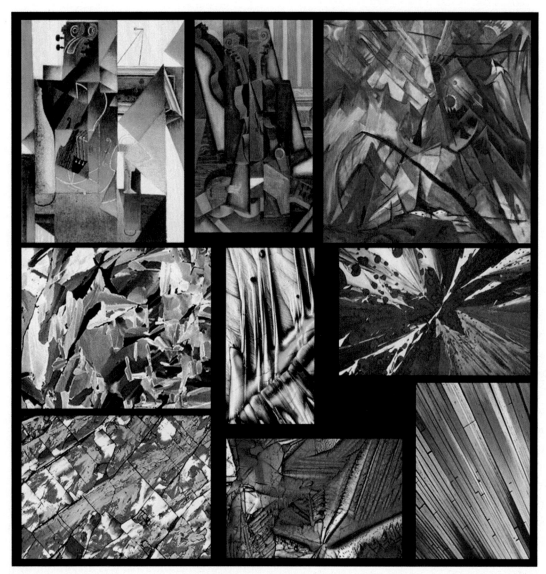

**FIGURE F-52.** (*From left to right, top row*) Paintings by the artists Juan Gris (1887–1927: the first two pictures are *Violin and Engraving, 1913* and *Violin and Guitar, 1913* respectively) and Franz Marc (1880–1916: *Tyrol*, 1914). (*middle row*) Polarized light photomicrographs showing glutamate, norepinephrine, and dopamine, respectively. (*bottom row*) Polarized light photomicrographs showing GABA, serotonin, and acetylcholine. Note the resemblance of the art and image of the neurotransmitters. Pictures of polarized light microscopy provided by Michael W. Davidson (Florida State University).

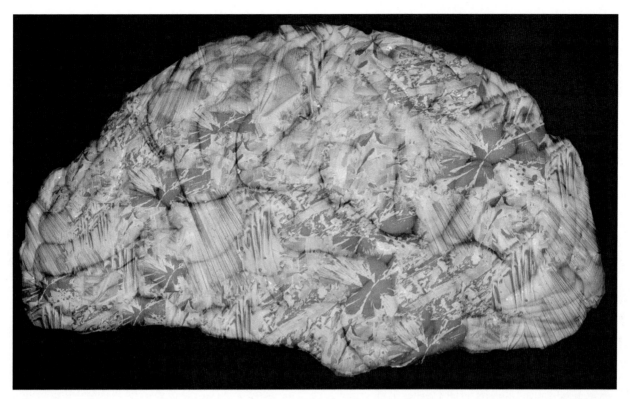

FIGURE F-53. Artistic representation of the human brain in which the colors represent the major neurotransmitters found in the brain (see **Fig. F-52**).

## ➤ BIBLIOGRAPHY

Alonso-Nanclares, L., Gonzalez-Soriano, J., Rodriguez, J. R., and DeFelipe, J. (2008) Gender differences in human cortical synaptic density. *Proc. Natl. Acad. Sci. USA* 105, 14615–14619.

Álvarez-Leefmans, F. J. (1987) La teoría celular en el tiempo: relato histórico que muestra que los hechos son los tiranos de la razón y los instrumentos sus cómplices. In *Teorías y hechos sobre la vida. Las células*, ed. J. Muñoz, 9–73. Mexico D.F.: Consejo Nacional de Fomento Educativo (SEP).

Alzheimer, A. (1911) Über eigenartige Krankheitsfälle des späteren Alters. *Z. gesamte Neurol. Psychiatr.* 4, 356–385.

Araque, A., Carmignoto, G., and Haydon, P. G. (2001) Dynamic signaling between astrocytes and neurons. *Ann. Rev. Physiol.* 63, 95–813.

Barker, L. F. (1899) *The nervous system and its constituent neurones*. New York: Appleton.

Benavides-Piccione, R., Arellano, J. I., and DeFelipe, J. (2005) Catecholaminergic innervation of pyramidal neurons in the human temporal cortex. *Cereb. Cortex* 15, 1584–1592.

Bennett, M. V. (2000) Electrical synapses, a personal perspective (or history). *Brain Res. Brain Res. Rev.* 32, 16–28.

Bennett, M. V., and Zukin, R. S. (2004) Electrical coupling and neuronal synchronization in the mammalian brain. *Neuron* 41, 495–511.

Bentivoglio, M. (1999) The discovery of the Golgi apparatus. *J. Hist. Neurosci.* 8, 202–208.

Bidder, F. H., and Kupffer, C. (1857) *Untersuchungen über die Textur des Rückenmarks und die Entwicklung seiner Formelemente*. Leipzig: Breitkopf & Härtel.

Bonne, C. (1906) L'écorce cérébrale. Développment, morphologie et connexions des cellules nerveuses. *Revue Générale d'Histologie*, vol. 2. Paris: A. Storck.

Brazier, M. A. B. (1988) *A history of neurophysyology in the 19th century*. New York: Raven Press.

Clarke, E., and Jacyna, L. S. (1987) *Nineteenth-century origins of neuroscientific concepts*. Berkeley: University of California Press.

Clarke, E., and O'Malley, C. D. (1968) *The human brain and spinal cord. A historical study illustrated by writings from antiquity to the twentieth century*. Berkeley: University of California Press.

Colonnier, M. (1966) The structural design of the neocortex. In *Brain and concious experience*, ed. J. C. Eccles, 1–23. Berlin: Springer-Verlag.

Crous, J. (1878) *Tratado elemental de anatomía y fisiología normal y patológica del sistema nervioso*. Valencia, Spain: Librería de Pascual Aguilar.

Cullheim, S., and Kellerth, J. O. (1976) Combined light and electron microscopic tracing of neurons, including axons and synaptic terminals, after intracellular staining with horseradish peroxidase. *Neurosci. Lett.* 2, 307–313.

DeFelipe, J. (2002a) Sesquicentennial of the birthday of Santiago Ramón y Cajal (1852–2002), the father of modern neuroscience. *Trends Neurosci.* 25, 481–484.

DeFelipe, J. (2002b) Cortical interneurons: From Cajal to 2001. *Prog. Brain Res.* 136, 215–238.

DeFelipe, J. (2006) Brain plasticity and mental processes: Cajal again. *Nat. Rev. Neurosci.* 7, 811–817.

DeFelipe, J. (2009) Cajal's place in the history of neuroscience. In *Encyclopedia of neuroscience*, vol. 2, ed. L. R. Squire, 497–507. Oxford, England: Academic Press.

DeFelipe, J., and Jones, E. G. (1988) *Cajal on the cerebral cortex*. New York: Oxford University Press.

DeFelipe, J., and Jones, E. G. (1991) *Cajal's degeneration and regeneration of the nervous system*. New York: Oxford University Press.

DeFelipe, J., and Jones, E. G. (1992) Santiago Ramón y Cajal and methods in neurohistology. *Trends Neurosci.* 15, 237–246.

Deiters, O. F. K. (1865) *Untersuchungen über Gehirn und Rückenmark des Menschen und der Säugethiere.* Ed. M. Schultze. Vieweg: Braunschweig.

Del Río-Hortega, P. (1920) La microglia y su transformación en células en bastoncito y cuerpos gránulo-adiposos. *Trabajos del Laboratorio de Investigaciones Biológicas de la Universidad de Madrid* 18, 37–82.

Del Río-Hortega, P. (1928) Tercera aportación al conocimiento morfológico e interpretación funcional de la oligodendroglia. *Mem. Real Soc. Esp. Hist. Nat.* 14, 5–122.

Del Río-Hortega, P. (1933) Arte y artificio de la ciencia histológica. *Rev. Resid. Estudiantes, Madrid* 4, 191–206.

Demoor, J. (1896) La plasticité morphologique des neurones cérébraux. *Arch. Biol. Bruxelles* 14, 723–752.

De Robertis, E. (1959) Submicroscopy morphology of the synapse. *Int. Rev. Cytol.* 8, 61–96.

De Robertis, E., and Bennett, H. S. (1955) Some features of the submicroscopic morphology of synapses in frog and earthworm. *J. Biophys. Biochem. Cytol.* 1, 47–58.

Dogiel, A. S. (1893) Zur Frage über das Verhalten der Nervenzellen zu einander. *Arch. Anat. Physiol. Anat. Abt.* 429–434.

Dogiel, A. S. (1899) Ueber den Bau der Ganglien in den Geflechten des Darmes und der Gallenblase des Menschen und der Säugethiere. *Arch. Anat. Entwicklungsgesch.* 130–158.

Dustin, A. (1905) Contribution à l'étude de l'influence de l'âge et de l'activité fonctionnelle sur le neurone. *Bull. Soc. Roy. Sc. Med. Nat. Bruxelles* 63, 292–295.

Dymecki, S. M., and Kim, J. C. (2007) Molecular neuroanatomy's "three Gs": A primer. *Neuron* 54, 17–34.

Fairén, A. (2005) Pioneering a golden age of cerebral microcircuits: The births of the combined Golgi-electron microscope methods. *Neuroscience* 136, 607–614.

Feng, G., Mellor, R. H., Bernstein, M., Keller-Peck, C., Nguyen, Q. T., Wallace, M., Nerbonne, J. M., Lichtman, J. W., and Sanes, J. R. (2000) Imaging neuronal subsets in transgenic mice expressing multiple spectral variants of GFP. *Neuron* 28, 41–51.

Fischer, O. (1912) Ein weiterer Beitrag zur Klinik und Pathologie der presbyophrenen Demenz. *Z. Gesamte Neurol. Psychiatr.* 12, 99–135.

Flesch, M., and Koneff, H. (1886) Bemerkungen über die Struktur der Ganglienzellen. *Neurol. Centralbl.* 5, 145–147.

Forel, A. H. (1887) Einige hirnanatomische Betrachtungen und Ergebnisse. *Arch. Psychiat. Nervenkr.* 18, 162–198.

Forel, A. H. (1890–1891) Ueber das Verhältniss der experimentellen Atrophie und Degenerationsmethode zur Anatomie und Histologie des Centralnervensystems, *Ursprung des ix., x. und xii. Hirnnerven. Festschrift zur Feier des Fünfzigjährigen Doktorjubiläums der Herren Prof. Dr Karl. v. Nägeli u Prof. A. v. Kölliker,* 37–50.

Foster, M., and Sherrington, C. S. (1897) *A text-book of physiology. Part III: The central nervous system.* London: Macmillan.

Fragnito, O. (1907) Le Fibrille e la sostanza fibrillogena nelle cellule ganglionari dei vertebrati. *Ann. Nevrol.* 25, 209–224.

Fuxe, K., Dahlström, A., Höistad, M., Marcellino, D., Jansson, A., Rivera, A., Diaz-Cabiale, Z., Jacobsen, K., Tinner-Staines, B., Hagman, B., Leo, G., Staines, W., Guidolin, D., Kehr, J., Genedani, S., Belluardo, N., and Agnati, L. F. (2007) From the Golgi-Cajal mapping to the transmitter-based characterization of the neuronal networks leading to two modes of brain communication: Wiring and volume transmission. *Brain Res. Rev.* 55, 17–54.

Gerlach, J. von (1872) Über die struktur der grauen Substanz des menschlichen Grosshirns. *Zentralbl. med. Wiss.* 10, 273–275.

Giepmans, B. N., Adams, S. R., Ellisman, M. H., and Tsien, R. Y. (2006) The fluorescent toolbox for assessing protein location and function. *Science* 312, 217–224.

Golgi, C. (1873) Sulla struttura della sostanza grigia del cervello (Comunicazione preventiva). *Gaz. Med. Ital. Lombardia* 33, 244–246.

Golgi, C. (1875) *Sulla fina struttura del bulbi olfattorii.* Reggio-Emilia: Stefano Calderini.

Golgi, C. (1885) Sulla fina anatomia degli organi centrali del sistema nervoso. *Riv. Sper. Fremiat. Med. Leg. Alienazioni Ment.* 11, 72–123.

Golgi, C. (1929) La dottrina del neurone. Teoria e fati. In *Opera Omnia.* Vol. IV. *Scritti su argomenti varii.* Chapter 30 (Nobel Prize Lecture), 1259–1291. Milano: Ulrico Hoepli.

Grainger, R. D. (1829) *Elements of general anatomy, containing an outline of the organization of the human body.* London: S. Highley.

Gray, E. G. (1959a) Electron microscopy of synaptic contacts on dendrite spines of the cerebral cortex. *Nature* 183, 1592–1593.

Gray, E. G. (1959b) Axo-somatic and axo-dendritic synapses of the cerebral cortex: An electron microscopic study. *J. Anat.* 93, 420–433.

Held, H. (1897a) Beiträge zur Structur der Nervenzellen und ihrer Fortsätze. Zweite Abhandlung. *Arch. Anat. Phys. (Anat. Abt.)* 204–294.

Held, H. (1897b) Beiträge zur Structur der Nervenzellen und ihrer Fortsätze. Dritte Abhandlung. *Arch. Anat. Phys. (Anat. Abt.)* 273–312.

Held, H. (1902) Ueber den Bau der grauen und weissen Substanz. *Arch. Anat. Phys. (Anat. Abt.)* 189–224.

Held, H. (1904) Zur weiterer Kenntniss der Nervenendfüsse und zur Struktur der Sehzellen. *Abhandl. math-phys. Kl. königl. sächs. Ges. Wissensch.* 29, 143–185.

Held, H. (1905) Zur Kenntniss einer neurofibrillären Continuität im Centralnervensystem der Wirbelthiere. *Arch. Anat. Phys. (Anat. Abt.)* 55–78.

Hendry, S. H. C., Jones, E. G., DeFelipe, J., Schmechel, D., Brandon, C., and Emson, P. C. (1984) Neuropeptide-containing neurons of the cerebral cortex are also GABAergic. *Proc. Natl. Acad. Sci. USA* 81, 6526–6530.

Hensen, V. (1864) Zur Entwickelung des Nervensystems. *Arch. Pathol. Anat. Physiol. Klin. Med.* 30, 176–186.

His, W. (1886) Zur Geschichte des menschlichen Rückenmarks und der Nervenwurzeln. *Abhandl. Math.- Phys. Klass. Königl. Sächs. Gesellsch. Wiss.* 13, 147–209; 477–513.

His, W. (1889) Die Neuroblasten und deren Entstehung im embryonalen Mark, *Abhandl. Math.- Phys. Klass. Königl. Sächs. Gesellsch. Wiss.* 15, 313–372.

Hodge, C. F. (1888) Some effects of stimulating ganglion cells. *Am. J. Psychol.* 1, 479–486.

Hodge, C. F. (1889) Physiologie des centralen und sympathischen Nervensystems. *Centralbl. Physiol.* 3, 40–401.

Hodge, C. F. (1892) A microscopical study of changes due to functional activity in nerve cells. *J. Morphol.* 7, 95–168.

Hodgkin, T., and Lister, J. J. (1827) Notice of some microscopical observations of the blood and animal tissues. *PM* 2, 130–138.

Holmgren, E. (1900) Studien in der Feineren Anatomie der Nervezellen. *Anat. Hefte* 15, 1–88.

Hormuzdi, S. G., Filippov, M. A., Mitropoulou, G., Monyer, H., and Bruzzone, R. (2004) Electrical synapses: A dynamic signaling system that shapes the activity of neuronal networks. *Biochim. Biophys. Acta* 1662, 113–137.

Hubbard, E. M. (2007) Neurophysiology of synesthesia. *Curr. Psychiatry Rep.* 9, 193–199.

Hughes, A. (1959) *A history of cytology.* New York: Abelard-Schuman.

Jankowska, E., Rastad, J., and Westman, J. (1976) Intracellular application of horseradish peroxidase and its light and electron microscopical appearance of spinocervical tract cells. *Brain Res.* 105, 557–562.

Jones, E. G. (1975) Varieties and distribution of non-pyramidal cells in the somatic sensory cortex of the squirrel monkey. *J. Comp. Neurol.* 160, 205–268.

Jones, E. G. (1994) The neuron doctrine. *J. Hist. Neurosci.* 3, 3–20.

Jones, E. G. (2006) The impossible interview with the man of the neuron doctrine. *J. Hist. Neurosci.* 15, 326–340.

Jones, E. G. (2007) Neuroanatomy: Cajal and after Cajal. *Brain Res. Rev.* 55, 248–255.

Jones, E. G., and Hartman, B. K. (1978) Recent advances in neuroanatomical methodology. *Annu. Rev. Neurosci.* 1, 215–296.

Kölliker, A. von (1852) *Handbuch der Gewebelehre des Menschen.* Leipzig: Engelmann.

Korybutt-Daszkiewicz, B. (1889) Wird der thätige Zustand des Centralnervensystems von mikroskopisch wahrzunehmenden Veränderungen begleitet? *Arch. Mikrosk. Anat.* 33, 51–70.

Kuhlman, S. J., and Huang, Z. J. (2008) High-resolution labeling and functional manipulation of specific neuron types in mouse brain by Cre-activated viral gene expression. *PLoS ONE* 3, e2005.

Kuypers, H. G., Bentivoglio, M., Catsman-Berrevoets, C. E., and Bharos, A. T. (1980) Double retrograde neuronal labeling through divergent axon collaterals, using two fluorescent tracers with the same excitation wavelength which label different features of the cell. *Exp. Brain Res.* 40, 383–392.

Lambert, M. (1893) Note sur les modifications produites par l'excitation électrique dans les cellules nerveuses des ganglions sympathiques. *Compt. Rend. Soc. Biol.* 45, 879–881.

Lichtman, J. W., Livet, J., and Sanes, J. R. (2008) A technicolour approach to the connectome. *Nat. Rev. Neurosci.* 9, 417–422.

Livet, J., Weissman, T. A., Kang, H., Draft, R. W., Lu, J., Bennis, R. A., Sanes, J. R., and Lichtman, J. W. (2007) Transgenic strategies for combinatorial expression of fluorescent proteins in the nervous system. *Nature* 450, 56–62.

Lotmar, F. (1918) Beiträge zur Histologie der akuten Myelitis und Encephalitis, sowie verwandter Prozesse. In *Histologische und histopathologische Arbeiten über die Grosshirnrinde*, eds. F. Nissl and A. Alzheimer, 245– 432, vol 6. Jena: Gustav Fischer.

Lugaro, E. (1895) Sulle modificazioni delle cellule nervose nei diversi stati funzionali. *Sperimentale* 49, 159–193.

Lund, J. S. (1973) Organization of neurons in the visual cortex, area 17, of the monkey Macaca mulatta. *J. Comp. Neurol.* 147, 455–496.

Maestre de San Juan, A. (1879) *Tratado de histología normal y patológica.* Madrid: Moya y Plaza.

Mann, G. (1894) Histological changes induced in sympathetic, motor, and sensory nerve cells by functional activity. *J. Anat. Physiol.* 29, 100–108.

Marek, K. W., and Davis, G. W. (2003) Controlling the active properties of excitable cells. *Curr. Opin. Neurobiol.* 13, 607–611.

Marin-Padilla, M. (1969) Origin of the pericellular baskets of the pyramidal cells of the human motor cortex: A Golgi study. *Brain Res.* 14, 633–646.

Marinesco, G. (1904) Recherches sur la structure de la partie fibrillaire des cellules nerveuses à l'état normal et pathologique. *Rev. Neurol.* 12, 405–428.

Marinesco, G. (1906) Recherches sur les changements des neurofibrilles consécutifs aux différents troubles de nutrition. *Névraxe* 8, 147–173.

Marinesco, G., and Minea, J. (1912) Untersuchungen über die "senilen Plaques." *Monatsschr. Psychiatr. Neurol.* 31, 79–133.

Martín-Araguz, A. (2006) Neurocodicología. La neurología en el arte de la miniatura medieval. In *Arte y Neurología*, ed. A. Martín-Araguz, 57–78. Madrid: Saned.

Martínez-Murillo, J. M. (2004). *La pintura, el dibujo y la fotografía creativa de Santiago Ramón y Cajal* (Tesis doctoral). Universidad Complutense, Facultad de Bellas Artes, Madrid.

Mazzarello, P. (1999) *The hidden structure: A scientific biography of Camillo Golgi.* Oxford, England: Oxford University Press.

Merico, G. (1999) Microscopy in Camillo Golgi's times. *J. Hist. Neurosci.* 8, 113–120.

Nieuwenhuys, R. (1994) The neocortex: An overview of its evolutionary development, structural organization and synaptology. *Anat. Embryol.* 190, 307–337.

Palade, G. E., and Palay, S. L. (1954) Electron microscope observations of interneuronal and neuromuscular synapses. *Anat. Rec.* 118, 335–336.

Palay, S. L. (1956) Synapses in the central nervous system. *J. Biophys. Biochem. Cytol. Suppl.* 2, 193–202.

Pergens, E. (1896) Action de la lumière sur la rétine. *Ann. Soc. Roy. Sc. Méd. Nat. Bruxelles* 5, 389–421.

Peters, A., Palay, S. L., and Webster, H. (1991) *The fine structure of the nervous system. Neurons and their supporting cells.* New York: Oxford University Press.

Purkinje, J. E. (1838) Bericht über die Versammlung deutscher Naturforscher und Ärzte in Prag im September, 1837. pt. 3, sec. 5, A. *Anatomisch-physiologische Verhandlungen* 177–180.

Ramón-Jiménez, J. (1942) *Españoles de tres mundos.* Buenos Aires: Losada.

Ramón y Cajal, S. (1888) Estructura de los centros nerviosos de las aves. *Rev. Trim. Histol. Norm. Patol.* 1, 1–10.

Ramón y Cajal, S. (1889a) *Manual de histología normal y de técnica micrográfica.* Valencia, Spain: Librería de Pascual Aguilar.

Ramón y Cajal, S. (1889b) Conexión general de los elementos nerviosos. *La Medicina Práctica* 88, 341–346.

Ramón y Cajal, S. (1891) Significación fisiológica de las expansiones protoplásmicas y nerviosas de las células de la substancia gris. *Rev. Ciencias Méd., Barcelona* 17, 673–679; 715–723.

Ramón y Cajal, S. (1893) *Manual de histología normal y de técnica micrográfica.* Second edition. Valencia, Spain: Librería de Pascual Aguilar.

Ramón y Cajal, S. (1894) Consideraciones generales sobre la morfología de la célula nerviosa. *La Veterinaria Española* 37, 257–260; 273–275; 289–291.

Ramón y Cajal, S. (1896) Estructura del protoplasma nervioso. *Rev. Trim. Micrográf. Madrid* 1, 83–113.

Ramón y Cajal, S. (1897) Leyes de la morfología y dinamismo de las células nerviosas. *Rev. Trimest. Micrográf.* 2, 1–28.

Ramón y Cajal, S. (1901–1902) Estudios sobre la corteza cerebral humana. IV. Estructura de la corteza cerebral olfativa del hombre y mamíferos. *Trab. Lab. Invest. Biol. Univ. Madrid* 1, 1–140.

Ramón y Cajal, S. (1903a) Sobre un sencillo proceder de impregnación de las fibrillas interiores del protoplasma nervioso. *Arch. Lat. Med. Biol.* 1, 1–6.

Ramón y Cajal, S. (1903b) Un sencillo método de coloración del retículo protoplásmico y sus efectos en los diversos centros nerviosos de vertebrados e invertebrados. *Trab. Lab. Invest. Biol. Univ. Madrid* 2, 129–221.

Ramón y Cajal, S. (1904a) Variaciones morfológicas, normales y patológicas del retículo neurofibrilar. *Trab. Lab. Invest. Biol. Univ. Madrid* 3, 9–15.

Ramón y Cajal, S. (1904b) Variaciones morfológicas del retículo nervioso de invertebrados y vertebrados sometidos a la acción de condiciones naturales (nota preventiva). *Trab. Lab. Invest. Biol. Univ. Madrid* 3, 287–297.

Ramón y Cajal, S. (1904c) Neuroglia y neurofibrillas del Lumbricus. *Trab. Lab. Invest. Biol. Univ. Madrid* 3, 277–285.

Ramón y Cajal, S. (1899–1904) *Textura del sistema nervioso del hombre y de los vertebrados.* Madrid: Moya. This book was revised and extended in the French version *Histologie du système nerveux de l'homme et des vertébrés,* trans. L. Azoulay. Paris: Maloine, 1909, 1911. English translations: *Histology of the nervous system of man and vertebrates,* trans. N. Swanson and L. W. Swanson. New York: Oxford University Press, 1995; *Texture of the nervous system of man and the vertebrates* (an annotated and edited translation of the original Spanish text with the additions of the French version by P. Pasik and T. Pasik). New York: Springer Wien, 2000–2001.

Ramón y Cajal, S. (1909–1911) *Histologie du système nerveux de l'homme et des vertébrés,* trans. L. Azoulay. Paris: Maloine.

Ramón y Cajal, S. (1912) *La fotografía de los colores. Fundamentos científicos y reglas prácticas.* Madrid: Moya.

Ramón y Cajal, S. (1913) Contribución al conocimiento de la neuroglia del cerebro humano. *Trab. Lab. Invest. Biol. Univ. Madrid* 11, 255–315.

Ramón y Cajal, S. (1914) *Manual de histología normal y de técnica micrográfica.* 6ª edición. Madrid: Imprenta y Librería de Nicolás Moya.

Ramón y Cajal, S. (1913–1914) *Estudios sobre la degeneración y regeneración del sistema nervioso.* Madrid: Moya. Reprinted and edited with additional translations by J. DeFelipe and E. G. Jones: *Cajal's degeneration and regeneration of the nervous system.* New York: Oxford University Press, 1991.

Ramón y Cajal, S. (1917) *Recuerdos de mi vida, Vol.2. Historia de mi labor científica.* Madrid: Moya.

Ramón y Cajal, S. (1933) ¿Neuronismo o reticularismo? Las pruebas objetivas de la unidad anatómica de las células nerviosas. *Arch. Neurobiol.* 13, 217–291: 579–646. English translation: *Neuron theory or reticular theory? Objective evidence of the anatomical unity of nerve cells,* trans. M. Ubeda-Purkiss and C. A. Fox. Madrid: *Consejo Superior de Investigaciones Científicas,* 1954.

Ramón y Cajal, S., and Tello, J. F. (1933) *Histology.* Baltimore: Williams Wood & Company.

Rebizzi, R. (1906) Su alcune variazione delle neurofibrille nella "hirudo medicinalis." *Riv. Patol. Nerv. Ment.* 11, 355–377.

Rezza, A. (1913) Alterazioni delle cellule gangliari del bulbo in un caso di demenza precoce con morte improvvisa. *Riv. Patol. Nerv. Ment.* 18, 426–429.

Robertson, J. D. (1953) Ultrastructure of two invertebrate synapses. *Proc. Soc. Exp. Biol. Med.* 82, 219–223.

Scheibel, M. E., and Scheibel, A. B. (1970) The rapid Golgi method: Indian summer or renaissance? In *Contemporary research methods in neuroanatomy,* eds. W. J. H. Nauta and S. O. E. Ebbesson, 1–11. New York: Springer.

Schleiden, M. J. (1838) Beiträge zur Phytogenesis. *Arch. Anat. Physiol. Wiss. Med.* 137–176.

Schüz, A., and Palm, G (1989) Density of neurons and synapses in the cerebral cortex of the mouse. *J. Comp. Neurol.* 286, 442–455.

Schwann, T. (1839) *Microscopic investigations on the accordance in the structure and growth of plants and animals.* London (English translation by the Sydenham Society, 1847).

Shepherd, G. M. (1991) *Foundations of the neuron doctrine.* New York: Oxford University Press.

Shepherd, G. M. (2004) *The neuron doctrine.* In *Encyclopedia of neuroscience*, third edition, eds. G. Adelman, H. Barry, and B. H. Smith. New York: Elsevier.

Sherrington, C. S. (1947) *The integrative action of the nervous system.* Cambridge: Cambridge University Press.

Sholl, D. A. (1956) *The organization of the cerebral cortex.* London: Methuen.

Simarro, L. (1900) Nuevo método histológico de impreganación por las sales fotográficas de plata. *Rev. Trim. Micrográf. Madrid* 5, 45–71.

Skirboll, L., Hökfelt, T., Norell, G., Phillipson, O., Kuypers, H. G., Bentivoglio, M., Catsman-Berrevoets, C. E., Visser, T. J., Steinbusch, H., Verhofstad, A., Cuello, A. C., Goldstain, M., and Brownstein, M. (1984) A method for specific transmitter identification of retrogradely labeled neurons: Immunofluorescence combined with fluorescence tracing. *Brain Res.* 320, 99–127.

Somjen, G. G. (1988) Nervenkitt: Notes on the history of the concept of neuroglia. *Glia* 1, 2–9.

Somogyi, P. (1990) Synaptic connections of neurones identified by Golgi impregnation: Characterization by immunocytochemical, enzyme histochemical, and degeneration methods. *J. Electron Microsc. Tech.* 15, 332–351.

Spielmeyer, W. (1922) *Histopathologie des Nervensystems.* Erster Band: Allgemeiner Teil. Berlin: J. Springer.

Szentágothai, J. (1969) Architecture of the cerebral cortex. In *Basic mechanisms of the epilepsies*, eds. H. Jasper, A. A. Ward, and A. Pope, 13–28. Boston: Little Brown.

Tello, F. (1903) Sobre la existencia de neurofibrillas gigantes en la médula espinal de los reptiles. *Trab. Lab. Invest. Biol. Univ. Madrid* 2, 223–225.

Tello, J. F. (1904) Las neurofibrillas en los vertebrados inferiores. *Trab. Lab. Invest. Biol. Univ. Madrid* 3, 113–151.

Tello, J. F. (1935) *Cajal y su labor histológica.* Madrid: Universidad Central.

Tsien, R. Y. (1998) The green fluorescent protein. *Annu. Rev. Biochem.* 67, 509–544.

Turner, W. (1890) The cell theory, past and present. *J. Anat. Physiol.* 24, 253–287.

Valentin, G. G. (1836) Über den Verlauf und die letzten Ende der Nerven. *Nova Acta Phys.-Med. Acad. Caes. Leopold.-Carol. Nat. Curiosorum, Breslau* 18, 51–240.

Valverde, F. (1970) The Golgi method: A tool for comparative structural analysis. In *Contemporary research methods in neuroanatomy*, eds. W. J. H. Nauta and S. O. E. Ebbesson, 11–31. New York: Springer.

Van der Loos, H. (1967) The history of the neuron. In *The neuron*, ed. H. Hydén, 1–47. Amsterdam: Elsevier.

Vas, F. (1892) Studien über den Bau des Chromatins in der sympathischen Ganglienzelle. *Arch. Mikrosk. Anat.* 40, 375–389.

Virchow, R. (1846) Über das granulierte Ansehen der Wandungen der Gerhirnventrikel. *Allg. Z. Psychiatr.* 3, 424–450.

Virchow, R. (1858) Die Cellularpathologie in ihrer Begründung auf physiologische und pathologische Gewebenlehre. Berlin: August Hirschwald. (Cellular pathology as based upon physiological and pathological histology: Twenty lectures delivered in the Pathological Institute of Berlin during the months of February, March, and April, 1858. Translated from the second edition of the original by Frank Chance. London: John Churchill, 1860)

von Gudden, B. (1870) Experimentaluntersuchungen über das peripherische und centrale Nervensystem. *Arch. Psychiat. Nervenkr.* 2, 693–723.

Waldeyer-Hartz, W. von (1891) Über einige neuere Forschungen im Gebiete der Anatomie des Centralnervensystems. *Dtsch. Med. Wschr.* 17, 1213–1218; 1244–1246; 1267–1269; 1287–1289; 1331–1332; 1352–1356.

Waller, A. V. (1850) Experiments on the section of the glosso-pharyngeal and hypoglossal nerves of the frog, and observations of the alterations produced thereby in the tructure of their primitive fibers. *Phil. Trans. Roy. Soc. Lond.* 140, 423–429.

Waller, A. V. (1852) Sur la reproduction des nerfs et sur la structure et les fonctions des ganglions spinaux. *Arch. Anat. Physiol. (Liepzig)* 11, 392–401.

White, E. L. (1989) *Cortical circuits: Synaptic organization of the cerebral cortex. Structure, function and theory.* Boston: Birkhäuser.

PART II

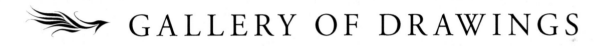 GALLERY OF DRAWINGS

# THE BENEDICTINE PERIOD: THE EARLY DAYS

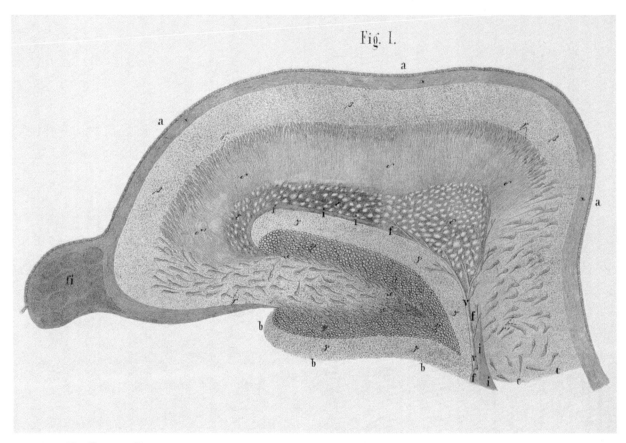

**FIGURE I.** Kupffer, 1859. Hippocampus.

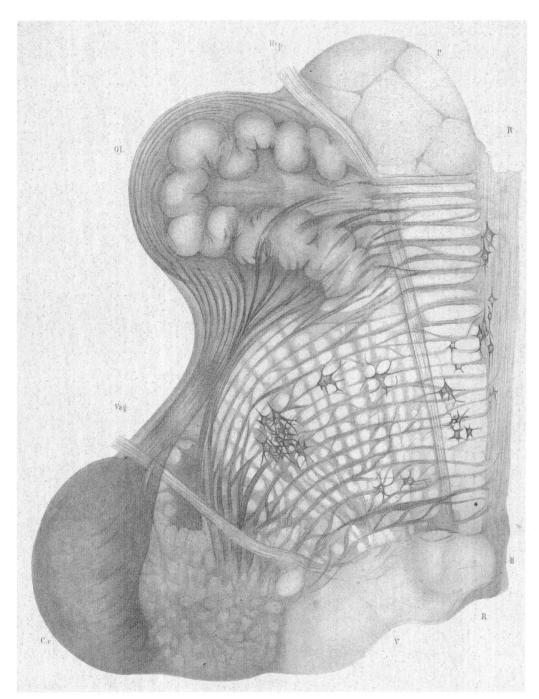

**FIGURE 2.** Deiters, 1865. Human medulla oblongata, I.

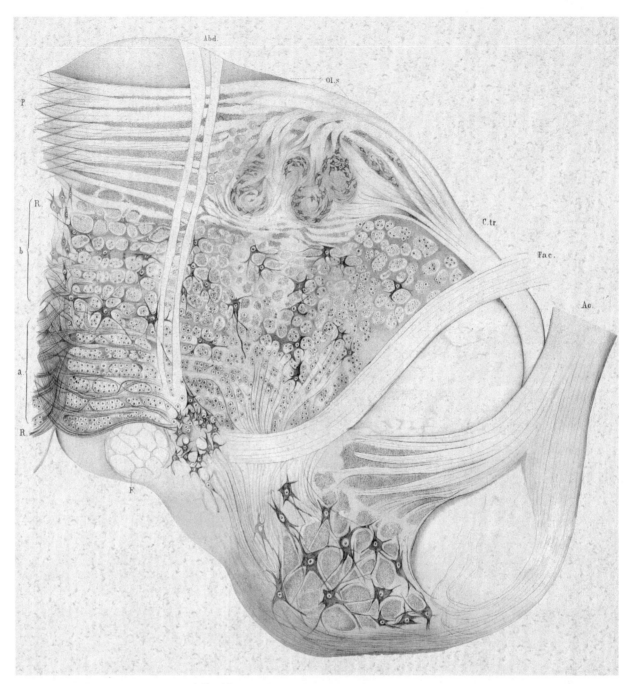

**FIGURE 3.** Deiters, 1865. Human medulla oblongata, II.

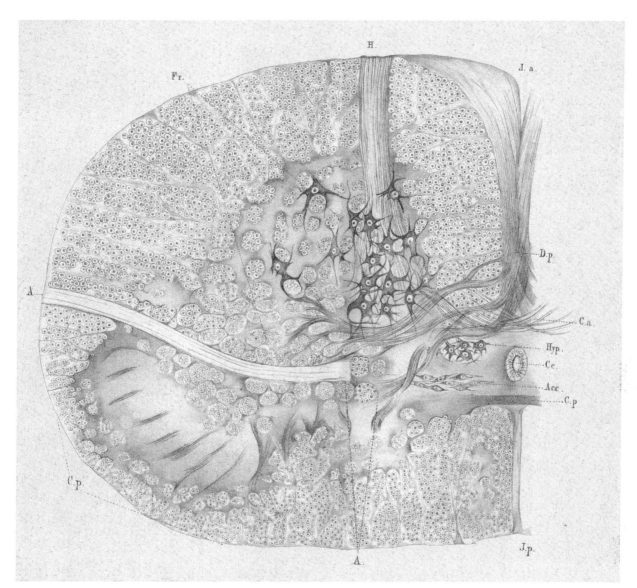

**FIGURE 4.** Deiters, 1865. Human medulla oblongata, III.

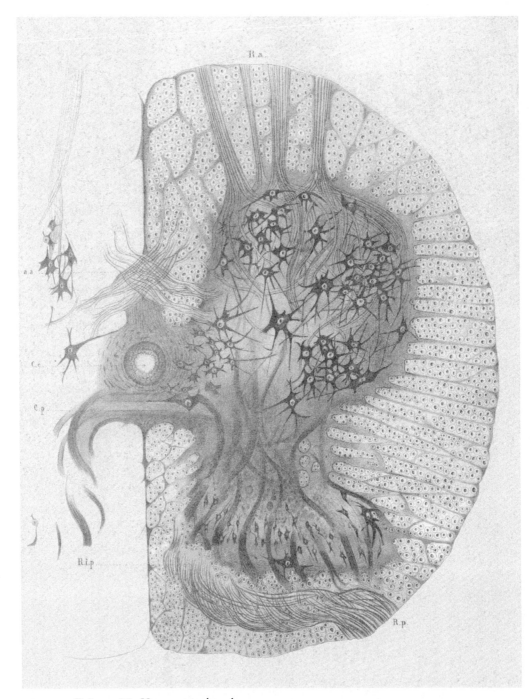

**FIGURE 5.** Deiters, 1865. Human spinal cord.

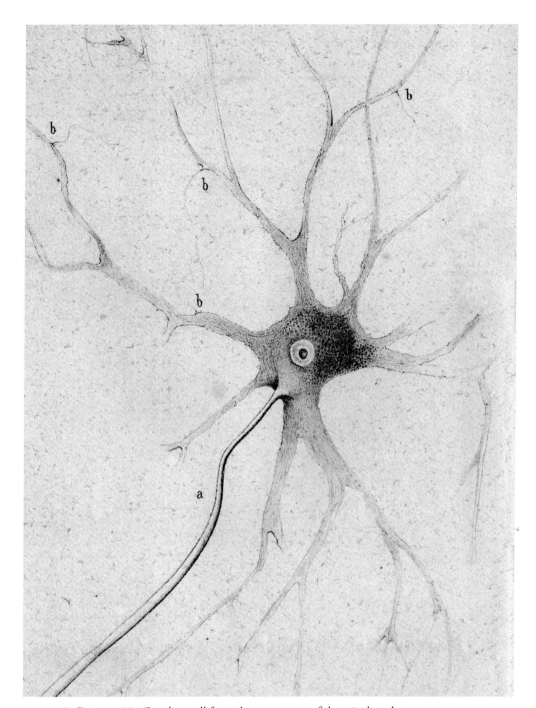

**FIGURE 6.** Deiters, 1865. Ganglion cell from the gray matter of the spinal cord.

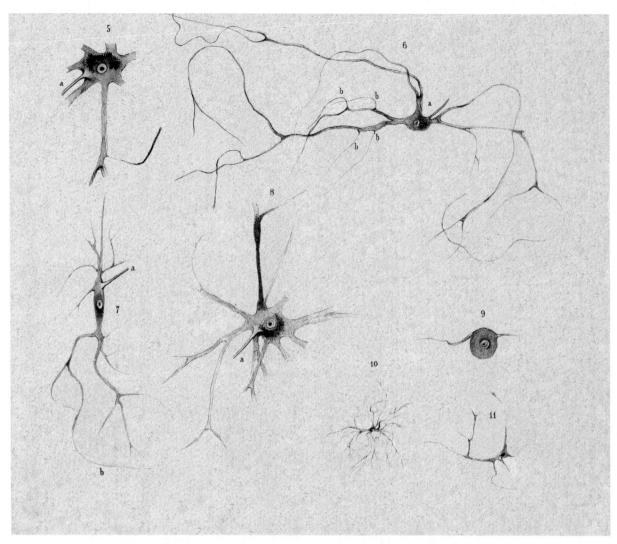

**FIGURE 7.** Deiters, 1865. Cells from the gray and white matter.

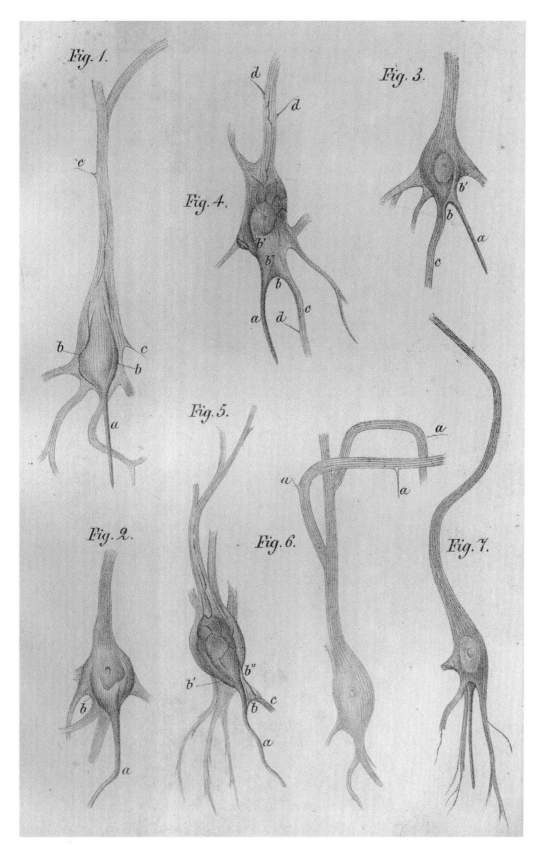

**FIGURE 8.** Butzke, 1872. Pyramidal cells of the cerebral cortex.

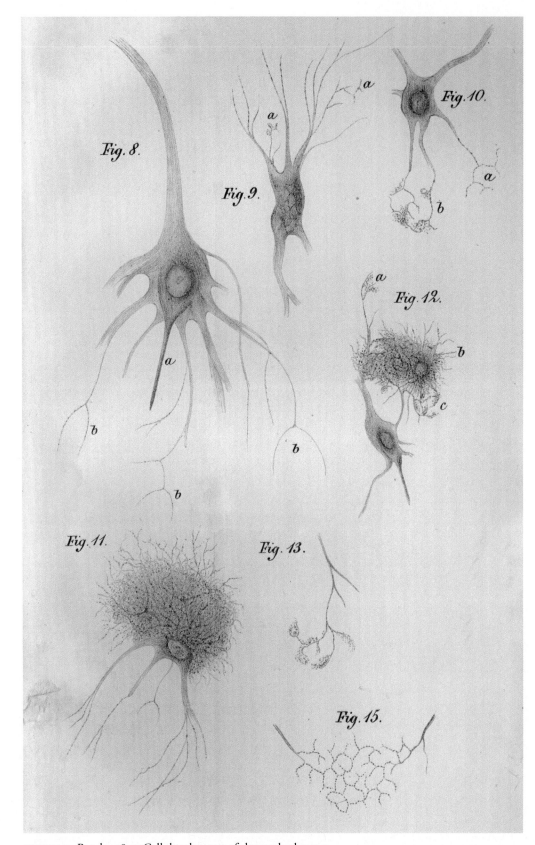

**FIGURE 9.** Butzke, 1872. Cellular elements of the cerebral cortex.

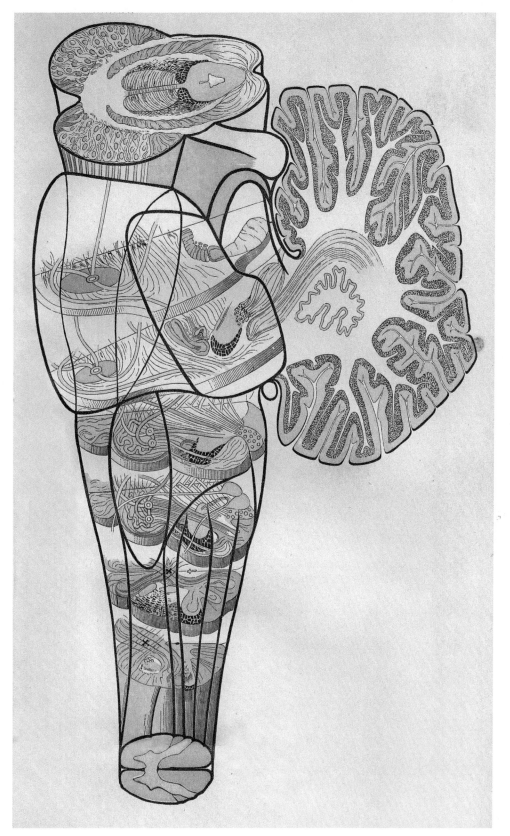

FIGURE 10. Meynert, 1874. Diagram of the structure of the human brain stem.

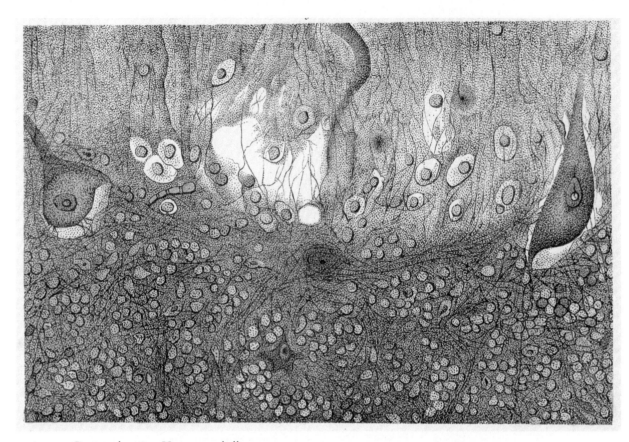

**FIGURE 11.** Denissenko, 1877. Human cerebellum.

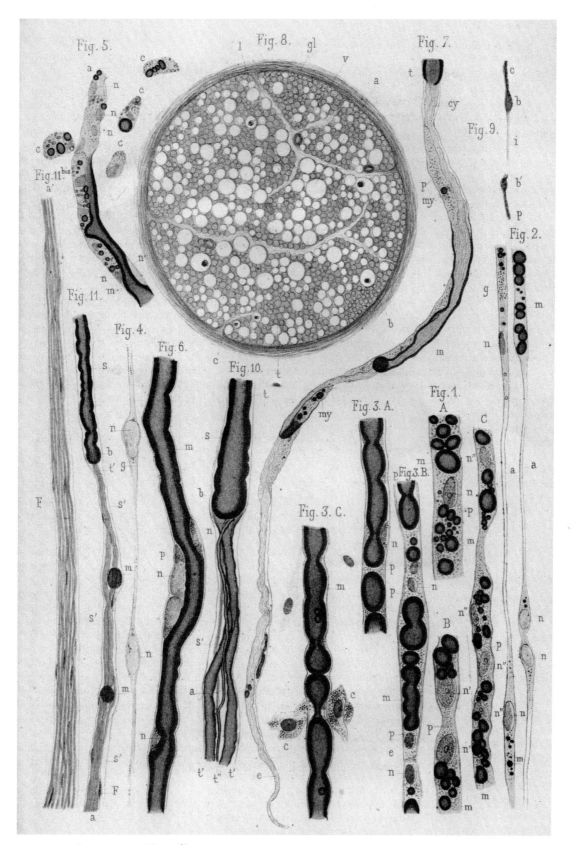

**FIGURE 12.** Ranvier, 1878. Nerve fibers.

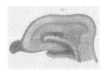

### FIGURE 1.

Kupffer, 1859.
Hippocampus.

FIG. 1. Segmentum transversam e cornu Ammonis cuniculi petitum, circiter ceuties amplificatum. a.a.a. Hujus organi superficies libera epithelio obtecta, quae in ventriculi lateralis cavum spectat. b.b.b. Gyrus in hemisphaerii superficie interna situs, qui fasciae dentatae apud bominem respondet. c.c.c. Transitus cornus Ammonis folii superioris in gyrum hippocampi; af. af. folium superius (cornus Ammonis.). bf.bf. folium inferius (cornus Ammonis.). f'. Introitus fissurae inter fasciam dentatam et gyrum hippocampi. f. Continuatio hujus flssurae inter ambo cornus Ammonis folia. fi. Fimbria. α. Stratum fibrarum nervearum. β. Stratum moleculare primum. γ. Stratum cellulosum . γ'γ'. Cellulae dispersae in cornus Ammonis folio inferiore et in eo loco ubi hujus organi folium superius in gyrum hippocampi transit. δδ. Stratum a peripheria ad cetrum striatum. δ'. Decussatio processuum cellularum. εε. Stratum reticulare. ζζζ. Stratum moleculare secundum. ηηη. Stratum granulosum. ف ى ى. Fibrae e granis prodeuntes. ii. Fibrae e strato reticulari prodenntes, quae in gyri hippocampi superfieiem tendunt. vv. Vas sauguiferum. Kupffer, G. (1859) De cornus ammonis textura disquisitiones praecipue in cuniculis institutae. *Dissertatio Inauguralis.* Typis Viduae J.C. Schünmanni et C. Mattieseni, Dorpati Livonorum [Figure 1].

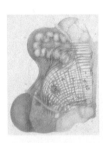

### FIGURE 2.

Deiters, 1865.
Human medulla oblongata, I.

FIG. 15. Durchschnitt der medulla oblongata des Menschen in der Höhe der Olive (Ol.) . *R.R* Raphe, Hyp. Nervus hypoglossus, Vag. Nervus vagus, deren Kerne in *V* und *H* liegen, aber in der Zeichnung nicht feiner ausgeführt sind. Den Haupttheil der Figur nimmt die Formatio reticularis ein mit ihren zerstreuten Ganglienzellen, und die Olive mit den zu ihr hinzutretenden Fasern des stratum zonale; *C. c* crura cerebelli ad medullam oblongatam; *P* Pyramidenstrang. Deiters, O. F. K. (1865) *Untersuchungen über Gehirn und Rückenmark des Menschen und der Säugethiere*, ed. M. Schultze. Braunschweig, Germany: F. Vieweg und Sohn [Plate 6, Figure 15].

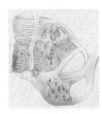

### FIGURE 3.

Deiters, 1865.
Human medulla oblongata, II.

FIG. 14. Querschnitt durch eine Hälfte der medulla oblongata dicht vor ihrem Uebergang in den pons Varolii, mit Wurzelbündeln des nervus abducens, facialis und acusticus. *E* Fasern der Pyramiden; *R R* Raphe, rechts davon das Balkenwerk der formatio reticularis, innerhalb deren in der oberen Partie *b* schmalere, in der unteren a breitere Nervenprimitivfasern liegen; OI (O₁. s.) Durchschnitt durch die obere Olive; *C. tr* Fasern des corpus trapezoides; *Cr.c* crura cerebelli ad medullam oblongatam mit den zahlreichen grossen Ganglienzellen, welche scheinbar zum Ursprung des Nervus acusticus *Ac* gehören; Fac. Nervus facialis; *F* derselbe Nerv im Querschnitt, Knie des facialis; Abd. Nervus abducens. Die Zeichnung ist nicht vollendet, so hätten z. B. bei *J* die Querschnitte der verschieden dicken Nervenfasern angegeben werden müssen, welche diese Stelle erfüllen. (Vergl. u. A. Seite 192, 231, 275.) Deiters, O. F. K. (1865) *Untersuchungen über Gehirn und Rückenmark des Menschen und der Säugethiere*, ed. M. Schultze. Braunschweig, Germany: F. Vieweg und Sohn [Plate 5, Figure 14].

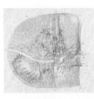

### FIGURE 4.

Deiters, 1865.
Human medulla oblongata, III.

FIG. 13. Querschnitt durch eine Hälfte der medulla oblongata in ihrem Anfange, mit Wurzelsträngen des nervus accessorius Willisii und hypoglossus. *J. a* vordere Incisur, zum Theil ausgefüllt durch die beginnende Pyramidenkreuzung *D. p; J. p* hintere Incisur; *C. a* vordere weisse Commissur; *C. p* hintere graue Commissur; C. c Centralcanal; *F. r* Formatio reticularis, die reticuläre Bindesubstanz, welche sich aus der Substanz der Vorderhörner hier entwickelt, und zunehmend nach und nach den grössten Theil der medulla oblongata einnimmt; *C.p* hinteres Horn, an seiner Basis auch bereits zu dem Balkenwerk der formatio reticularis aufgelöst; *A* nervus accessorius; *H* nervus hypoglossus; *A'* Querschnitt von Bündeln des Accessorius; *Acc.* Zellen des Accessoriuskernes; Hyp. Zellen des Hypoglossuskernes (S. 172 u. 220). Deiters, O. F. K. (1865) *Untersuchungen über Gehirn und Rückenmark des Menschen und der Säugethiere*, ed. M. Schultze. Braunschweig, Germany: F. Vieweg und Sohn [Plate 4, Figure 13].

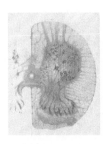

### FIGURE 5.

Deiters, 1865.
Human spinal cord.

FIG. 12. Querschnitt durch eine Hälfte des unteren Endes des Rückenmarkes vom Menschen. Wahrscheinlich Anfang des conus medullaris. *R. a* vordere Wurzelbündel, aus dem Vorderhorn entspringend, in dessen Innerem man die markhaltigen Nervenfasern zwischen den grossen Ganglienzellen verlaufen sieht; *R.p* hintere Wurzel, aus dem Hinterhorn hervorgehend, dessen Ganglienzellen blasser und, bis auf einige wenige, viel kleiner sind als die des Vorderhorns; *R. i . p* innerer Theil der hinteren Wurzel (Seite 139); *C. c* Canalis centralis mit seiner Auskleidung von Wimperepithel, von Bindesubstanz umgeben; *C . p* hintere graue Commissur; *C. a. a* vordere weise Commissur. Ringsum die grauen Hörner zeigen sich die Querschnitte der in verschiedenen Gegenden verschieden dicken markhaltigen Nervenfasern mit Axencylinder (Seite 135 ff). Deiters, O. F. K. (1865) *Untersuchungen über Gehirn und Rückenmark des Menschen und der Säugethiere*, ed. M. Schultze. Braunschweig, Germany: F. Vieweg und Sohn [Plate 3, Figure 12].

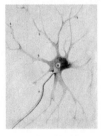

### FIGURE 6.

Deiters, 1865.
Ganglion cell from the gray matter of the spinal cord.

Isolirte Ganglienzellen aus der grauen Substanz des Rückenmarkes in 300 bis 400 maliger Vergrösserung dargestellt [table legend]. FIG.1. Eine grosse Ganglienzelle aus dem vorderen Horn mit möglichst vollständig erhaltenen Fortsätzen. In der Zellsubstanz ist dunkelgelbes Pigment abgelagert. a der Hauptaxencylinderfortsatz; b, b, b die von den Protoplasmafortsätzen entspringenden feinen Axencylinderfortsätze (Seite 56). Deiters, O. F. K. (1865) *Untersuchungen über Gehirn und Rückenmark des Menschen und der Säugethiere*, ed. M. Schultze. Braunschweig, Germany: F. Vieweg und Sohn [Plate 1, Figure 1].

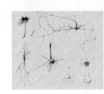

### FIGURE 7.

Deiters, 1865. Cells from the gray and white matter.

FIG. 5. Pigmentirte Ganglienzelle

aus dem vorderen Horn der grauen Substanz des Rückenmarkes. Von den Protoplasmafortsätzen ist nur einer länger gezeichnet, um den Ursprung des feinen Axencylinderfortsatzes b, der zu einer feinen markhaltigen Nervenfaser wird, zu zeigen. a Hauptaxencylinderfortsatz. FIG. 6. Mit allen Fortsätzen möglichst vollständig isolirte Ganglienzelle aus dem hinteren Horn der grauen Substanz des Rückenmarks. *a* Hauptaxencylinderfortsatz; *b* feine Axencylinderfortsätze, welche von Protoplasmafortsätzen entspringen (Seite 87). FIG. 7. Eine Zelle der gleichen Art, sensible Zelle aus dem Hinterhorn; *a* Hauptaxencylinderfortsatz, *b* feiner, gleich nach seinem Ursprung mit Mark sich umgebender Axencylinderfortsatz. FIG. 8. Eine grosse Zelle aus dem Hinterhorn, welche einer motorischen ähnlich sieht mit einem sehr stark pigmentirten Protoplasmafortsatz. *a* Hauptaxencylinderfortsatz (Seite 89). FIG. 9. Eigenthümliche kuglige Ganglienzelle, wie sie sich am Ursprung des Trochlearis finden, gewöhnlich nur mit einem, hier mit zwei Fortsätzen (Seite 91). FIGS. 10 und 11. Bindegewebszellen aus der weissen und grauen Substanz der Centralorgane, FIG 10 aus der grauen Substanz des Hypoglossuskernes (Seite 45). Deiters, O. F. K. (1865) *Untersuchungen über Gehirn und Rückenmark des Menschen und der Säugethiere*, ed. M Schultze, Braunschweig, Germany: F. Vieweg und Sohn [Plate 2, Figures 5–11].

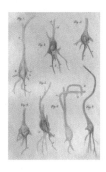

FIGURE 8.
Butzke, 1872.
Pyramidal cells of the cerebral cortex.

Die Objecte sind den frischen Gehirnen zum grössten Theil ausgewachsener Kälber, ausnahmsweise dem Schafe entnommen. Vergrösserung: Gundlach Immersion No. VII. Ocular II (Die von dem Herrn Verfasser gezeichneten Figuren sind auf zwei Drittel der Grösse reducirt auf den Tafeln wiedergegeben) [table legend]. FIG. 1. Grosse pyramidale Ganglienzelle aus der Grosshirnrinde des Kalbes mittelst Chloralhydrat isolirt (stets). Deutliche Längsstreifung der verzweigten Fortsätze. Kern nicht sichtbar. a. Deiters'scher Fortsatz, b,b. dunkle Linien, welche die Insertion dieses Fortsatzes in und auf der Ganglienzelle bezeichnen, c,c. feinste Ausläufer: die von Deiters als zweites

System echter Nervenfasern bezeichneten. FIG. 2. Gleiches Object. Chloralhydrat und Hyperosmiumsäure. Kern deutlich. a und b wie in Fig. 1. FIG. 3. Gleiches Präparat. Der Deiters'sche Fortsatz inserirt sich an den Fortsatz c; b Abzweigung auf den verzweigten Fortsatz; b' Abzweigung desselben auf und in die Ganglienzelle. FIG. 4. Gleiches Präparat. Der Deiters'sche Fortsatz inserirt sich an oder nahe an den verzweigten Fortsatz c und theilt sich in drei dunkle Linien, von denen b auf den Fortsatz c, b' und b" auf und in den Ganglienkörper übergehen. FIG. 5. Gleiches Präparat und gleiche Bedeutung der Buchstaben. (Aus dem Gehirne eines Schafes.). FIG. 6. Gleiches Präparat wie Fig. 4. Kern nicht zu sehen. Intensiv glänzende Zelle. Theilung des Spitzenfortsatzes; bei c Verdickung vor der Theilung. Jeder der drei Zweige nicht wesentlich dünner als der Stamm. FIG. 7. Pyramidenkörper mit colossal langem Spitzenfortsatz, der noch ungetheilt bleibt. Butzke, V. (1872) Studien über den feineren Bau der Grosshirnrinde. *Arch. Psychiat. Nervenk.* 3, 575–600 [Figures 1–7].

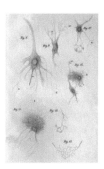

FIGURE 9.
Butzke, 1872.
Cellular elements of the cerebral cortex.

Die Objecte sind den frischen Gehirnen zum grössten Theil ausgewachsener Kälber, ausnahmsweise dem Schafe entnommen.
Vergrösserung: Gundlach Immersion No. VII. Ocular II (Die von dem Herrn Verfasser gezeichneten Figuren sind auf zwei Drittel der Grösse reducirt auf den Tafeln wiedergegeben) [table legend]. FIG. 8. Grosser Pyramidenkörper mit reicher Verzweigung der Basalfortsätze. a. Deiters Fortsatz. b. Terminalreiser. FIG. 9. Kleiner Ganglienkörper. Getheilte Fortsätze direct in Endreiser sich zerspaltend. Bei a setzen sich Endfäserchen an die Endreiser an. FIG. 10. Dito. Bei b sieht man Bruchstücke eines Endfäserchennetzes mit der anhaftenden feinkörnigen Zwischenmasse. FIG. 11. Kleiner Ganglienkörper. Verzweigte Fortsätze in Endreiser zerfallend. Anhaftend ein Stück Hirnfilzes. FIG. 12. Dito. Bei a selzt sich feinkörnige Zwischenmasse an. Bei b ein Stück anhaftenden Hirnfilzes mit einem eingesponnenen Gliakörperchen. Bei c Terminalreiser ein Endfäserchennetz ansetzend. FIG. 13. Ein verzweigter Fortsatz in Endreiser zerfallend, an diese

anschliessend Endfäserchen, die mit feinkörniger Zwischenmasse besetzt sind. FIG. 15. Schematische Erläuterung des Principes der Verbindung zwischen den Elementarcentren. Butzke, V. (1872) Studien über den feineren Bau der Grosshirnrinde. *Arch. Psychiat. Nervenk.* 3, 575–600 [Figures 8-13, 15].

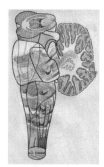

FIGURE 10.
Meynert, 1874.
Diagram of the structure of the human brain stem.

Der Grosshirnstamm. Diese Tafel ist das Seitenstück zu der nach Buchstaben erläuterten schematischen Abbildung des Grosshirnstammes der Taf. III, daher die einleitendee Bemerkungen der bezüglichen Tafelerklärung auch hierfür nachzulesen sind. Die Bedeutung der Farben ist: Roth stellt die graue Substanz, blau die centrifugal leitenden Bahnen, hellbraun die centripetal leitenden Bahnen, gelb die aus dem Kleinhirn hervortretenden Arme und Bündel dar. Die Continuität der dargestellen Bündel und grauen Substanz tritt durch gleichfarbige Uebereinanderlagerung ihrer Querschnitte vor Augen. Der graue Boden der Rautengrube ist die Brücke hindurch nicht dargestellt, weil dadurch die Continuität des Processus cerebelli ad cerebellum unklar geworden wäre. Das in der Hirnschenkelebene Taf. III mit vp bezeichnete Feld ist darum nicht blau gefärbt, weil gerade die fortlaufend durchgeführte Absetzung der Schleifenschichten, innerhalb der hintern Bahn des Stammes eine Grundlage der Orientirung abgibt. Auf folgende Unvollkommenheiten des Druckes mache ich aufmerksam: In der obersten, durch das verlängerte Mark gelegten Ebene, sollten die helibraunen Fäden (Taf. III fb fb) gleichmässig bis an ihr hinteres Ende gefärbt sein, und ist das in derselben Ebene über den Quintusdurchschnitt nach vorn hinaus reichende Roth wegzudenken. Der äussere Contour des Vaguskernes in der zweiten Oblongatenebene (Taf. III tr) sollte gerade, nicht convex sein, weil hierdurch der innere Acusticuskern weggeschnitten wird. Das Vorderhorn in der untersten Oblongatenebene (entsprechend Taf. IV FIG. 6 cra) ist schlecht begränzt. Als Hauptobjekt der ganzen Darstellung bedarf diese Tafel hier keiner weiteren Erklärung. Meynert, T. (1874) *Skizze des menschlichen Grosshirnstammes nach seiner Aussenform und seinem inneren Bau. Arch. Psychiatr. Nervenkr.* 4, 387–431 [Plate 5].

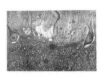

**FIGURE 11.**

Denissenko, 1877. Human cerebellum.

FIG. 6. Ein Schnitt durch das Kleinhirn des Menschen. 3: VIII. An der Grenze zwischen der molekulären und der Körnerschichte liegt eine Ganglienzelle; umgeben von einer grossen Menge von Nervenfasern, die nach allen Richtungen verlaufen. Die ellipsoiden Zellen mit ihren Haematoxylinkernen liegen höher. Hier liegen auch einige Ganglienzellen, die keine scharfen Umrisse besitzen. Linkerseits von der Purkinje 'schen Zelle liegt eine kleine Ganglienzelle. Der Kern und das Kernkörperchen der rechtsseitigen Purkinje 'schen Zelle besitzen Fortsätze. Die Haematoxylin- und Eosinzellen sind theils einzeln, theils in Gruppen angeordnet. Denissenko, G. (1877) Zur Frage über den Bau der Kleinhirnrinde bei verschiedenen Klassen von Wirbelthieren. *Arch. Mikrosk. Anat.* 14, 203–242 [Plate 14, Figure 6].

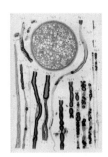

**FIGURE 12.**

Ranvier, 1878. Nerve fibers.

FIG. 1. A, B, C. Trois tubes nerveux du segment périphérique du sciatique du pigeon, le troisième jour après la section. Ces tubes, isolés après une heure de macération du nerf dans une solution d'acide osmique à 1 pour 100, ont été colorés au picrocarminate et conservés dans la glycérine substituée lentement au liquide colorant (Voy. p.4). A, portion médiane d'un segment interannulaire, présentant un seul noyau hypertrophié *n*, entouré d'une masse de protoplasma *p*. et de gouttes de myéline teintes par l'osmium, *m*. B, partie centrale d'un segment interannulaire, présentant deux noyaux *n' n'*, plongés dans une masse protoplasmique commune *p*. Entre les deux noyaux, le tube nerveux présente un léger rétrécissement. C, quatre noyaux *n" n" n" n"* se rencontrent dans un même segment interannulaire. Le protoplasma *p* qui les enveloppe n'est pas segmenté, et dans son intérieur sont également contenues des boules de myéline, *m*. FIG. 2. Deux tubes nerveux à myéline du segment périphérique du pneumogastrique du lapin, six jours après la section. Dissociation après macération dans une solution d'acide osmique à 1 pour 100; coloration au moyen du picrocarminate; couservation dans la glycérine. Les portions *a a* de ces tubes, qui ne sont occupées

ni par des gouttes de myéline ni par des noyaux, sont revenues sur elles-mêmes, et à leur niveau le tube nerveux est rétréci. *n n*, noyaux proliférés des segments interannulaires; *m m*, gouttes de myéline; *g*, granulations graisseuses (*Voy.* p. 9). FIG. 3. A, B, C. Trois Tubes nerveux du segment périphérique du sciatique du lapin, quatre jours après la section. Même mode de préparation que pour les tubes représentés figure 2 (*Voy.* p. 9). A. Le noyau *n* du segment, légèrement hypertrophié, comprime la myéline; autour de lui, le protoplasma *p*, s'étant accru, a refoulé en divers points la gaîne médullaire ou l'a complétement sectionnée. B, prolifération des noyaux *n* des segments interanuulaires; *e*. étranglement annulaire, effacé en partie par le gonflement du protoplasma *p*; *m*, gaîne médullaire fragmentée. C, tube nerveux dont la gaîne médullaire est déprimée ou sectionnée par l'accroissement du protoplasma, et de chaque côté duquel se voicent deux cellules du tissu connectif intrafasciculaire *c c* (*Voy.* p. 15). FIG. 4. Portion d'une fibre de Remak du segment périphérique du sciatique du lapin, cinq jours après la section. Mode de préparation indiqué à l'explication de la figure 2, *n n*, noyaux hypertrophiés et légèrement étranglés; *g*. granulations graisseuses (*Voy.* p. 14). FIG. 5. Un tube nerveux de l'extrémité du segment supérieur du sciatique du rat, trois jours après la section. La figure est retournée; en a se trouve l'extrémité ouverte du tube sectionné, dont le calibre est occupé en grande partie par des cellules limphatiques, dans lesquelles on distingue les noyaux *n*, les granulations graisseuses et les gouttes de myéline qu'elles contiennent. La gaîne médullaire m est déformée, rongée ou refoulée par les cellules lymphatiques. *n'*. noyau du segment interannulaire. *c c c c*. quatre cellules lymphatiques du tissu conjonctif intrafasciculaire, chargées de granulations graisseuses et de gouttes de myéline (*Voy.* p. 37). FIG. 6. Tube nerveux du bourgeon central du nerf sciatique du lapin, quatre jours après la section. La portion qui a été dessinée a été prise un peu au-dessus de l'extrémité sectionnée. Même mode de préparation que pour les tubes représentés dans les figures précédentes. *m*, gaîne médullaire refoulée en quelques points, mais non sectionnée par le protoplasma *p* et les noyaux proliférés *n n n* (*Voy.* p. 41). FIG. 7. Tube nerveux complétement isolé du bourgeon central du nerf sciatique du rat, trois jours après la section (*Voy.* p. 33). *t*, terminaison de la gaîne médullaire normale; *cy*, cylindre axe strié; *p*, protoplasma granuleux qui l'entoure; *m*, portion de la gaîne médullaire n'ayant subi qu'une résorption incomplète;

*my*, boules de myéline; *e*, extrémité libre du cylindre axe au niveau de la section. FIG. 8. Coupe transversale d'un des faisceaux du segmet périphérique du nerf sciatique du lapin, vingt-huit jours après la section. Le durcissement du nerf a été obtenu par une macération d'une semaine dans une solution d'acide chromique à 2 pour 100, un séjour de vingt-quatre heures dans l'eau pour enlever l'excès du réactif et de vingt-quatre heures dans l'alcool pour donner au nerf une consistance convenable. La coupe a été colorée au moyen du picrocarminate et elle a été montée dans le baume du Canada après avoir été déshydratée par l'alcool et éclaircie par l'essence de girofle. (*Voy.* p. 10). *gl*, gaîne lamelleusc; *v*, vaisseaux sanguins; *a*, gros tubes nerveux sans cylindre axe ; *b*, tubes nerveux encore munis d'un cylindre axe ; *t*, petits tubes nerveux sans cylindre axe, *c*, tissu conjonctif in trafasciculaire; *l*, lames intrafasciculaires. FIG. 9. Nerf pneumogastrique du lapin enlevé soixante jours après la section, vu à l'œil nu et dessiné à sa gradeur naturelle après macération de vingt.-quatre heures dans une solution d'acide osmique à 1 pour 100. *c*, segment central; *b*, bourgeon central; *i*. segment intermédiaire on cicatriciel; *b'*. bourgeon périphérique ; *p*, segment périphérique (*Voy.* p. 47). FIG. 10. Un gros tube nerveux à myéline du bourgeon central du nerf pneumogastrique du lapin, soixante-douze jours après la section, isolé après une macération de vingt-quatre heures dans une solution d'acide osmique à 1 pour 100. La gaîne médullaire du tube primitif *t* se termine par un bourgeon *b*, de l'extrémité duquel partent des tubes à myéline *t' t''* et des fibres sans myéline. *s*, gaîne de Schwann du tube primitif formant aux tubes qui en émanent une gaîne secondaire, *s'* (*Voy.* p. 61). FIG. 11 et 11 bis. Tube nerveux du bourgeon central du nerf sciatique du lapin, quatre-vingt-dix jours après la section. La figure 11 *bis* doit être reportée à la suite de la figure 11, de telle sorte que *a'* se continue avec *a* (*Voy*, p. 62). Ce tube nerveux a été isolé après une macération de vingt-quatre heures dans l'acide osmique à. 1 pour 100. *t*, tube nerveux primitif entouré de sa gaîne de Schwan *s*, et se terminant par un bourgeon de sa gaîne médullaire *b*. De l'extrémité de ce bourgeon part un tube secondaire *t'*, qui se divise et se subdivise pour donner un faisceau de tubes nerveux médullaires grêtes F, entouré d'une gaîne secondaire *s'*, émanation de la gaîne de Schwann; *m*, boules de myéline provenant de la gaîne médullaire de l'ancien tube. Ranvier, L. (1878) *Leçons sur l'histologie du système nerveux.* Savy, Paris (Plate 1, Figures 1–11).

# THE BLACK PERIOD: NEURONS, GLIA, AND THE ORGANIZATION OF THE NERVOUS SYSTEM

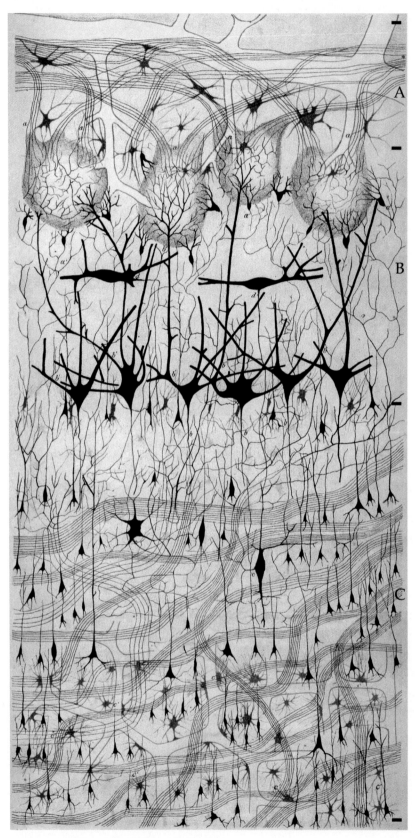

FIGURE 13. Golgi, 1875. Olfactory bulb of a dog.

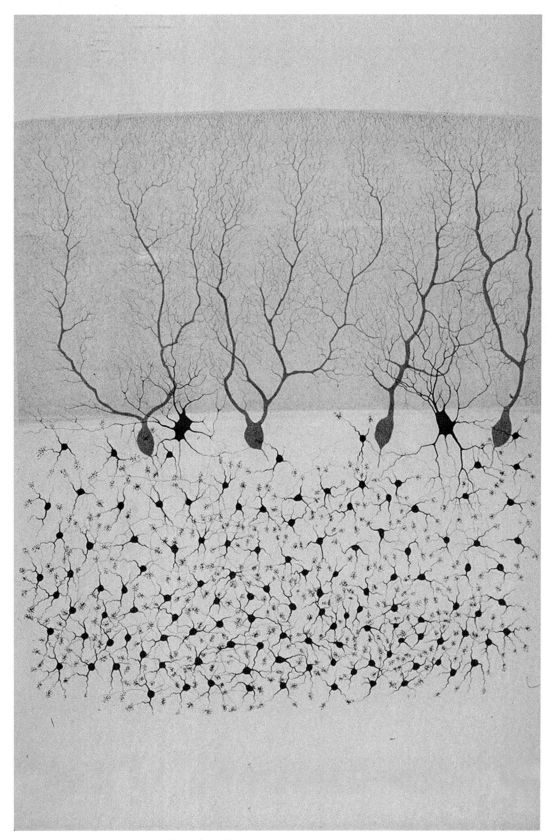

FIGURE 14. Golgi, 1882. Cerebellum of a rabbit.

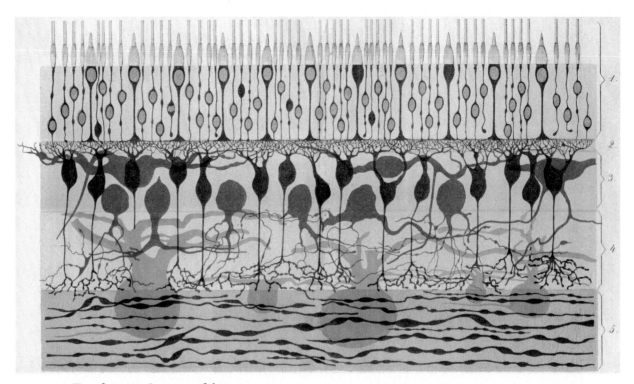

**FIGURE 15.** Tartuferi, 1887. Structure of the retina.

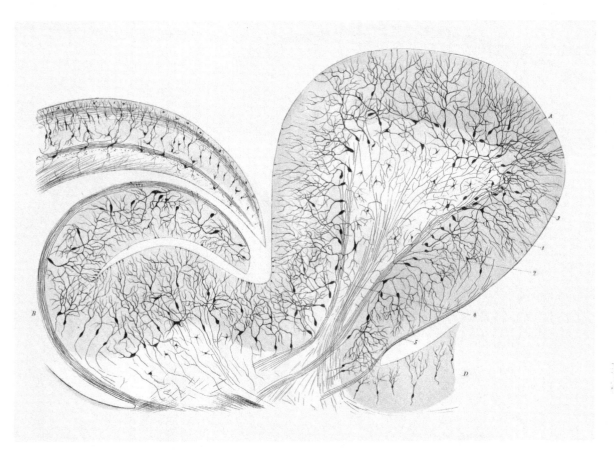

FIGURE 16. Fusari, 1887. Structure of the central nervous system of teleosts, I.

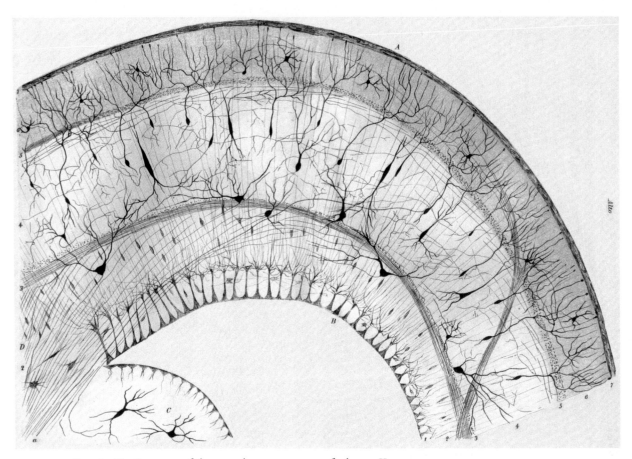

FIGURE 17. Fusari, 1887. Structure of the central nervous system of teleosts, II.

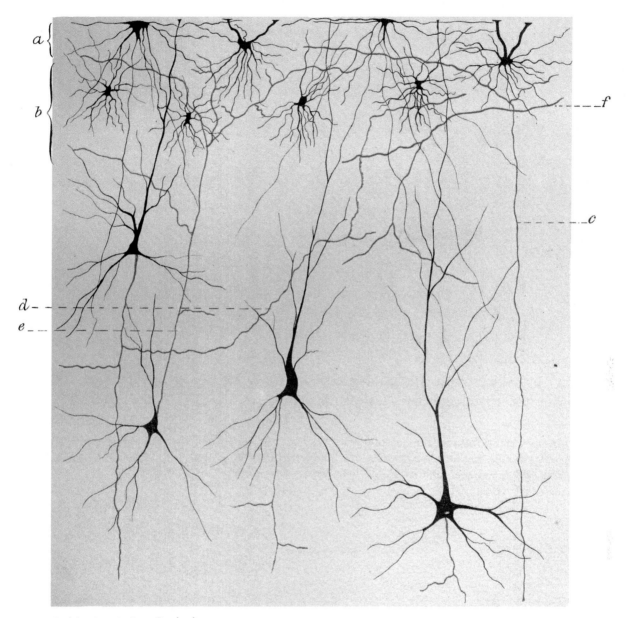

FIGURE 18. Martinotti, 1890. Cerebral cortex.

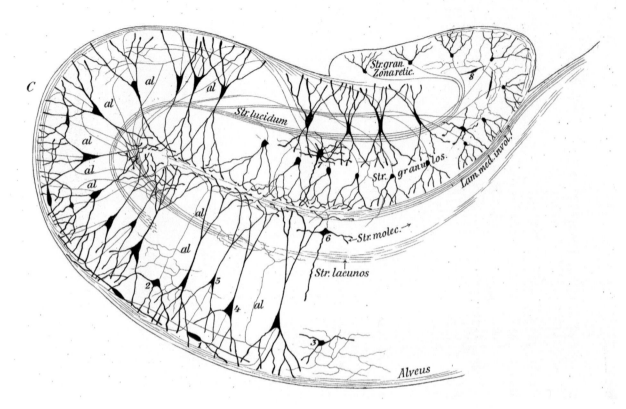

**FIGURE 19.** Schaffer, 1892. Structure of the hippocampus.

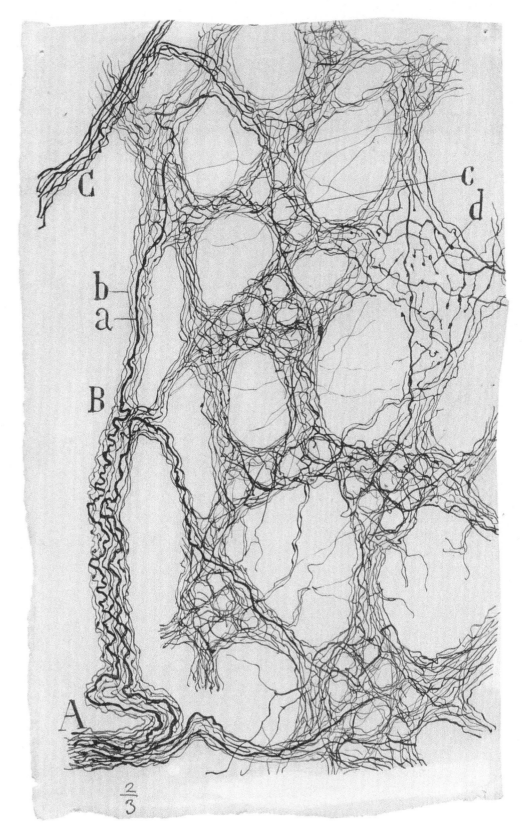

FIGURE 20. Ramón y Cajal, 1893. Auerbach plexus and ganglia of a mouse.

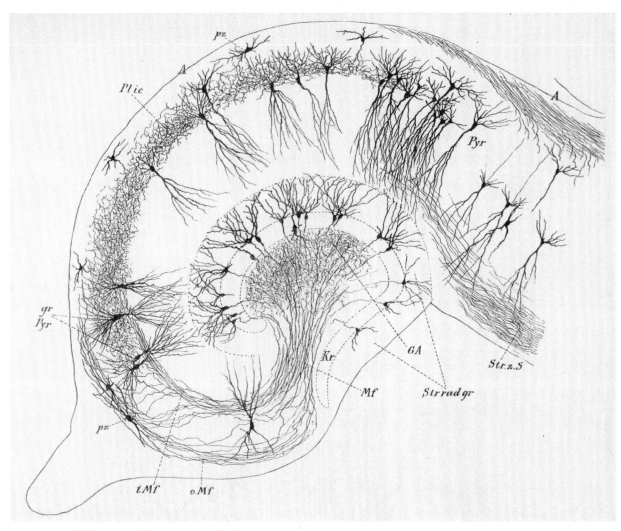

**FIGURE 21.** Kölliker, 1893. Hippocampus of a kitten.

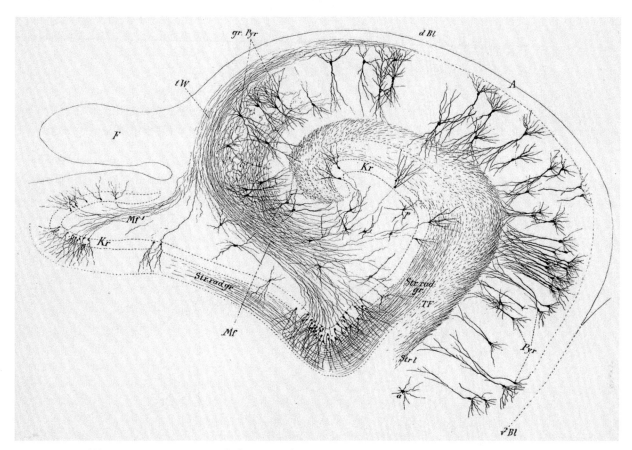

**FIGURE 22.** Kölliker, 1893. Hippocampus of a human embryo.

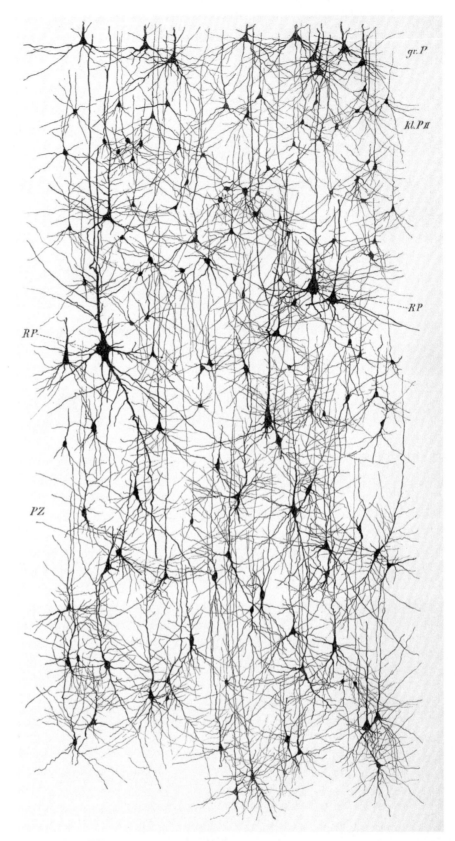

FIGURE 23. Kölliker, 1893. Human cerebral cortex.

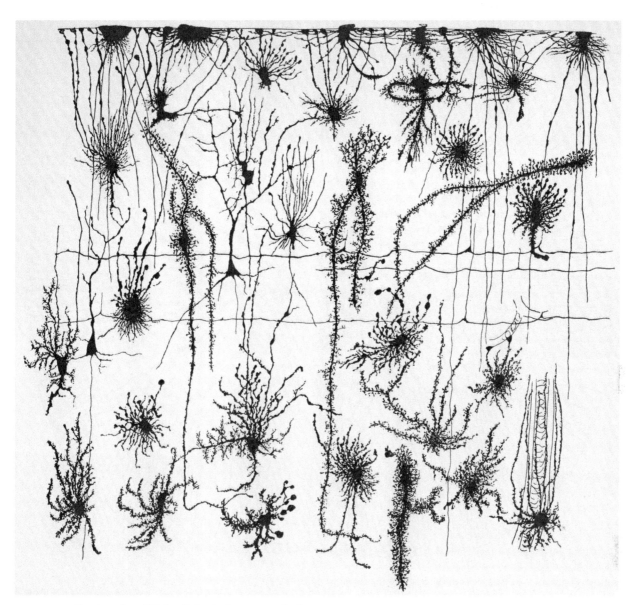

**FIGURE 24.** Retzius, 1894. Glial cells in the human cerebral cortex.

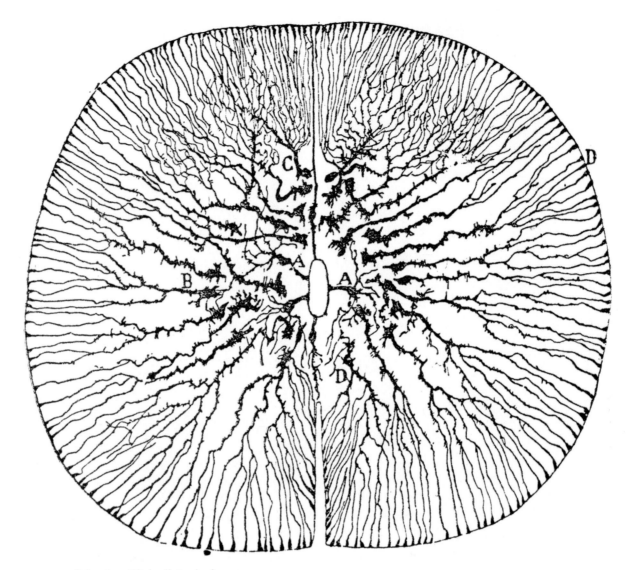

**FIGURE 25.** Sala, 1894. Glial cells in the frog.

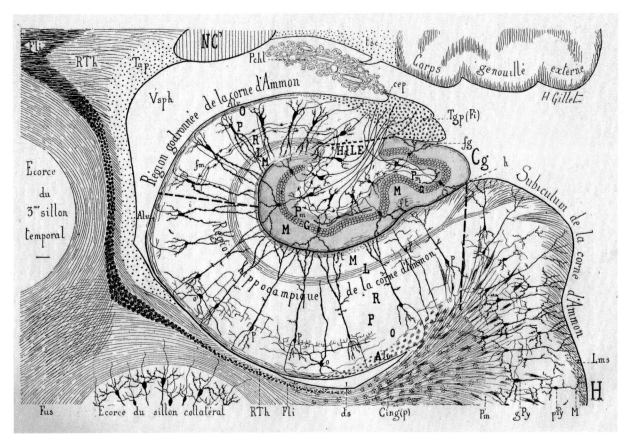

**FIGURE 26.** Dejerine, 1895. Human hippocampal formation.

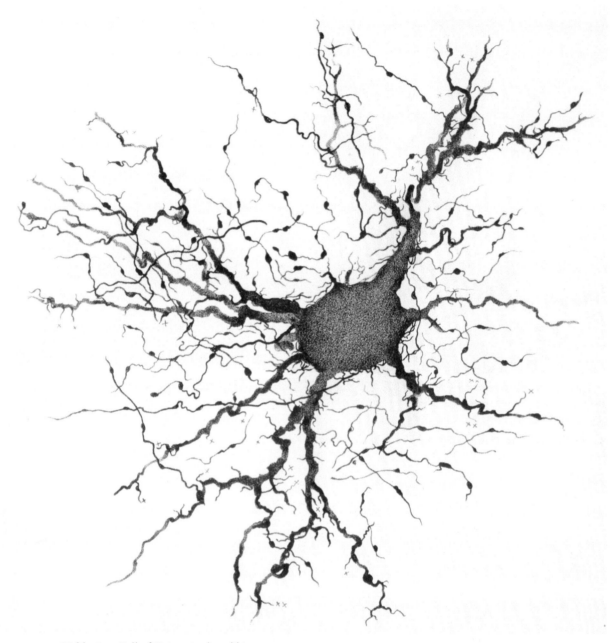

**FIGURE 27.** Held, 1897. Cell of Deiters in the rabbit.

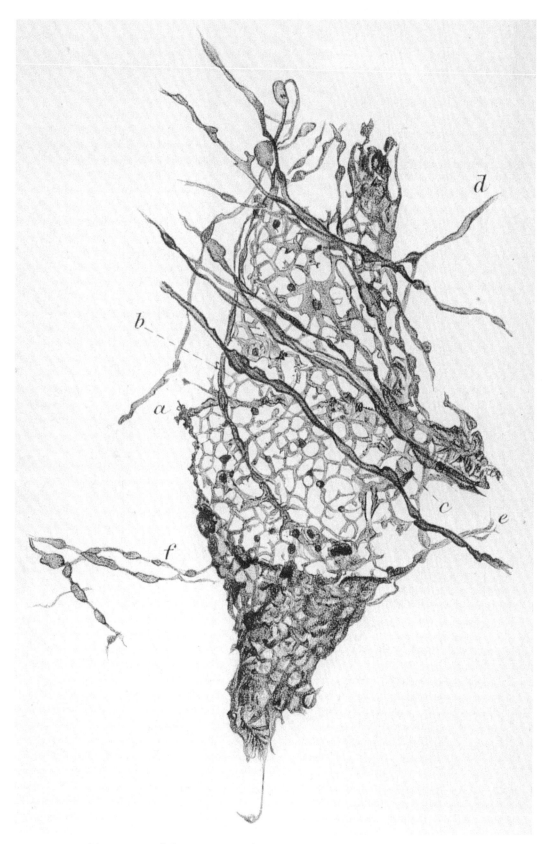

FIGURE 28. Held, 1897. Pericellular axon terminals.

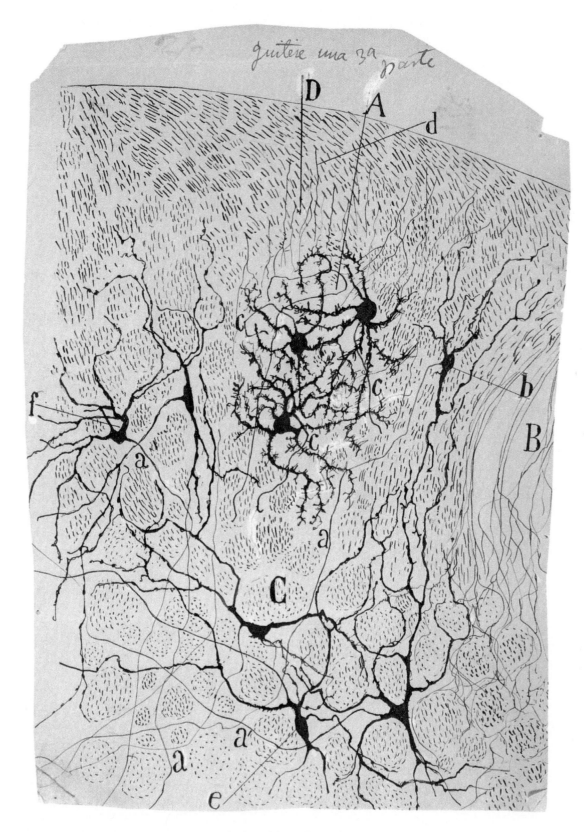

**FIGURE 29.** Ramón y Cajal, 1897. Neurons in the lateral funiculus.

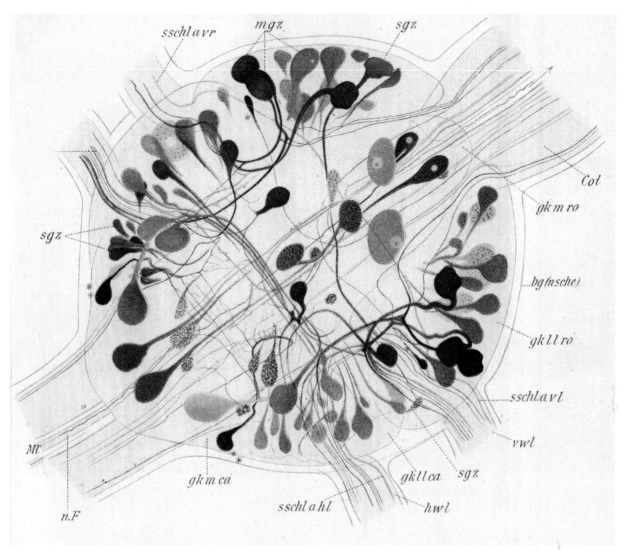

**FIGURE 30.** Apáthy, 1897. Ganglion cells in the leech.

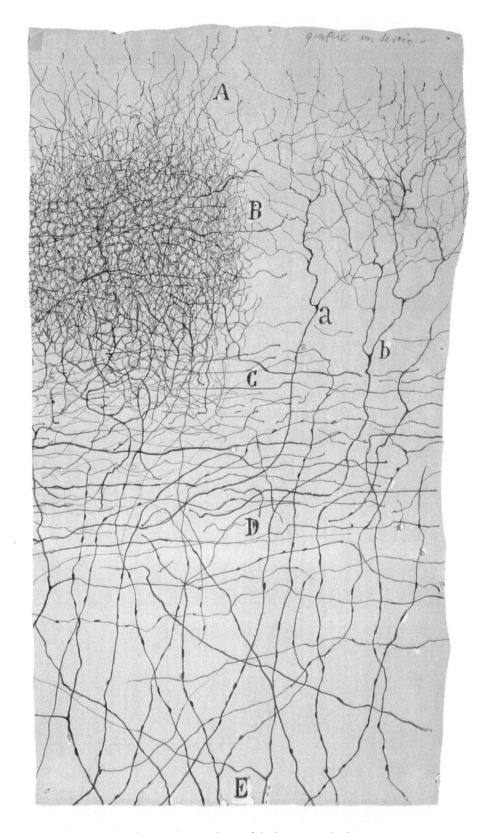

**FIGURE 31.** Ramón y Cajal, 1899. Sensory plexus of the human cerebral cortex.

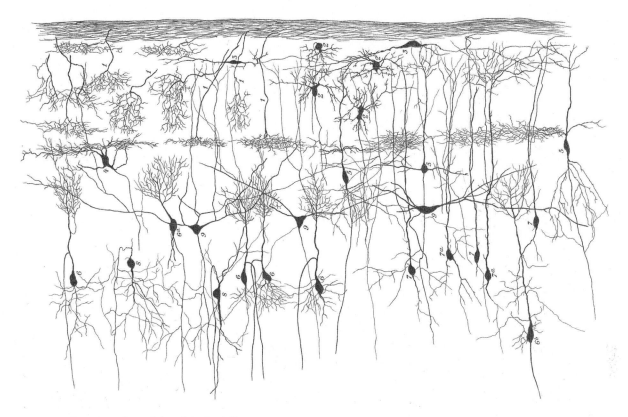

FIGURE 32. Ris, 1899. Optic lobe of the bird, I.

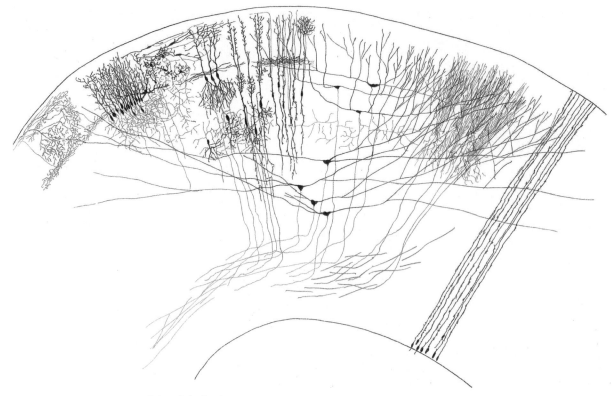

**FIGURE 33.** Ris, 1899. Optic lobe of the bird, II.

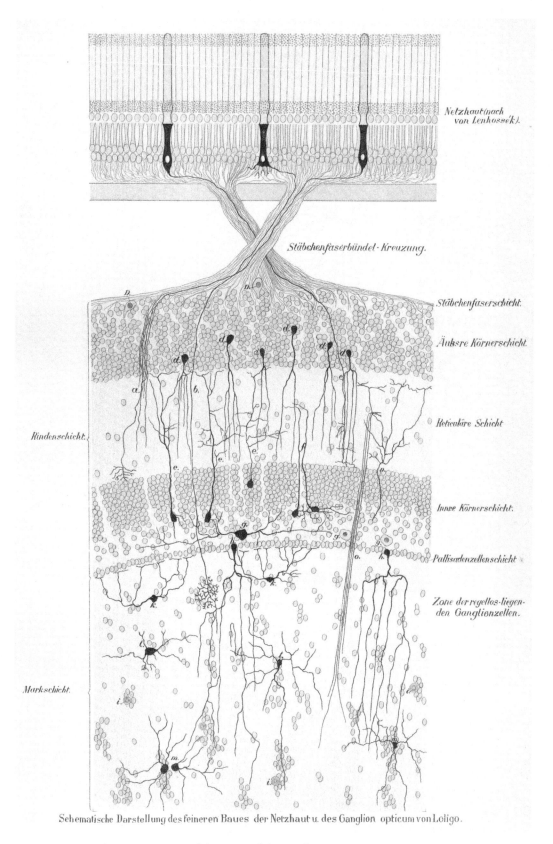

Netzhaut (nach von Lenhossék).

Stäbchenfaserbündel-Kreuzung.

Stäbchenfaserschicht.

Äussre Körnerschicht.

Reticuläre Schicht.

Rindenschicht.

Innre Körnerschicht.

Pallisadenzellenschicht.

Zone der regellos liegenden Ganglienzellen.

Markschicht.

Schematische Darstellung des feineren Baues der Netzhaut u. des Ganglion opticum von Loligo.

**FIGURE 34.** Kopsch, 1899. Diagram of the retina of the squid.

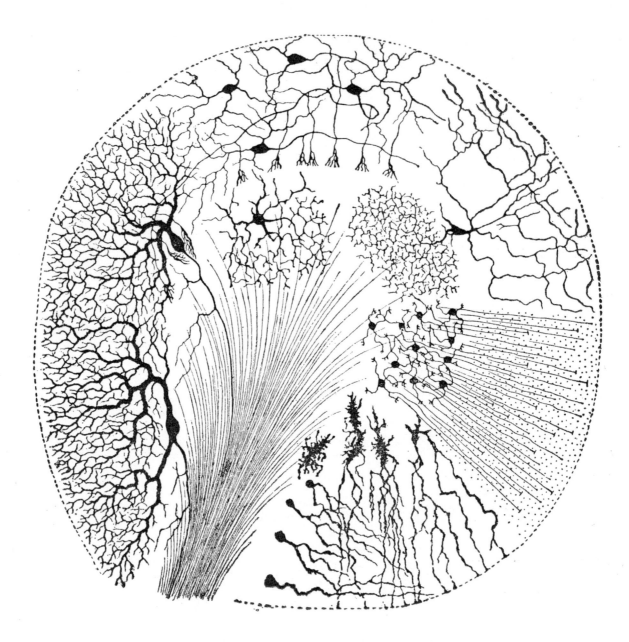

**FIGURE 35.** Van Gehuchten, 1900. Neuronal components of the cerebellar cortex.

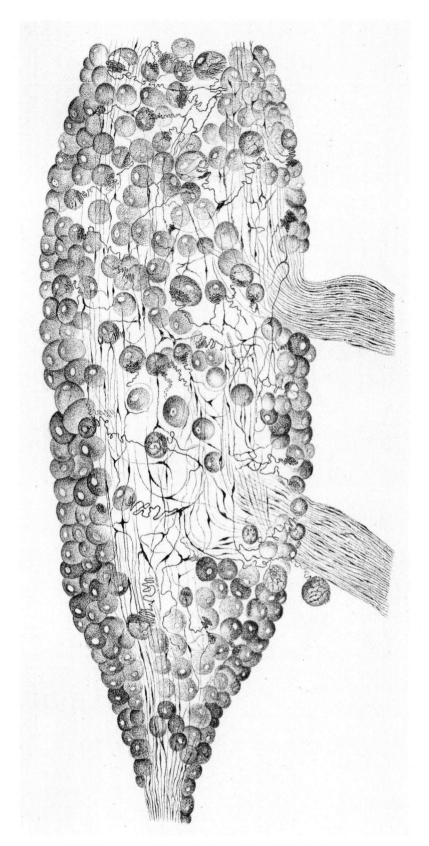

FIGURE 36. Smirnow, 1900. Sympathetic ganglion cells in the frog.

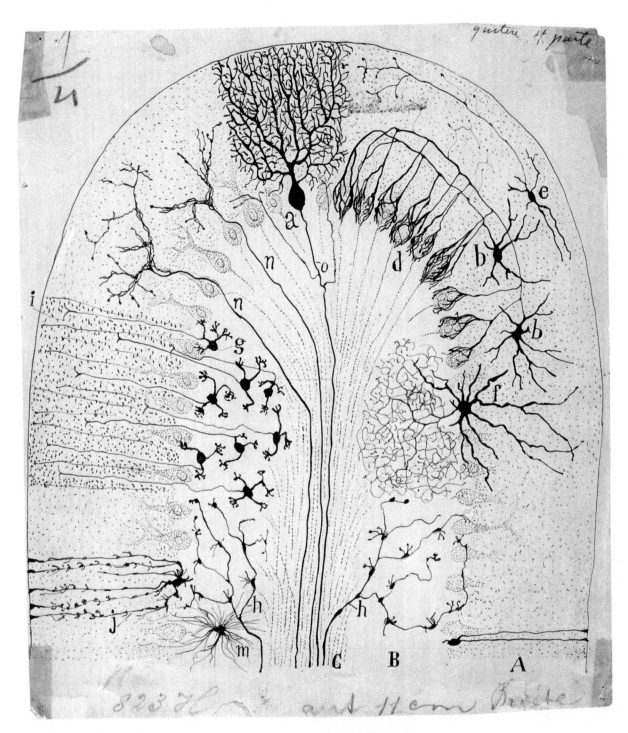

**FIGURE 37.** Ramón y Cajal, 1904. Schema of the structure of the mammalian cerebellum.

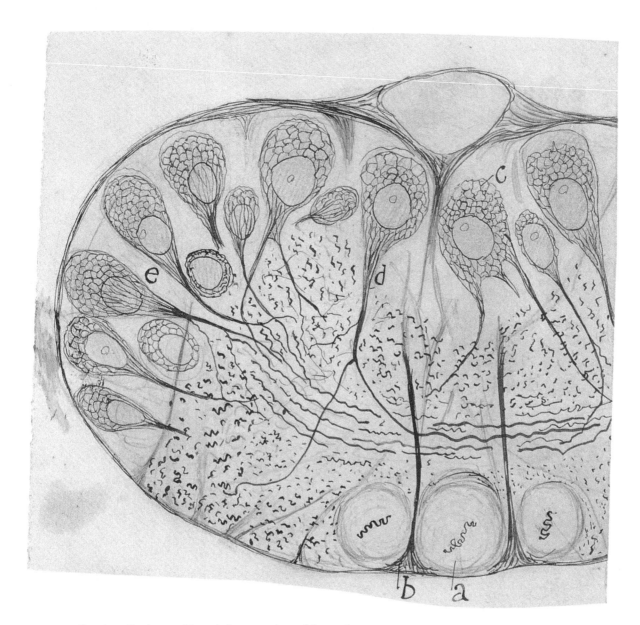

FIGURE 38. Ramón y Cajal, 1904. Ventral chain ganglion of the earthworm.

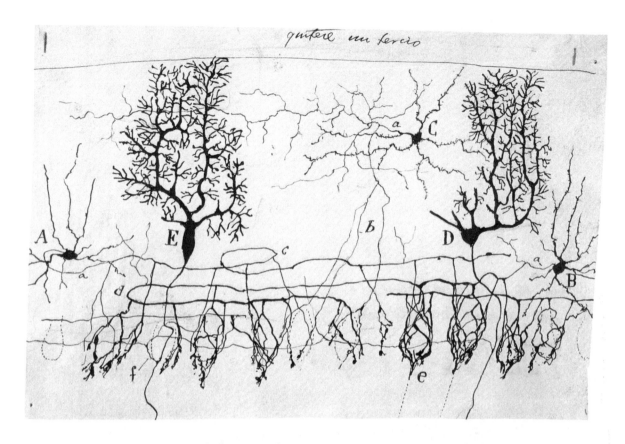

**FIGURE 39.** Ramón y Cajal, 1904. Cerebellar cortex of a guinea pig.

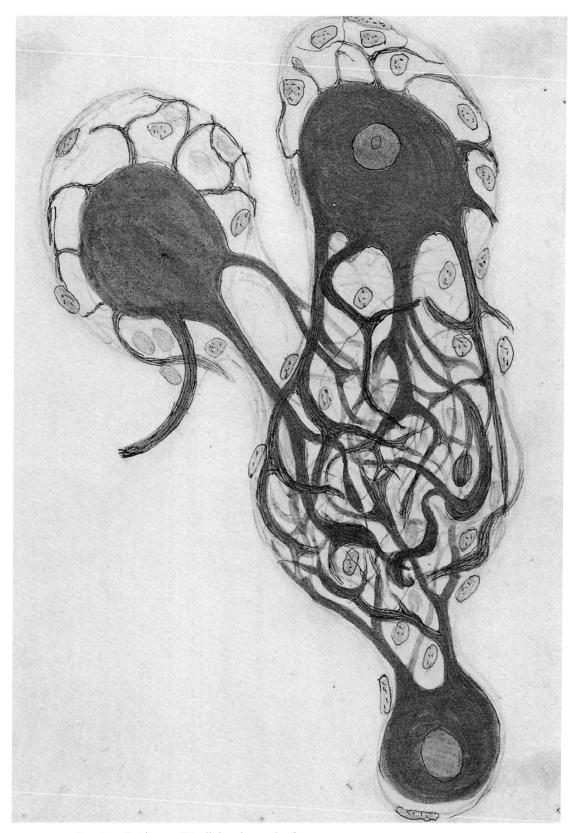

**FIGURE 40.** Ramón y Cajal, 1905. Tricellular glomerulus from a man.

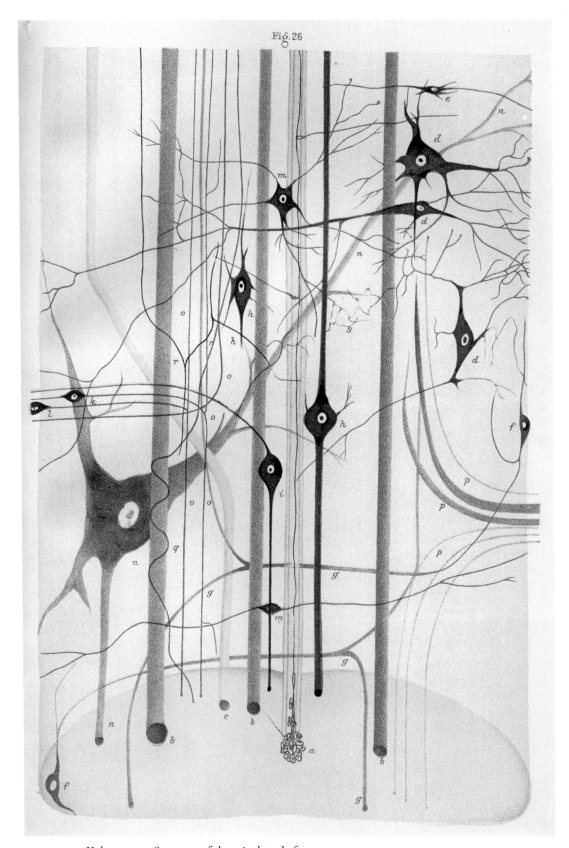

**FIGURE 41.** Kolmer, 1905. Structure of the spinal cord of ammocoetes.

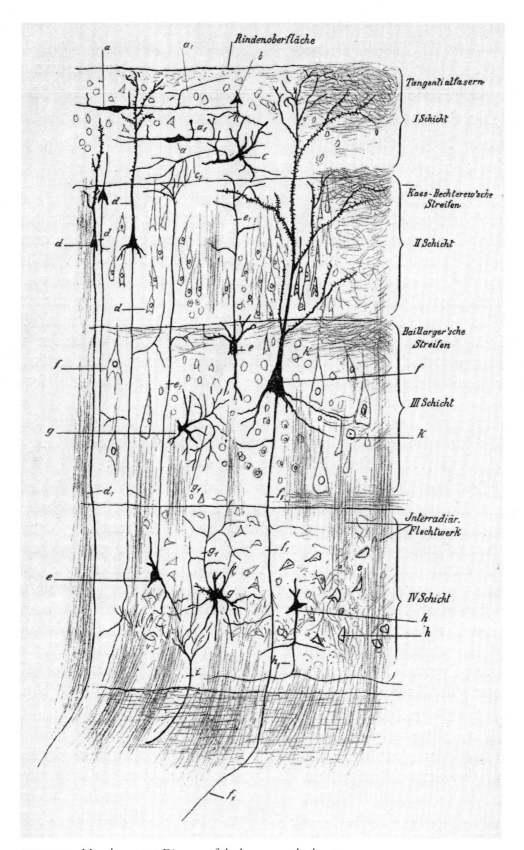

FIGURE 42. Monakow, 1905. Diagram of the human cerebral cortex.

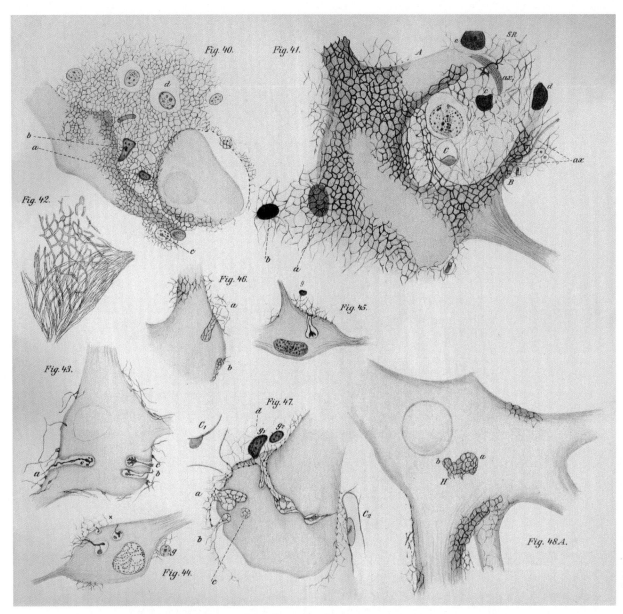

**FIGURE 43.** Economo, 1906. Normal structure of ganglion cells.

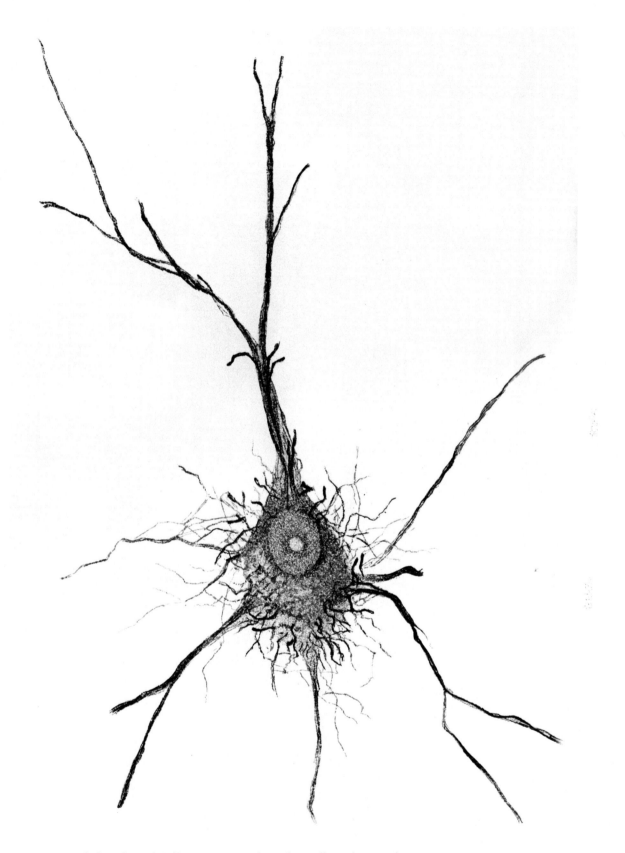

**FIGURE 44.** Bielschowsky and Gallus, 1913. Atypical ganglion cell in tuberous sclerosis.

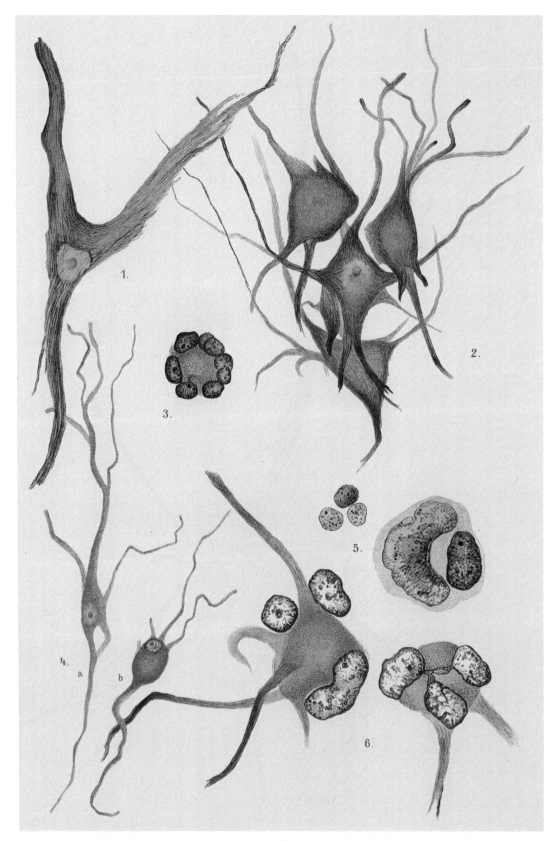

**FIGURE 45.** Bielschowsky and Gallus, 1913. Atypical cells in tuberous sclerosis, I.

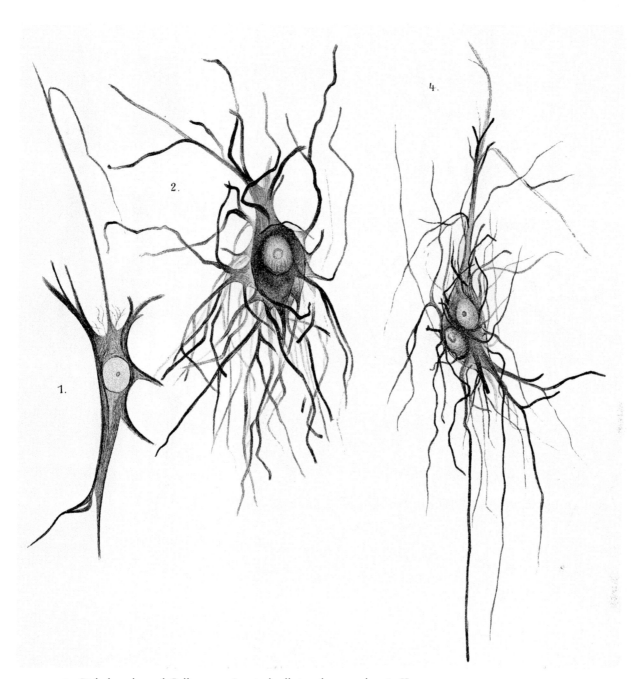

FIGURE 46. Bielschowsky and Gallus, 1913. Atypical cells in tuberous sclerosis, II.

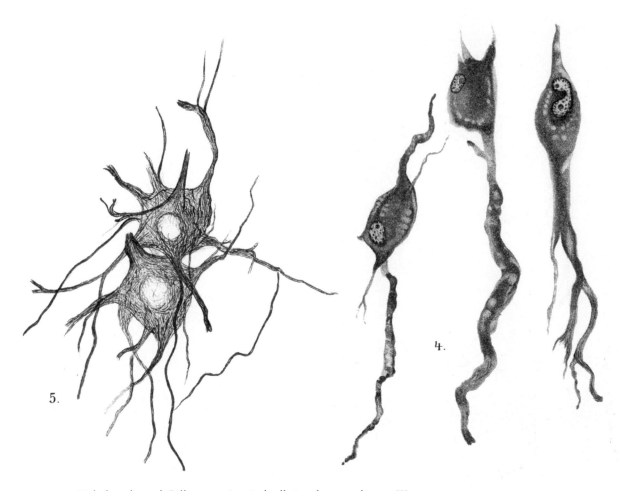

FIGURE 47. Bielschowsky and Gallus, 1913. Atypical cells in tuberous sclerosis, III.

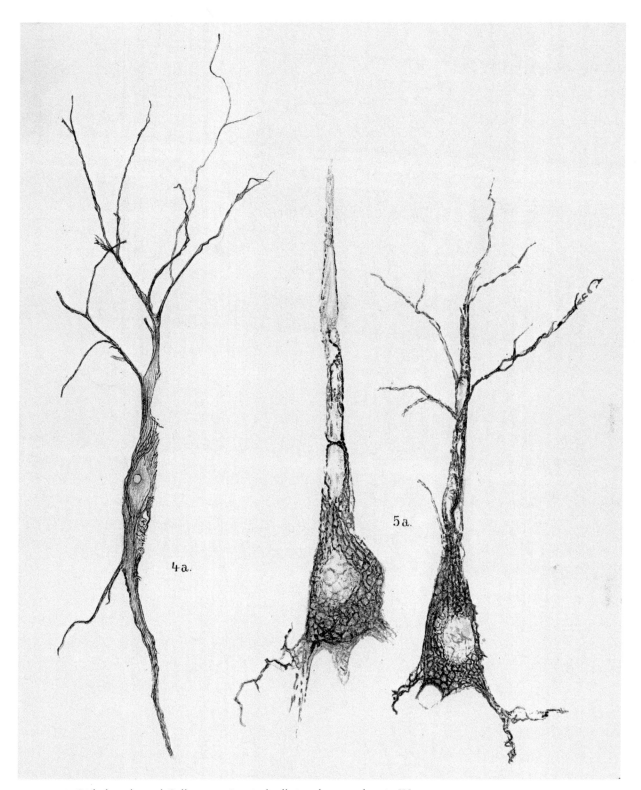

**FIGURE 48.** Bielschowsky and Gallus, 1913. Atypical cells in tuberous sclerosis, IV.

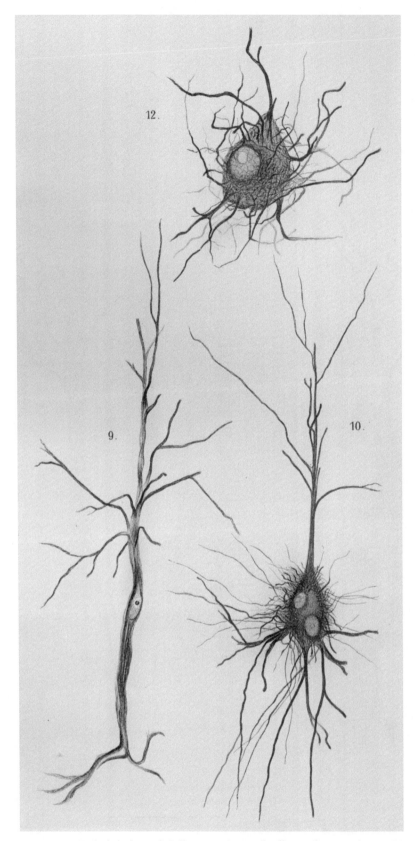

**FIGURE 49.** Bielschowsky and Gallus, 1913. Atypical cells in tuberous sclerosis, V.

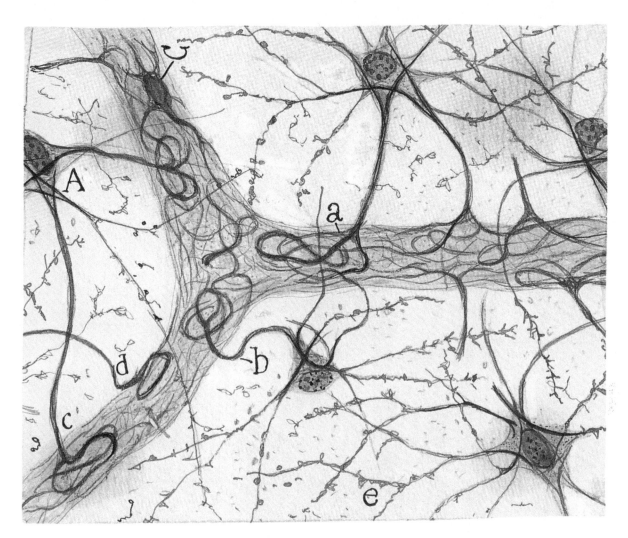

**FIGURE 50.** Ramón y Cajal, 1913. Cells of the cat Ammon's horn.

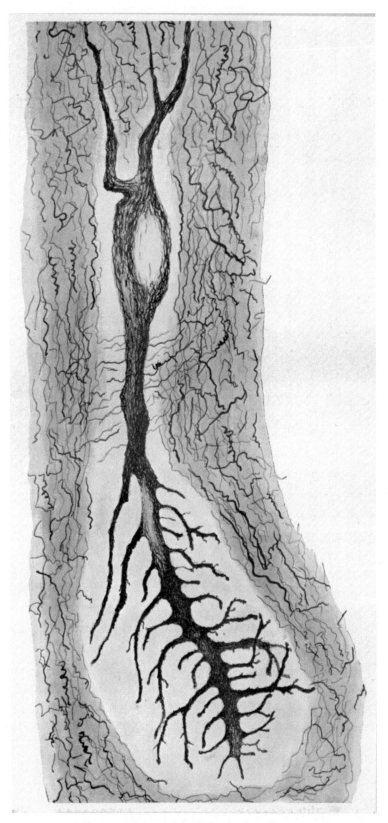

FIGURE 51. Lafora, 1914. Pyramidal cell dendritic neoformations in the senile dog.

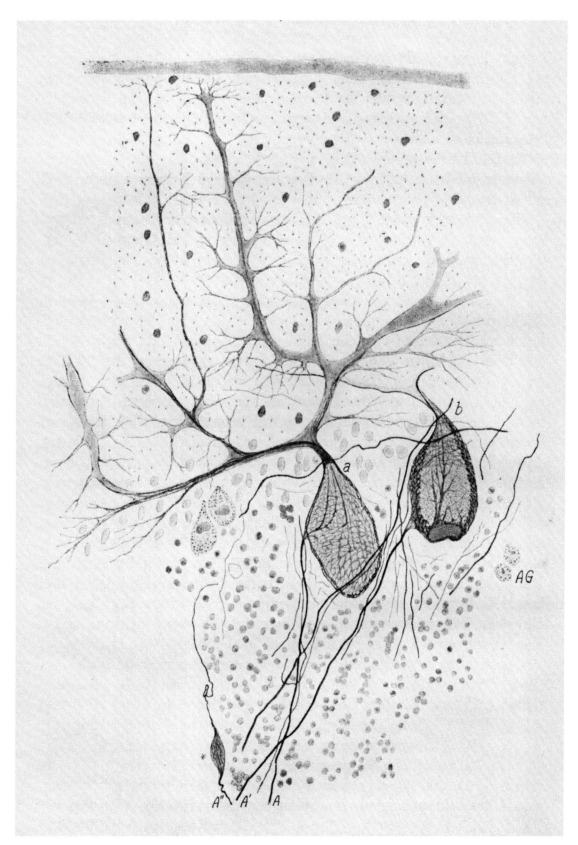

**FIGURE 52.** Schaffer, 1914. Structure of the cerebellar cortex.

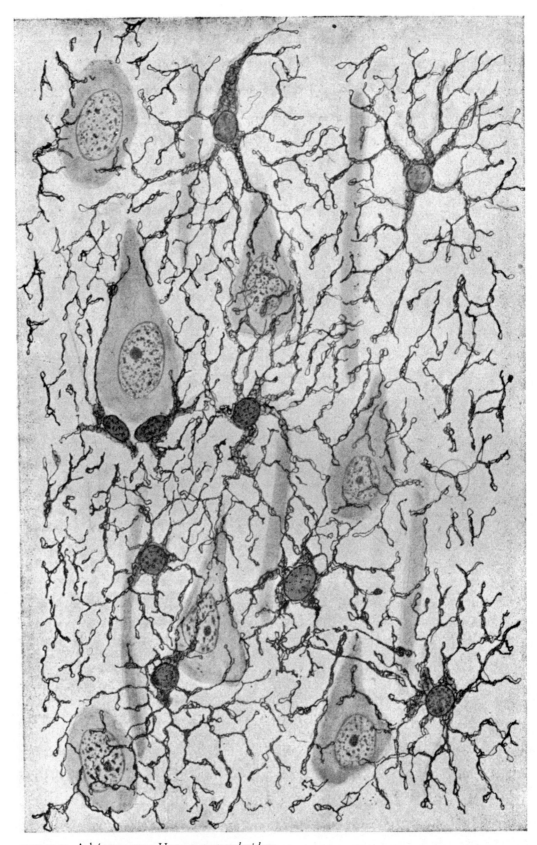

FIGURE 53. Achúcarro, 1914. Human *stratum lucidum*.

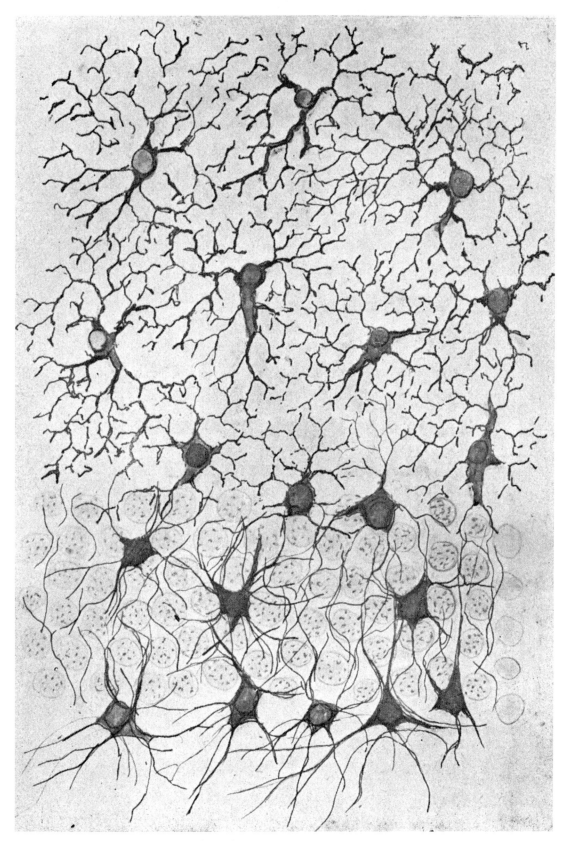

**FIGURE 54.** Achúcarro, 1914. Human *fascia dentata*.

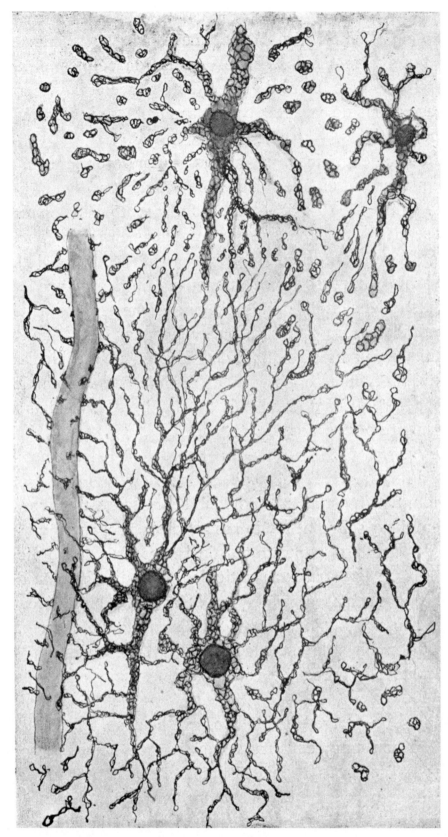

**FIGURE 55.** Achúcarro, 1914. Human *stratum radiatum.*

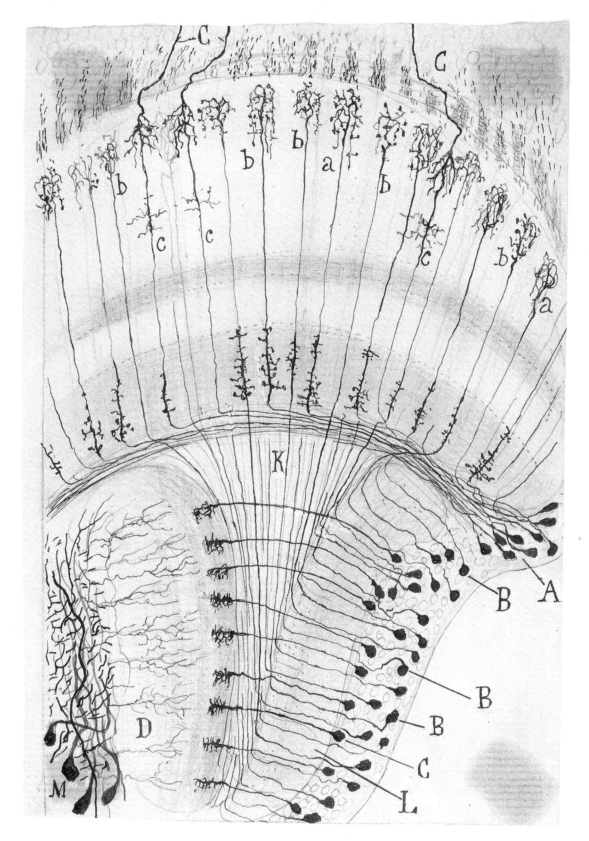

FIGURE 56. Ramón y Cajal and Sánchez y Sánchez, 1915. Retina and optic lobe of the horsefly.

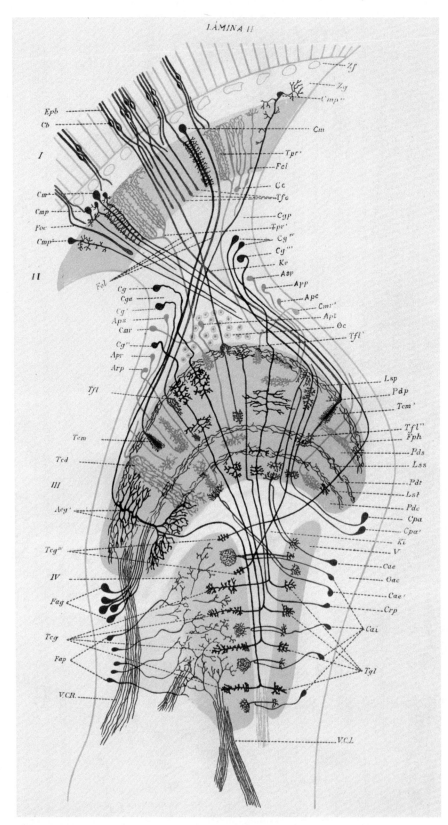

**FIGURE 57.** Ramón y Cajal and Sánchez y Sánchez, 1915. Schema of the retina and visual centers of the fly.

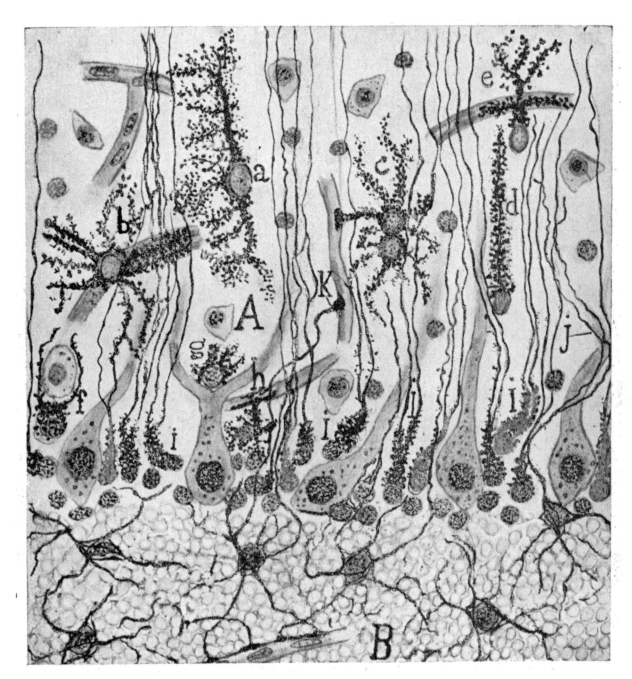

FIGURE 58. Ramón y Fañanás, 1916. Neuroglia in the rabbit cerebellum.

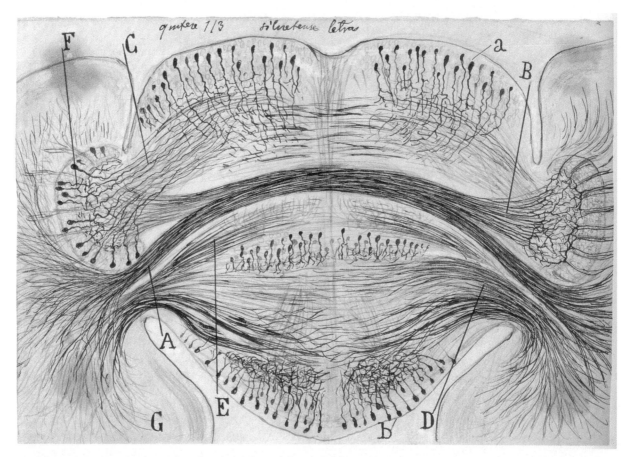

**FIGURE 59.** Ramón y Cajal, 1917. Cerebroid ganglion of the cuttlefish.

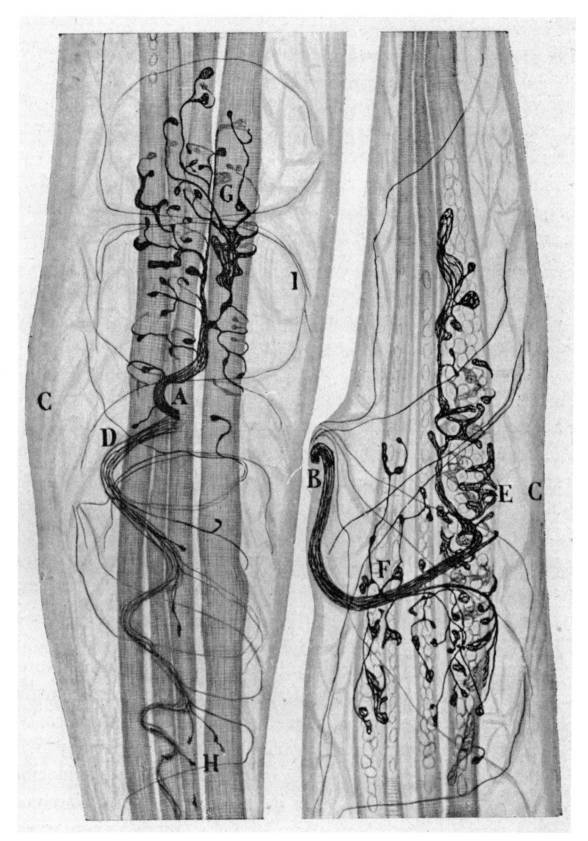

FIGURE 60. Tello, 1917. Human neuromuscular spindle.

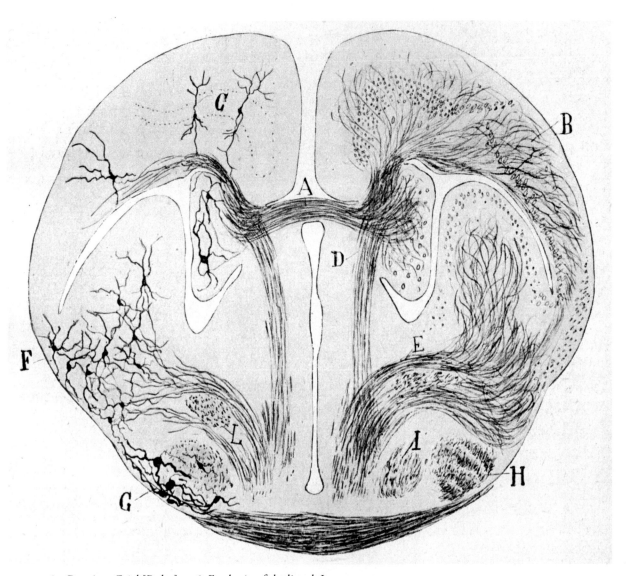

**FIGURE 61.** Ramón y Cajal [Pedro], 1918. Forebrain of the lizard, I.

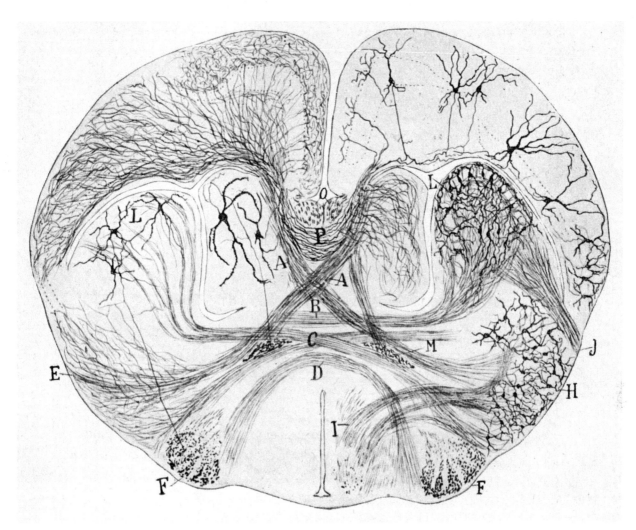

FIGURE 62. Ramón y Cajal [Pedro], 1918. Forebrain of the lizard, II.

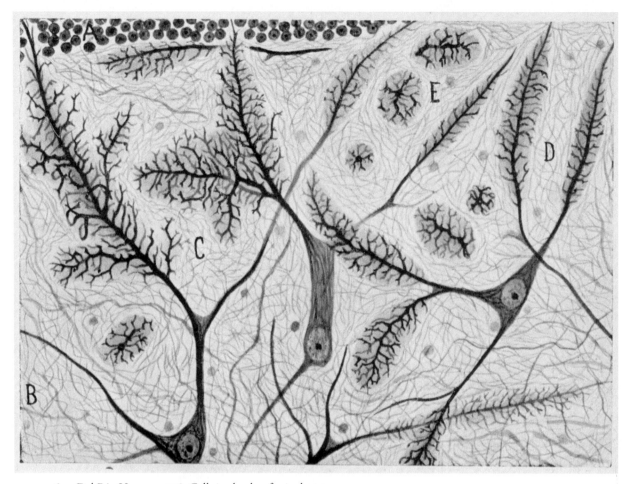

FIGURE 63.  Del Río-Hortega, 1918. Cells in the dog *fascia dentata*.

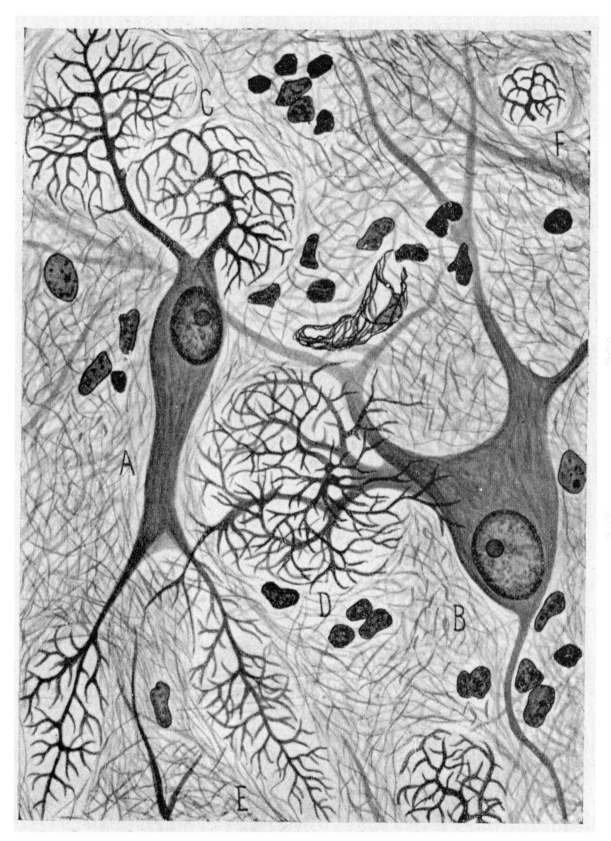

**FIGURE 64.** Del Río-Hortega, 1918. Cells in the horse *fascia dentata*.

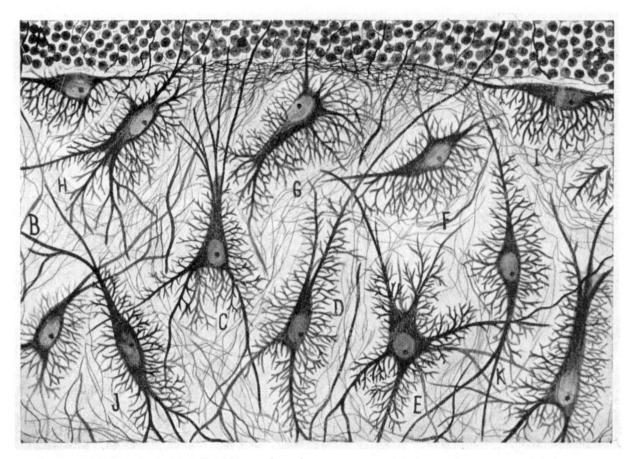

**FIGURE 65.** Del Río-Hortega, 1918. Cells in the ram *fascia dentata*.

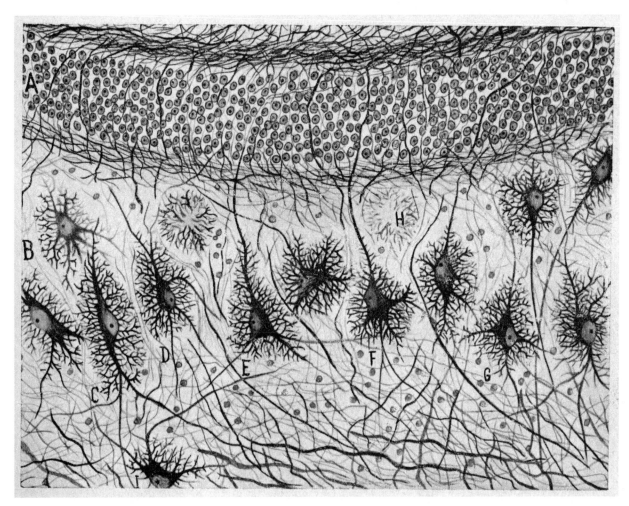

FIGURE 66. Del Río-Hortega, 1918. Cells in the bull *fascia dentata*.

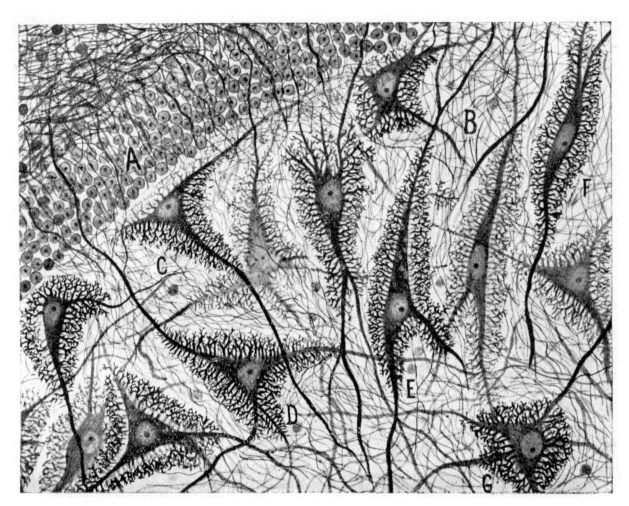

**FIGURE 67.** Del Río-Hortega, 1918. Cells in the ox *fascia dentata*.

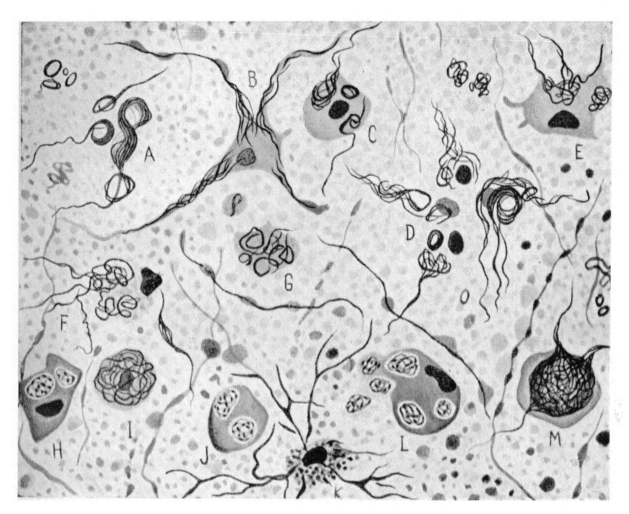

**FIGURE 68.** Del Río-Hortega, 1918–1919. Neuroglial cells of the aging human cerebral cortex.

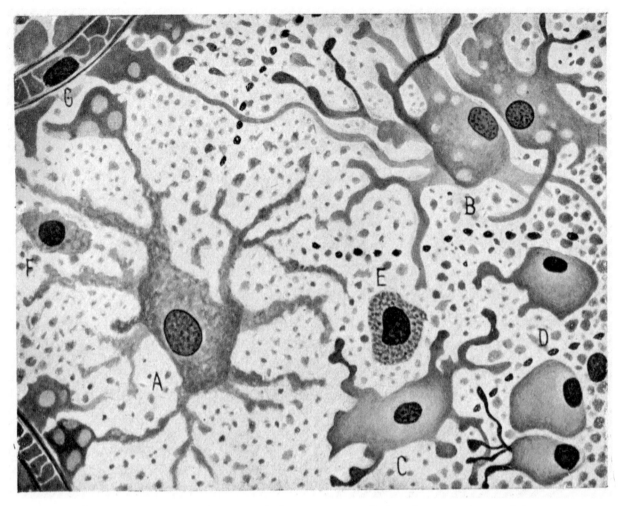

**FIGURE 69.** Del Río-Hortega, 1918–1919. Human cerebral cortex in a case of tuberculous meningo-encephalitis.

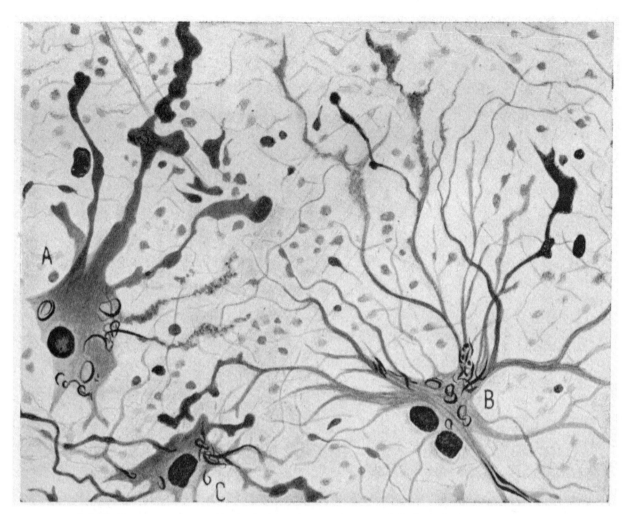

**FIGURE 70.** Del Río-Hortega, 1918–1919. Cerebral white substance in a case of paralytic dementia.

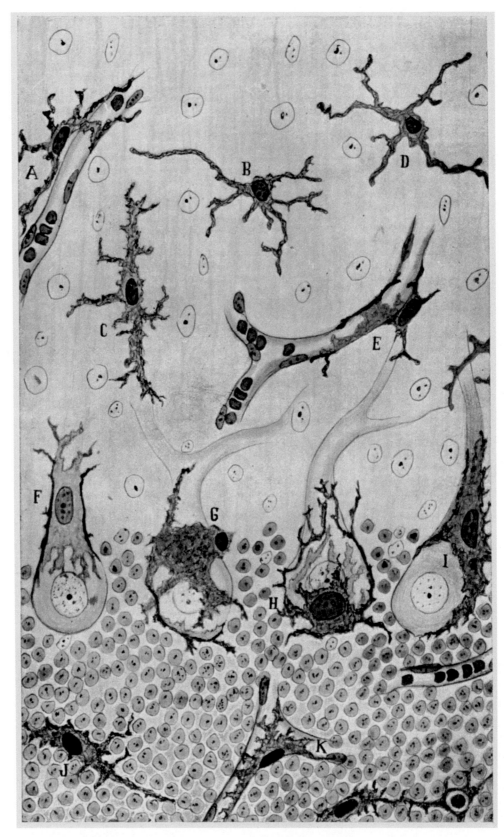

FIGURE 71. Collado, 1919. Cerebellar microglia of the rabbit with rabies.

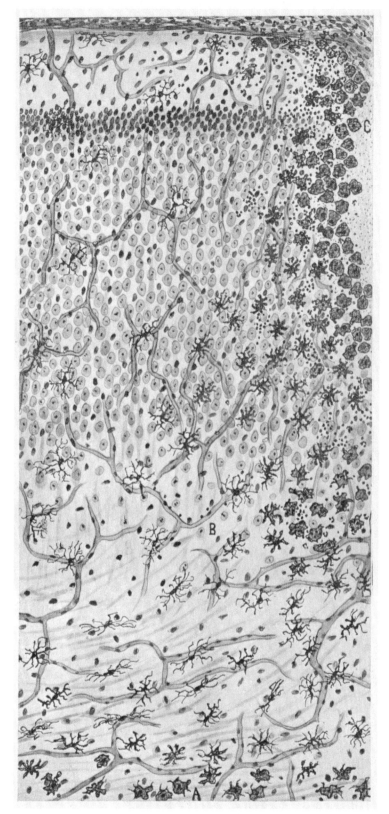

FIGURE 72. Del Río-Hortega, 1919. Migration and transformation of microglia in the vicinity of a cerebral injury.

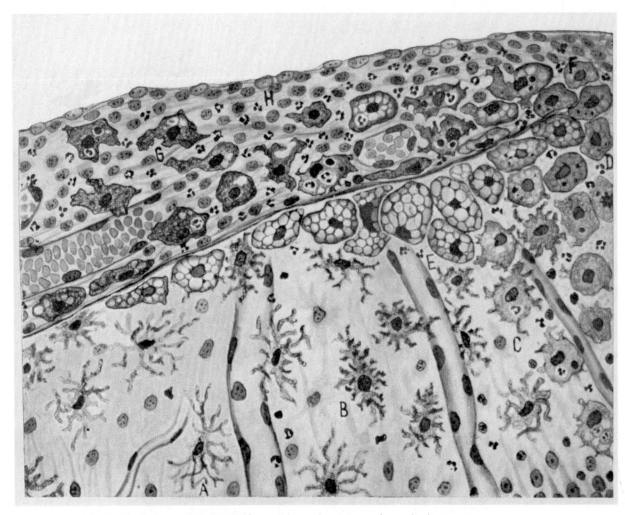

**FIGURE 73.** Del Río-Hortega, 1919. Migration of microglia in the vicinity of a cerebral injury.

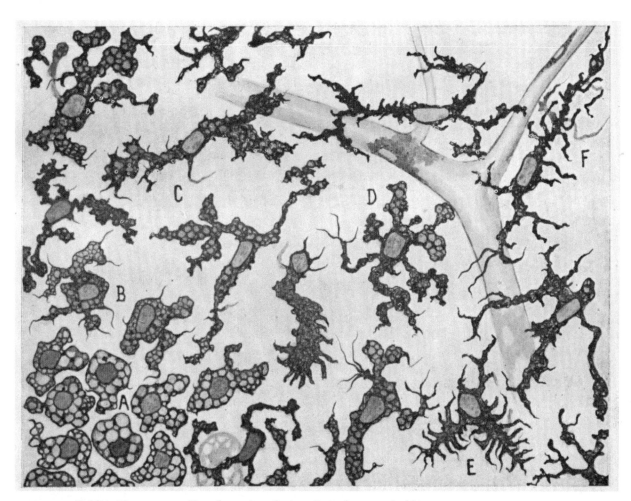

**FIGURE 74.** Del Río-Hortega, 1919. Transformation of microglia in the normal rabbit.

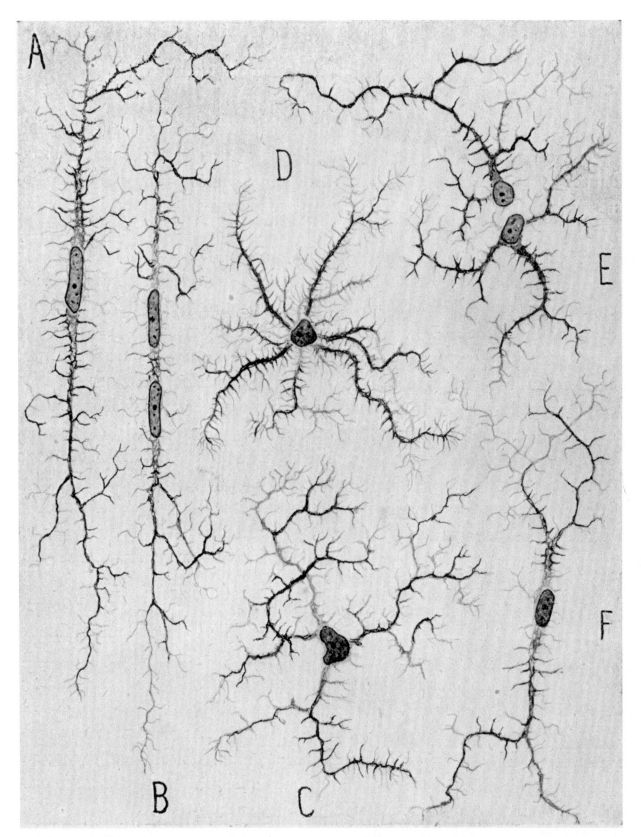

**FIGURE 75.** Del Río-Hortega, 1920. Human microglia.

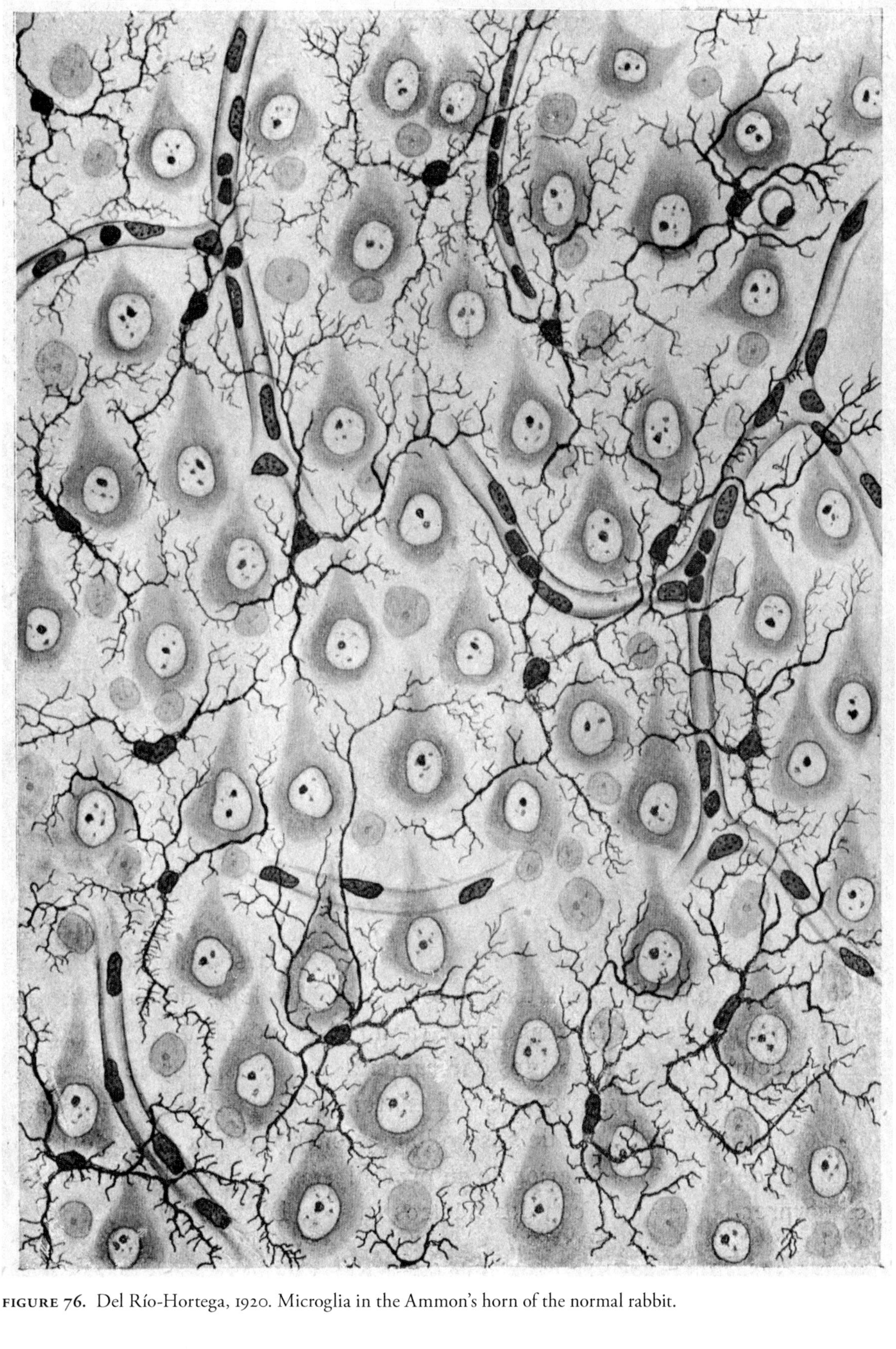

**FIGURE 76.** Del Río-Hortega, 1920. Microglia in the Ammon's horn of the normal rabbit.

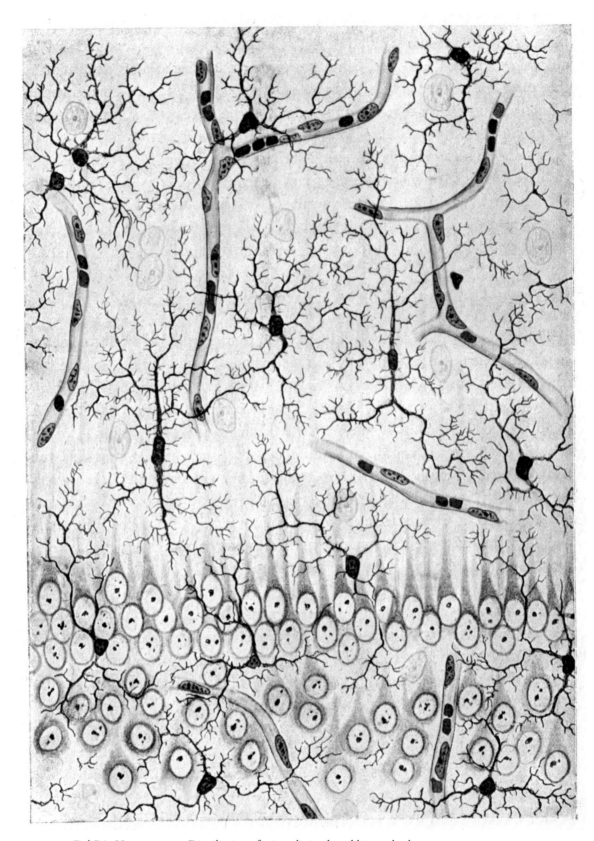

**FIGURE 77.** Del Río-Hortega, 1920. Distribution of microglia in the rabbit cerebral cortex.

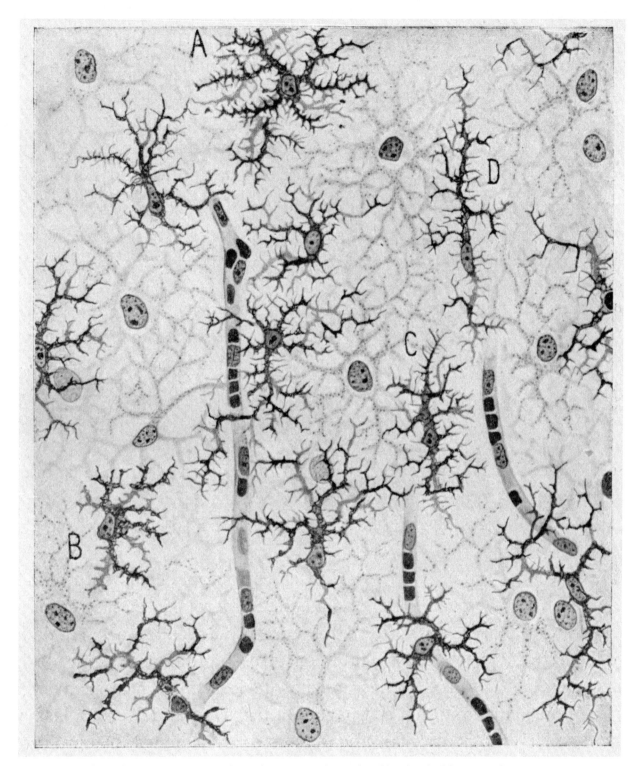

**FIGURE 78.** Del Río-Hortega, 1920. Microglia in the Ammon's horn of a rabbit that died from an infectious disease.

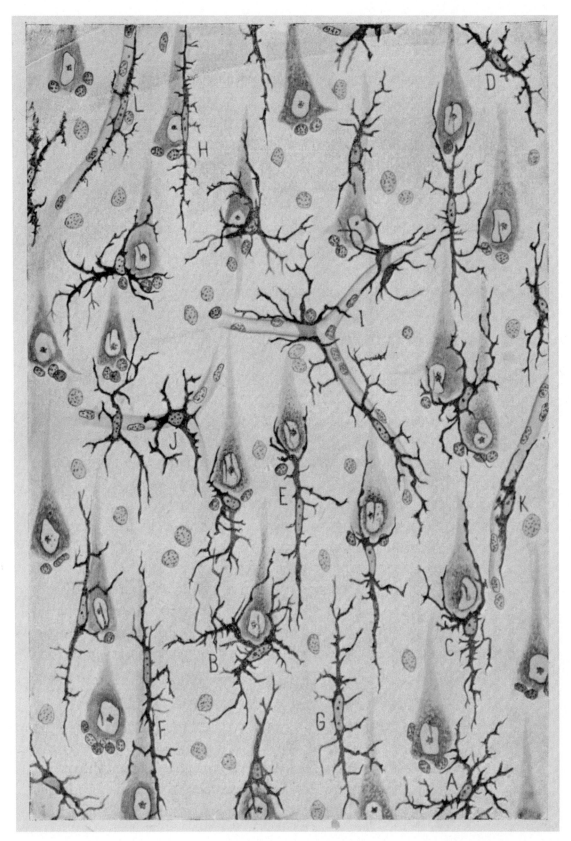

**FIGURE 79.** Del Río-Hortega, 1920. Microglia of the human cerebral cortex from a case of acute meningitis.

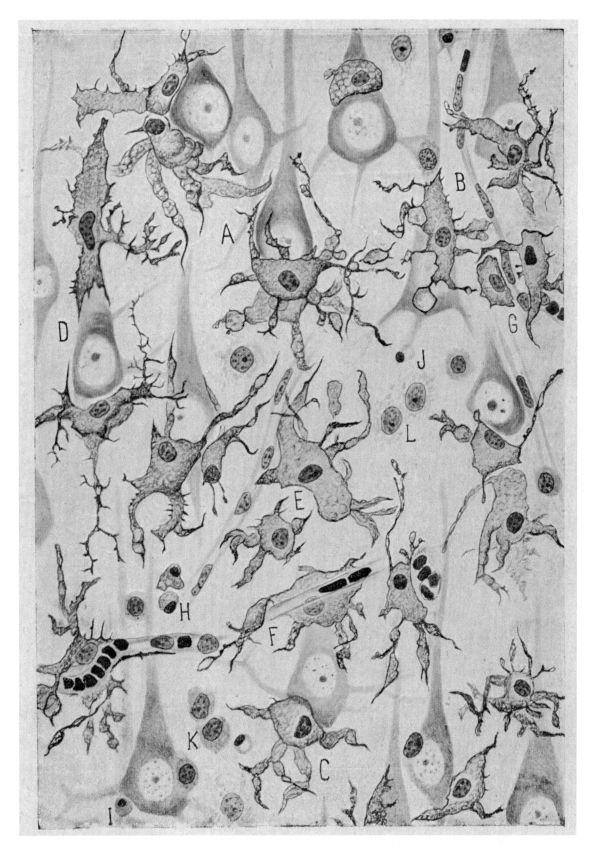

**FIGURE 80.** Del Río-Hortega, 1920. Microglia of the rabbit cerebral cortex in the vicinity of a wound.

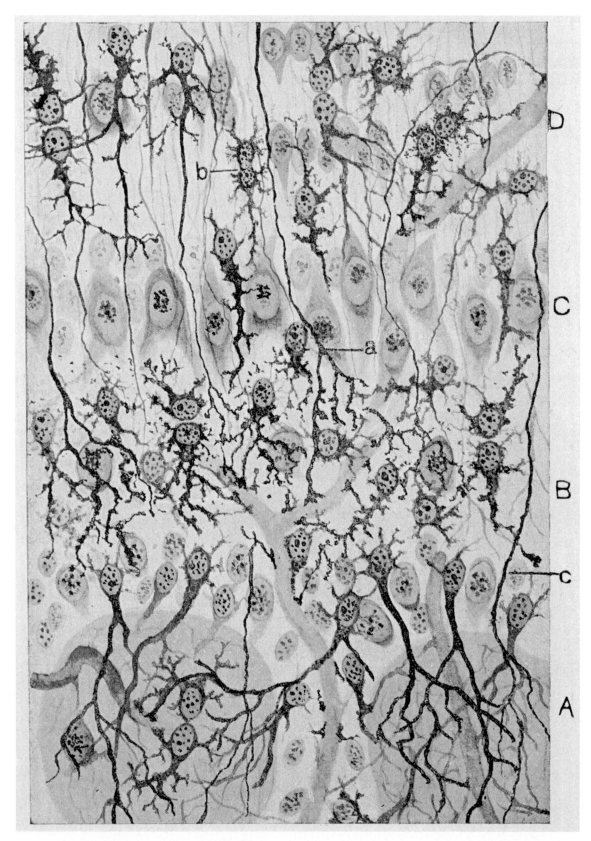

FIGURE 81. De Castro, 1920. Olfactory bulb of the cat.

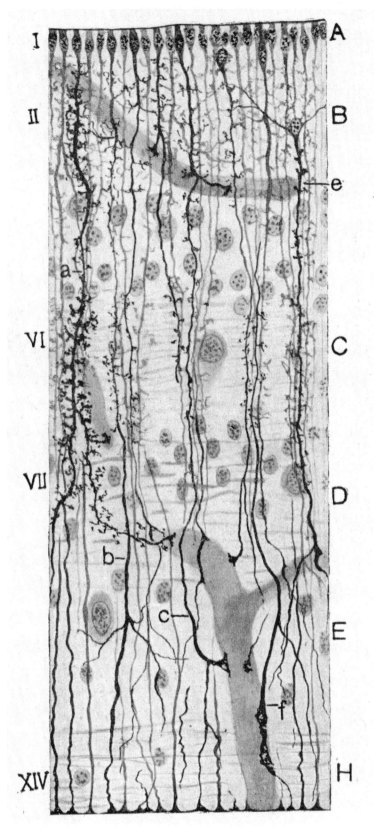

FIGURE 82. De Castro, 1920. Optic lobe of the lizard.

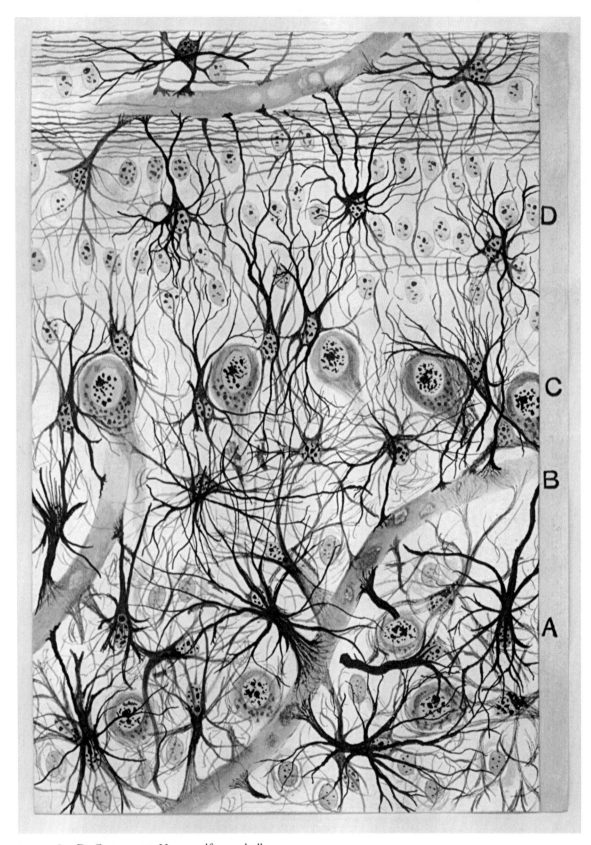

**FIGURE 83.** De Castro, 1920. Human olfactory bulb.

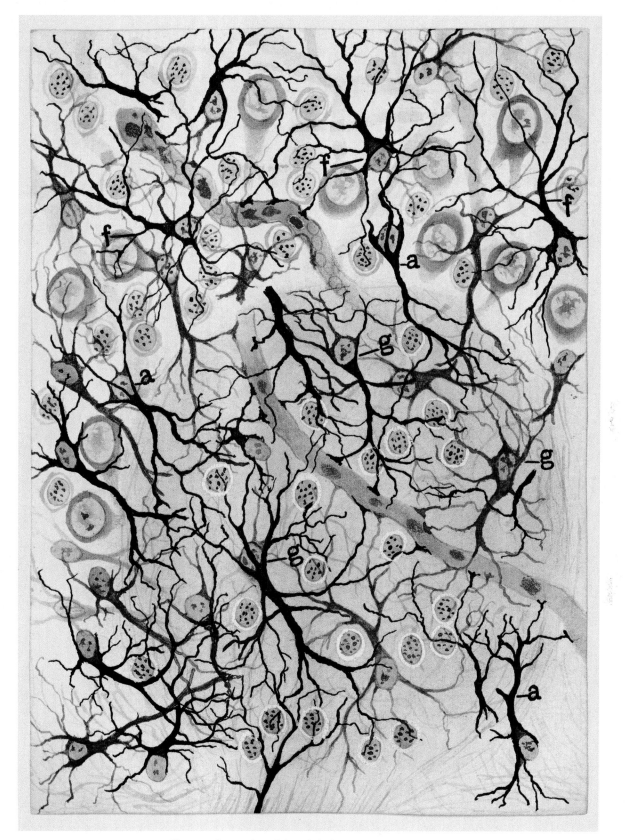

**FIGURE 84.** De Castro, 1920. Olfactory glomerulus of the adult dog.

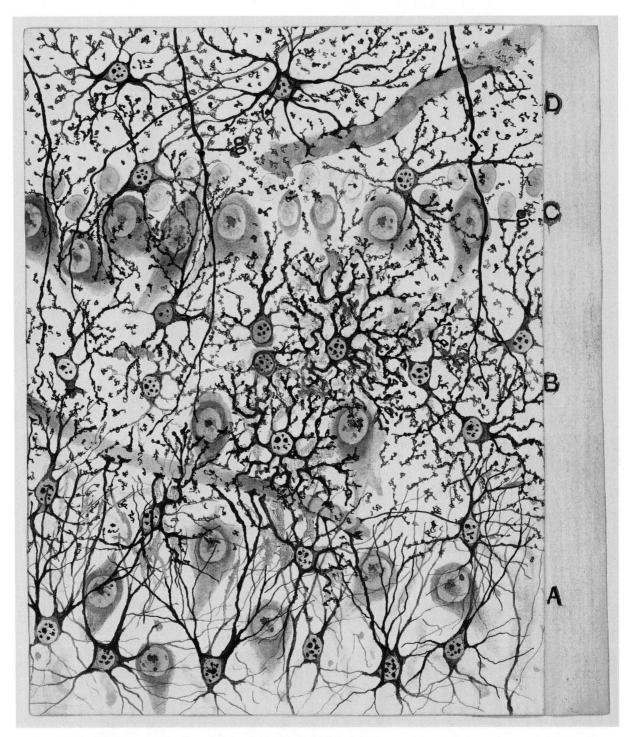

**FIGURE 85.** De Castro, 1920. Plexiform layer and mitral cells of the adult cat.

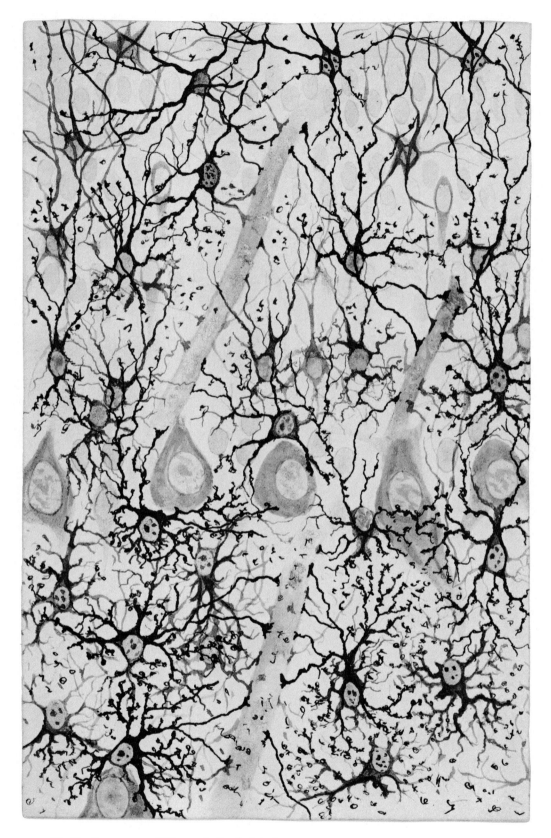

FIGURE 86. De Castro, 1920. Olfactory bulb of adult dog.

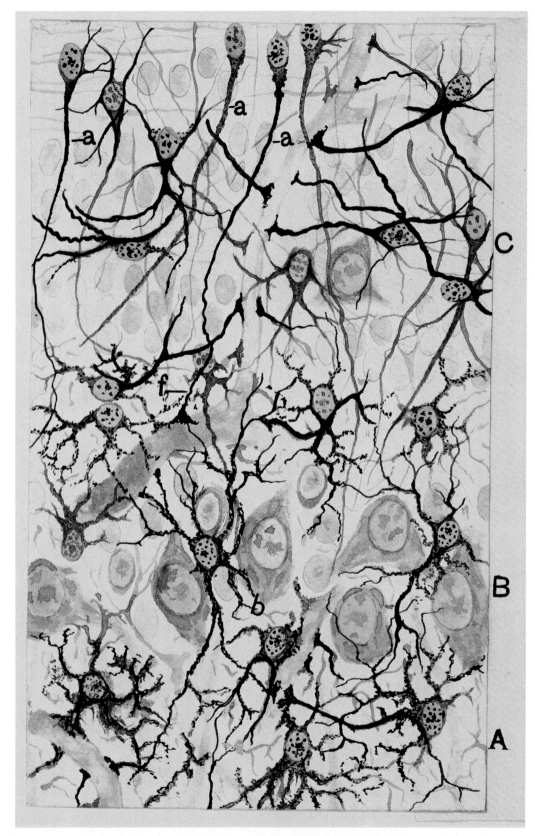

**FIGURE 87.** De Castro, 1920. Structure of neuroglia in the human cerebral cortex.

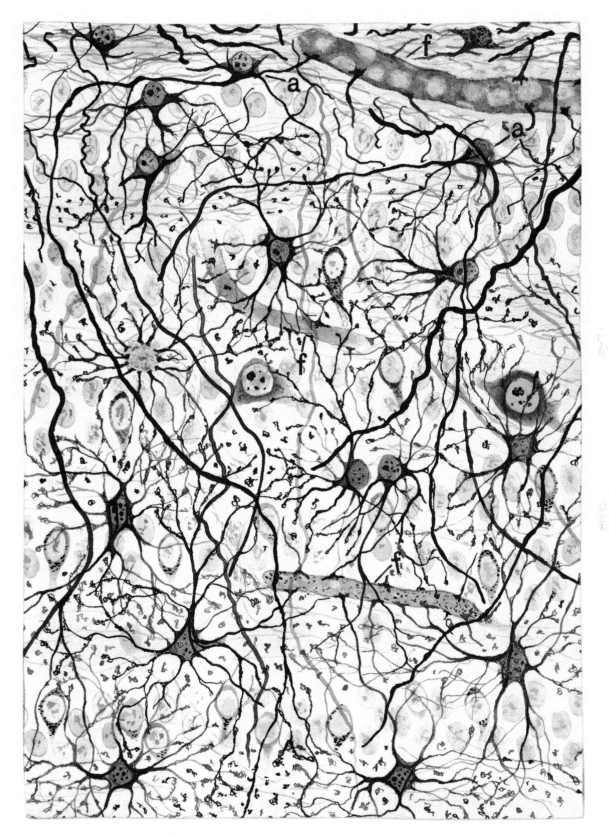

**FIGURE 88.** De Castro, 1920. Olfactory bulb of the cat.

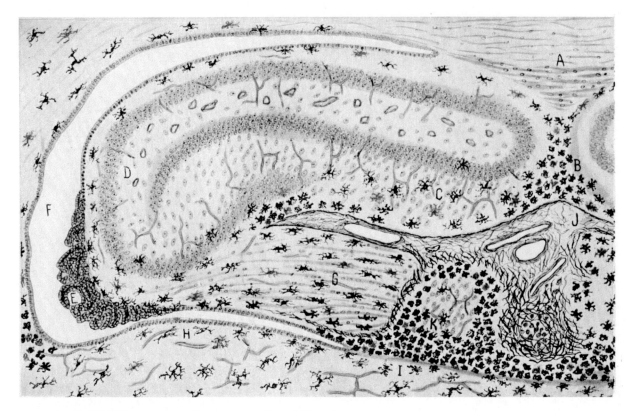

**FIGURE 89.** Del Río-Hortega, 1921. Cross-section of the rabbit brain.

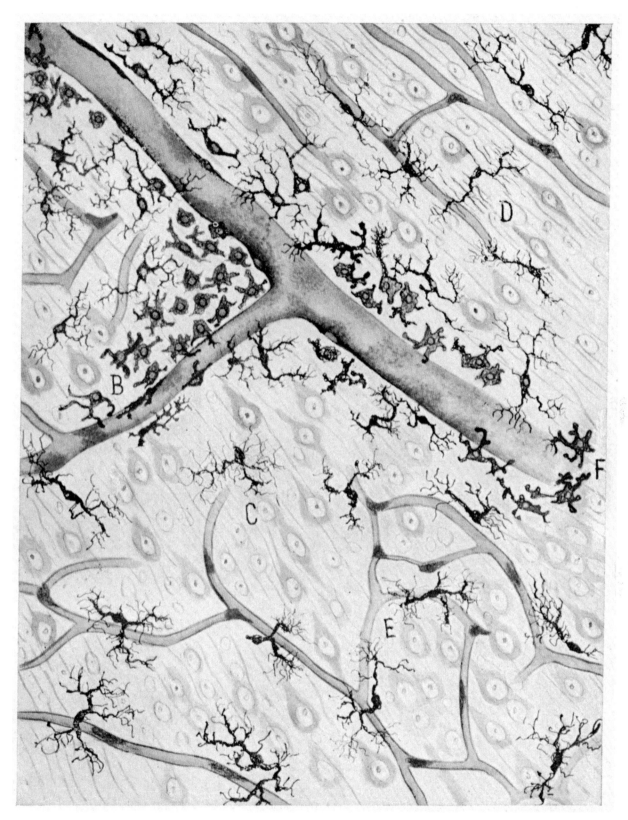

FIGURE 90. Del Río-Hortega, 1921. Perivascular microglia.

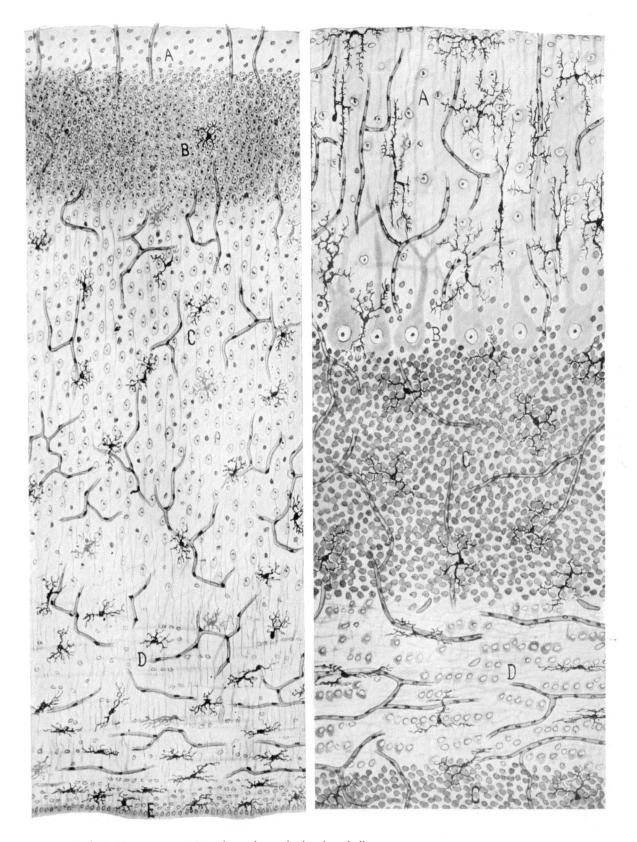

**FIGURE 91.** Del Río-Hortega, 1921. Microglia in the cerebral and cerebellar cortex.

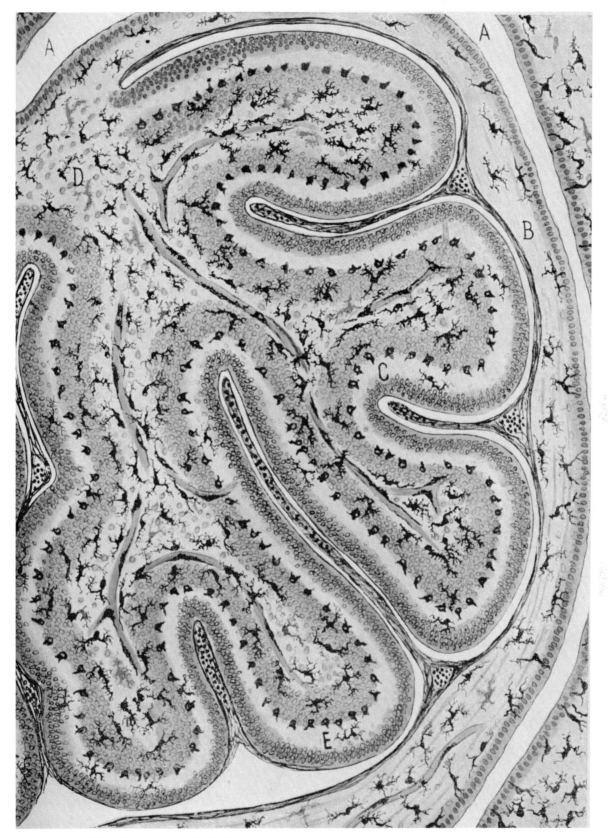

FIGURE 92. Del Río-Hortega, 1921. Cerebellar microglia.

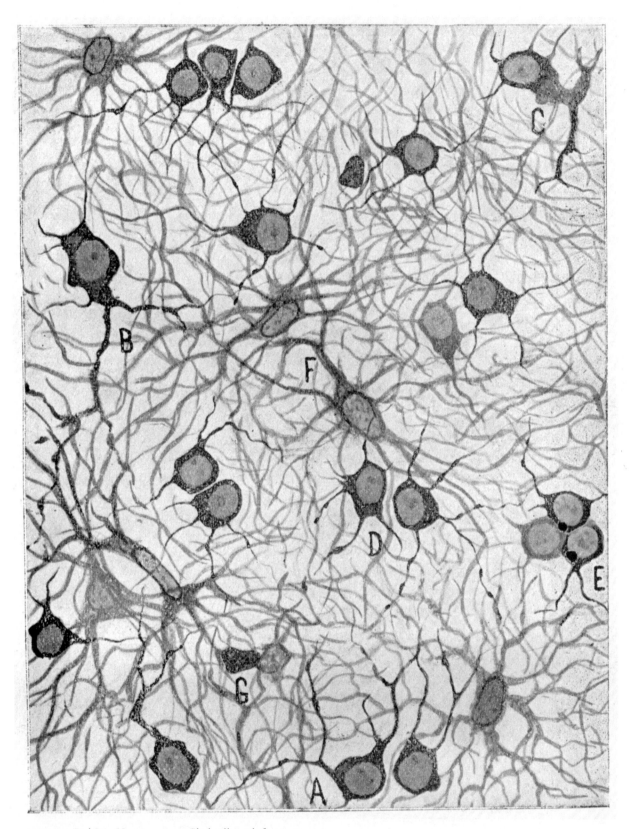

**FIGURE 93.** Del Río-Hortega, 1921. Glial cells with few processes.

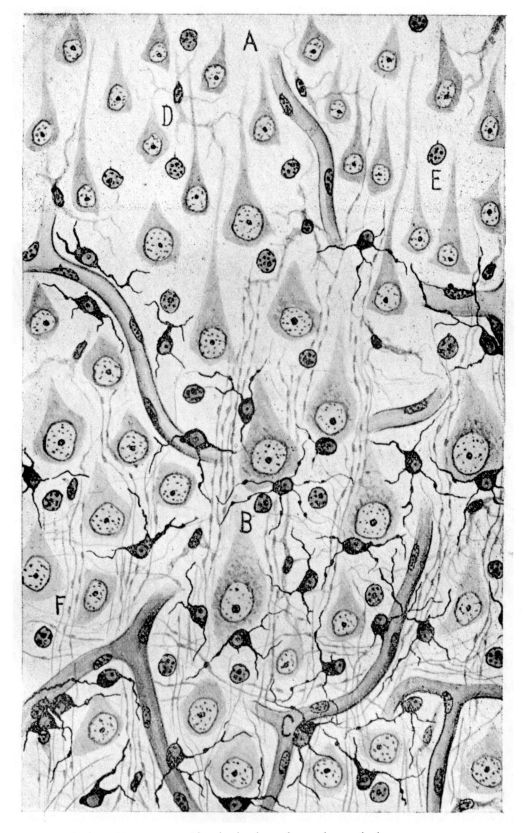

**FIGURE 94.** Del Río-Hortega, 1921. Oligodendroglia in the monkey cerebral cortex.

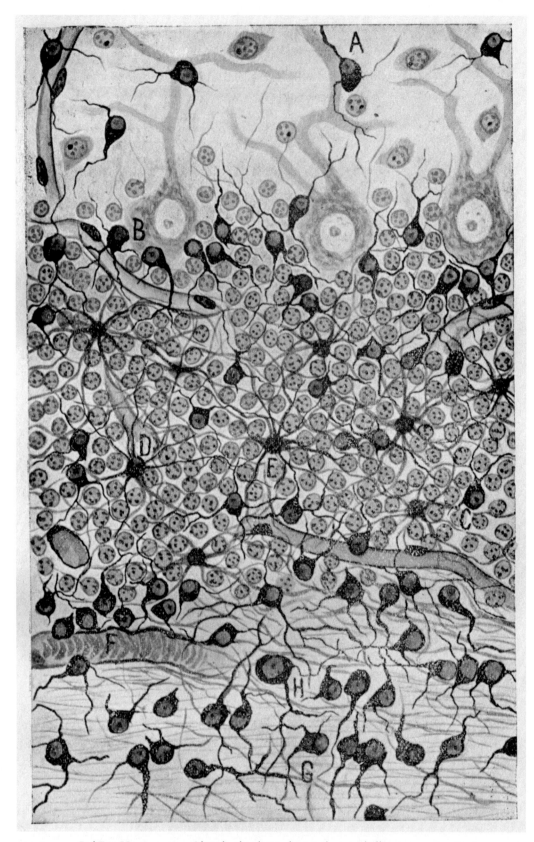

**FIGURE 95.** Del Río-Hortega, 1921. Oligodendroglia in the monkey cerebellar cortex.

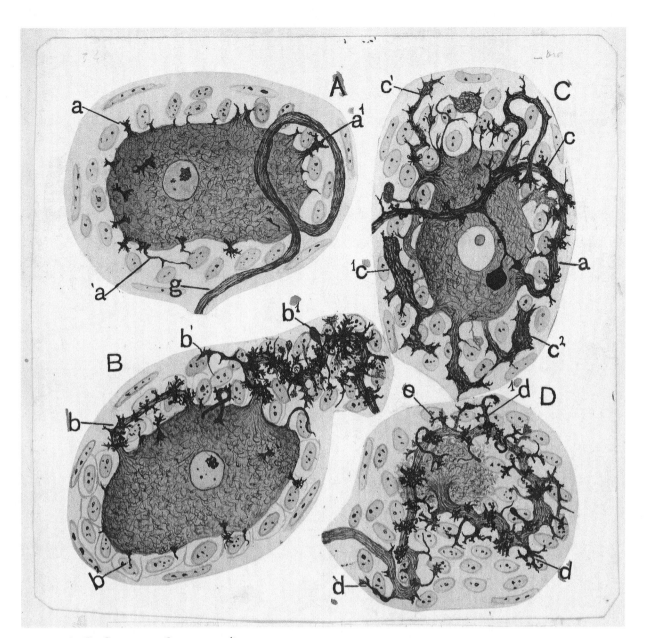

**FIGURE 96.** De Castro, 1921. Sensory ganglion neurons.

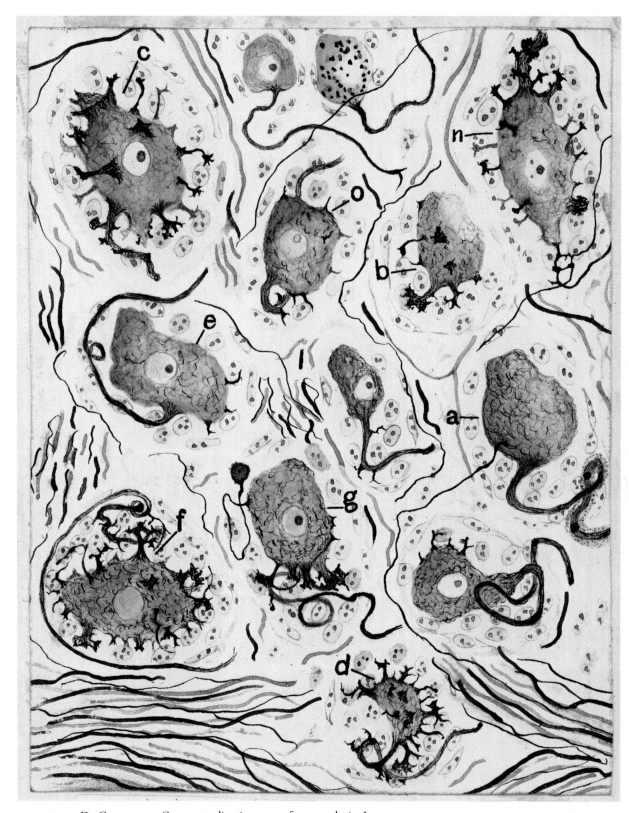

**FIGURE 97.** De Castro, 1921. Gasser ganglion in a case of osteomalacia, I.

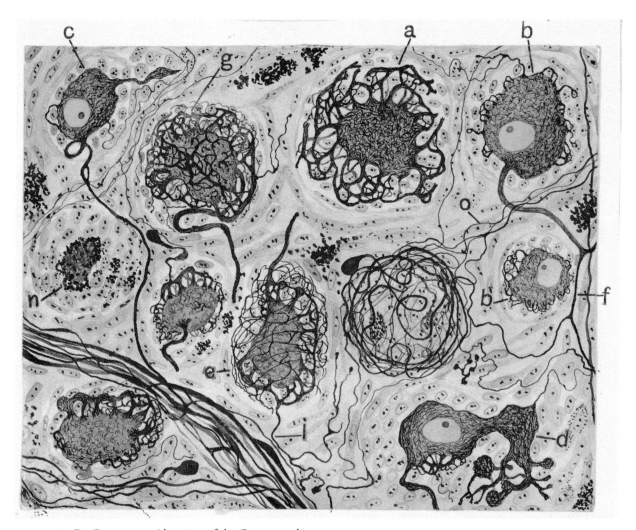

**FIGURE 98.** De Castro, 1921. Alteration of the Gasser ganglion.

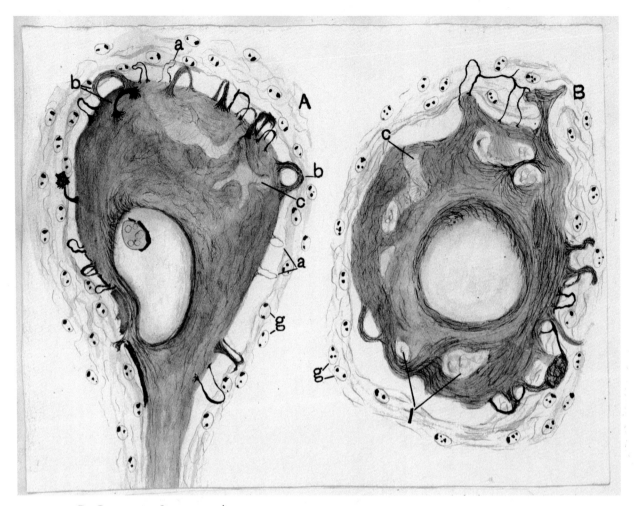

**FIGURE 99.** De Castro, 1921. Sensory ganglion neurons.

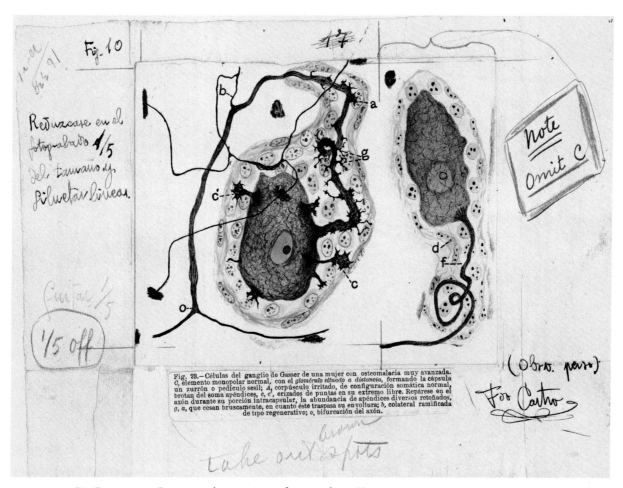

Fig-10
17
b
a
g
c'
c
o
d
f
Note
Omit C
Reduzcase en el fotograbado 1/5 del tamaño y siluetar líneas.
1/5 off
(Obra. paso)
For Castro
take out spots
Fig. 23.—Células del ganglio de Gasser de una mujer con osteomalacia muy avanzada. C, elemento monopolar normal, con el *glomérulo situado a distancia*, formando la cápsula un zurrón o pedículo sesil; A, corpúsculo irritado, de configuración somática normal, brotan del soma apéndices, c, c', erizados de puntas en su extremo libre. Repárese en el axón durante su porción intracapsular, la abundancia de apéndices diversos retoñados, g, a, que cesan bruscamente, en cuanto éste traspasa su envoltura; b, colateral ramificada de tipo regenerativo; o, bifurcación del axón.


FIGURE 100. De Castro, 1921. Gasser ganglion in a case of osteomalacia, II.

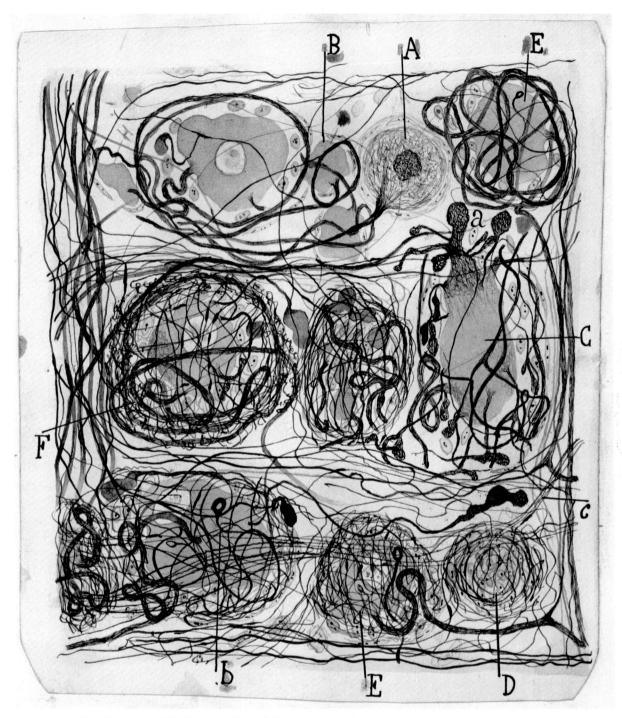

FIGURE 101. De Castro, 1921. Plexiform ganglion of the vagus nerve, I.

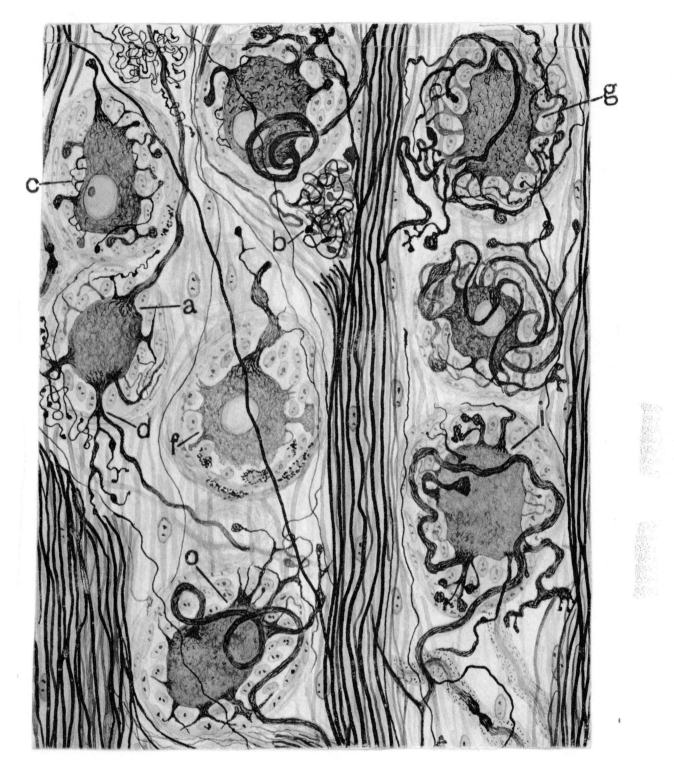

**FIGURE 102.** De Castro, 1921. Plexiform ganglion of the vagus nerve, II.

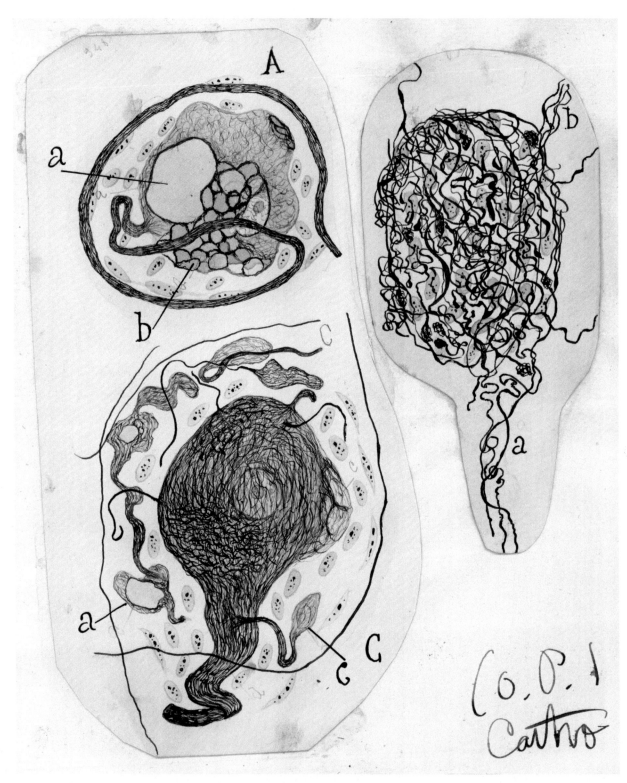

**FIGURE 103.** De Castro, 1921. Changes of sensory ganglion cells.

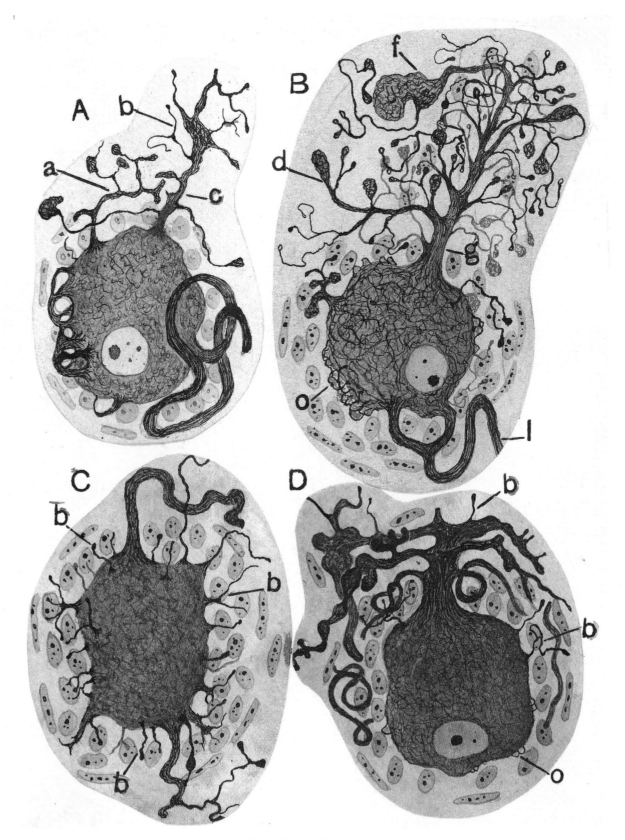

**FIGURE 104.** De Castro, 1921. Sensory ganglion cells: multipolar elements.

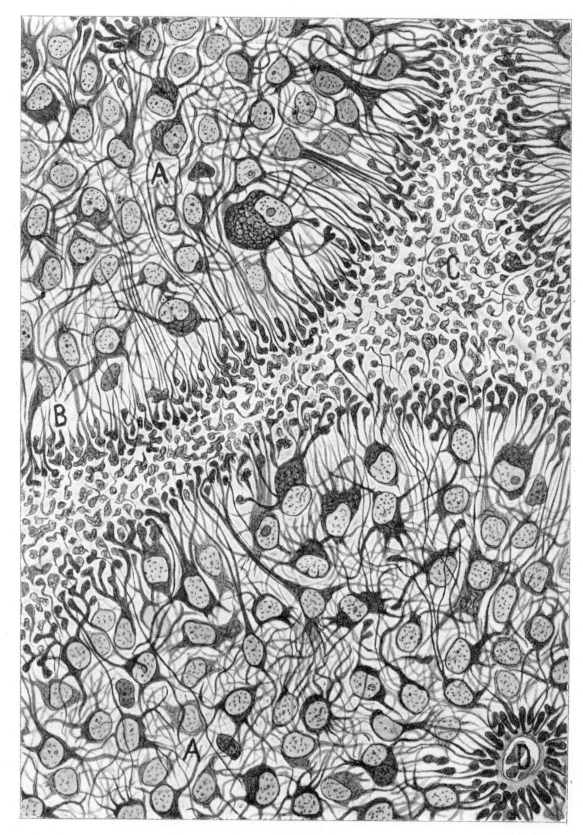

**FIGURE 105.** Del Río-Hortega, 1922. Structure of the pineal gland, I.

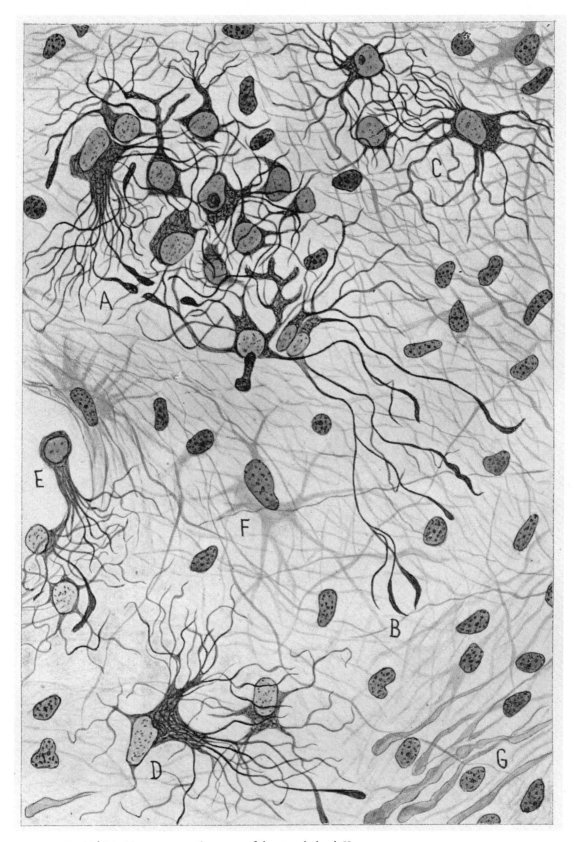

FIGURE 106. Del Río-Hortega, 1922. Structure of the pineal gland, II.

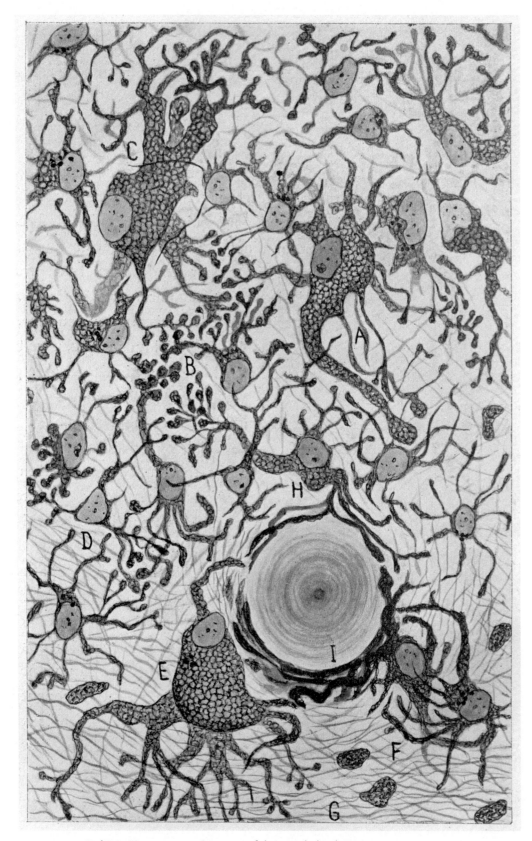

**FIGURE 107.** Del Río-Hortega, 1922. Structure of the pineal gland, III.

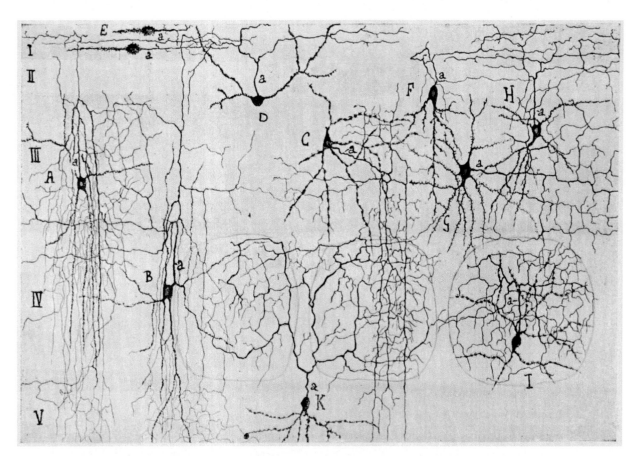

**FIGURE 108.** Lorente de Nó, 1922. Mouse cortical interneurons.

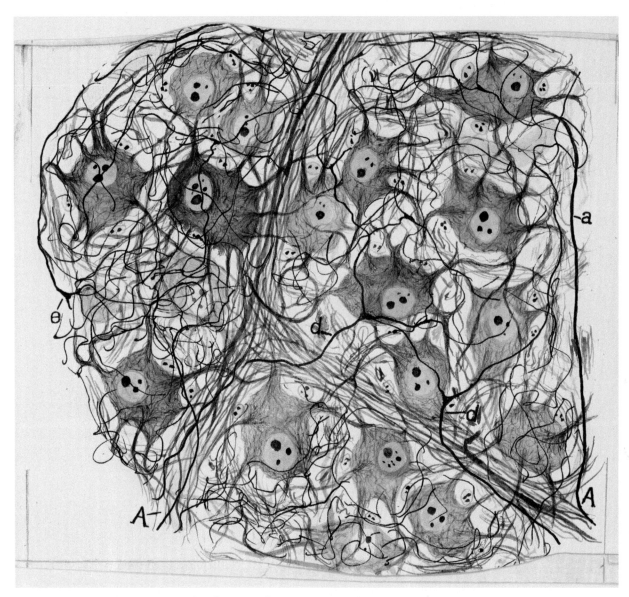

**FIGURE 109.** De Castro, 1922–1923. Semilunar ganglion.

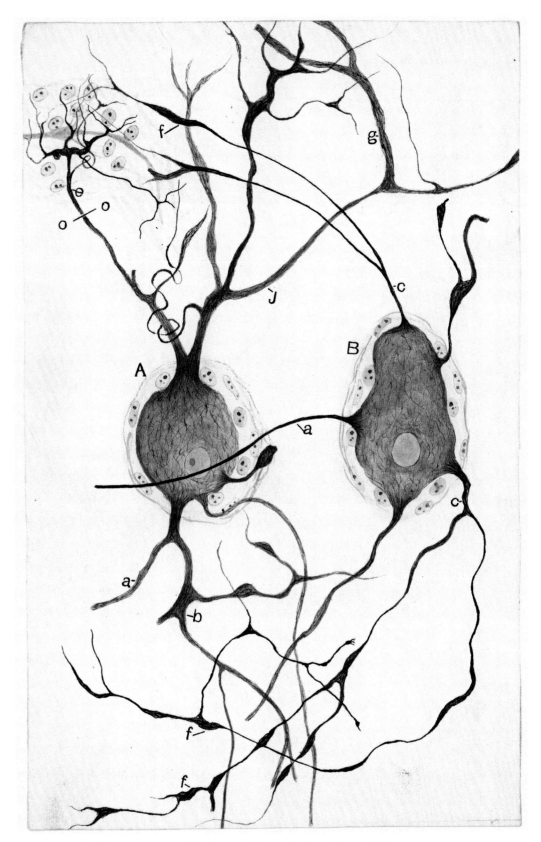

**FIGURE 110.** De Castro, 1922–1923. Human superior cervical ganglion cells, I.

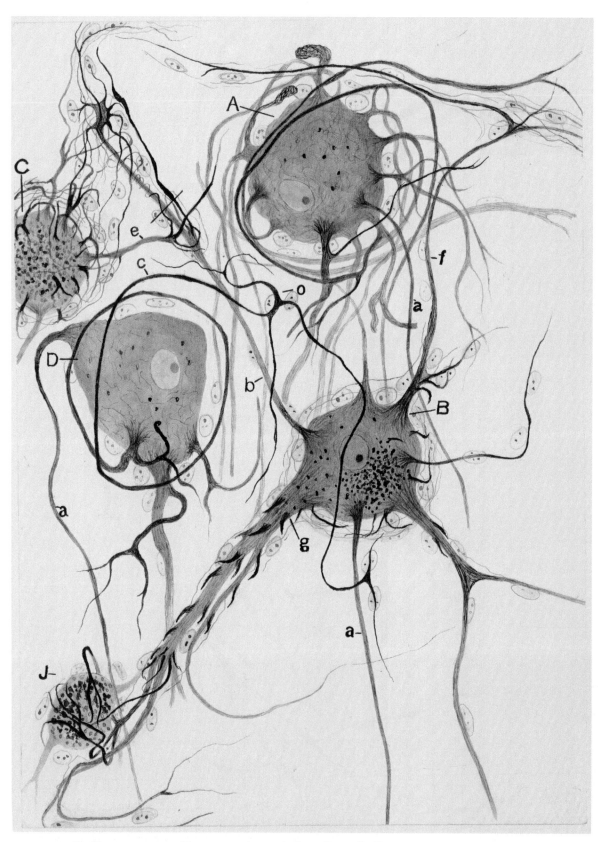

**FIGURE III.** De Castro, 1922–1923. Human superior cervical ganglion cells, II.

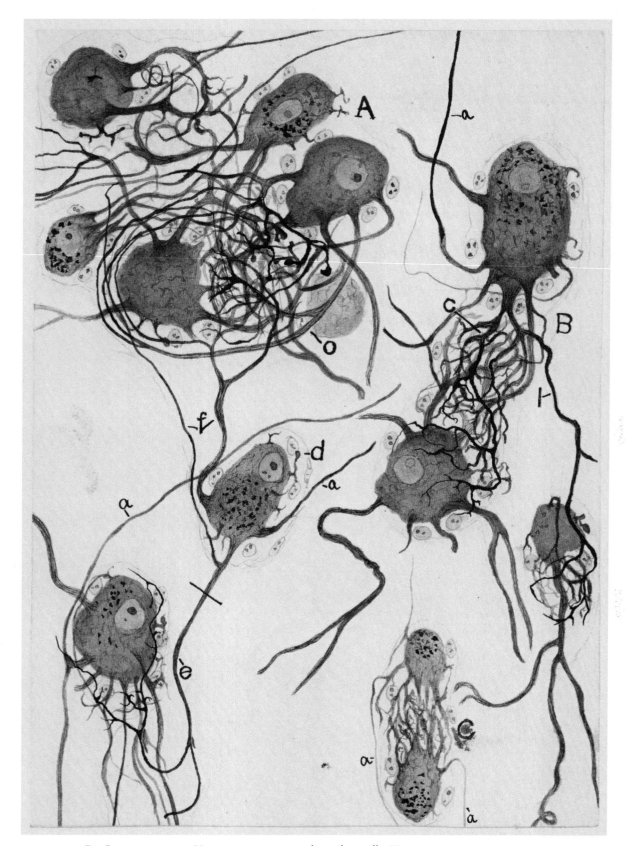

**FIGURE 112.** De Castro, 1922–1923. Human superior cervical ganglion cells, III.

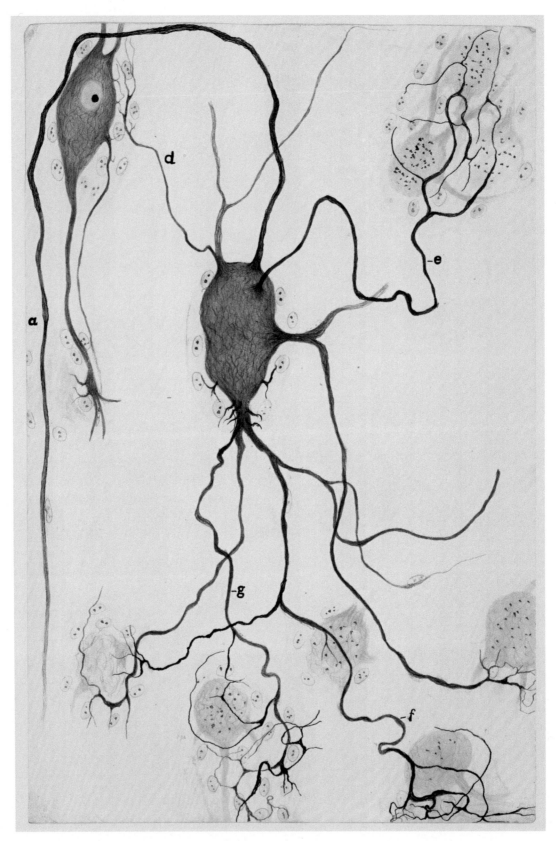

**FIGURE 113.** De Castro, 1922–1923. Human lumbar ganglion, I.

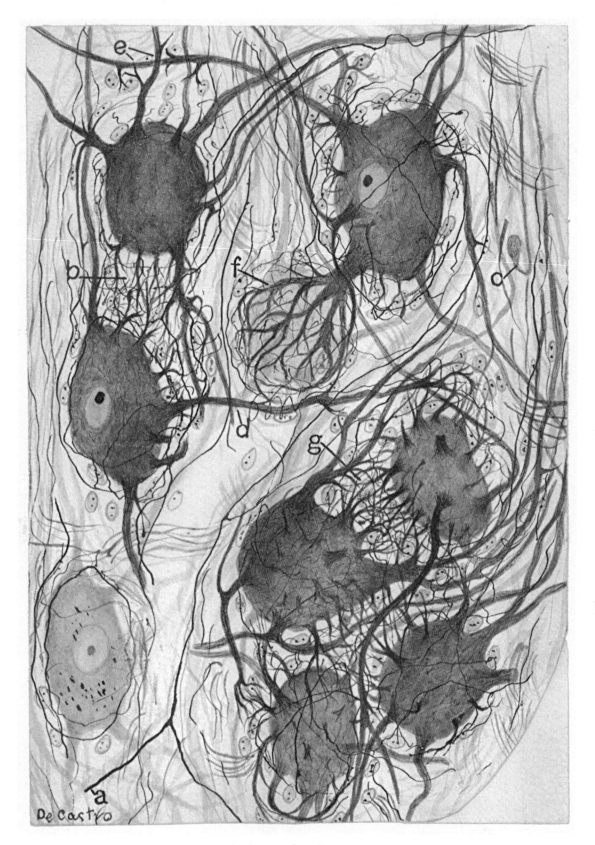

**FIGURE 114.** De Castro, 1922–1923. Human lumbar ganglion, II.

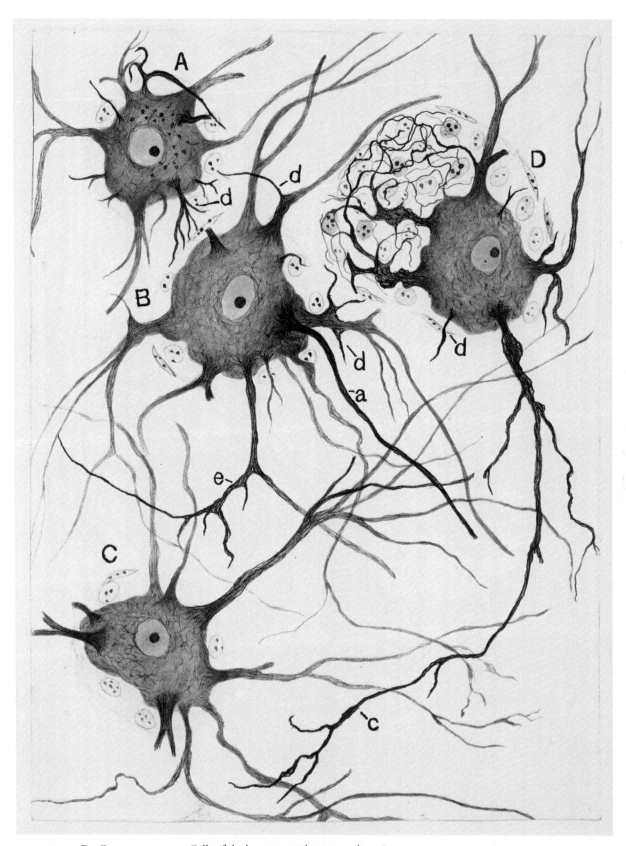

**FIGURE 115.** De Castro, 1922–1923. Cells of the human semilunar ganglion, I.

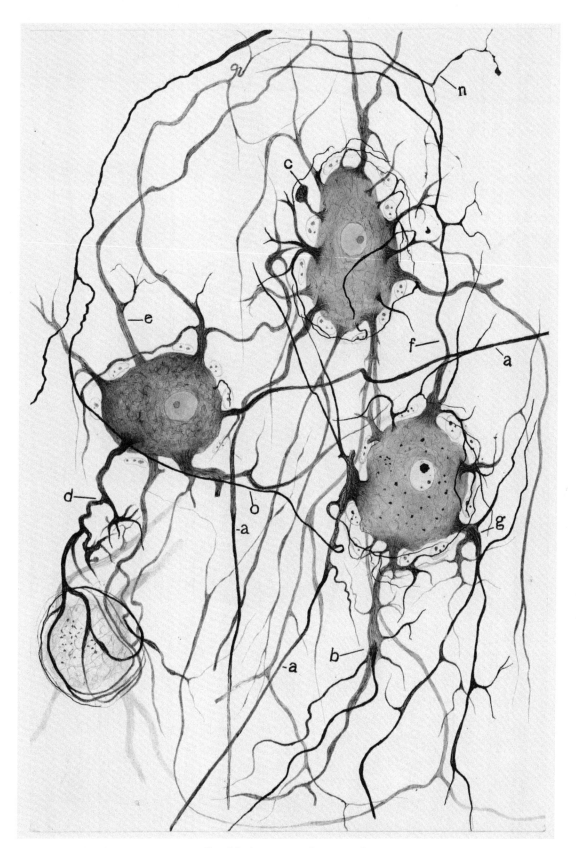

FIGURE 116. De Castro, 1922–1923. Cells of the human semilunar ganglion, II.

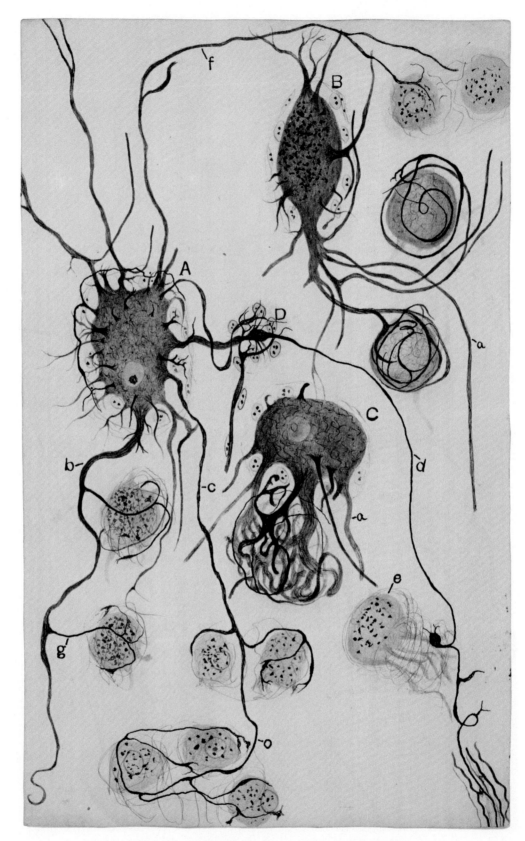

**FIGURE 117.** De Castro, 1922–1923. Cells of the human superior cervical ganglion.

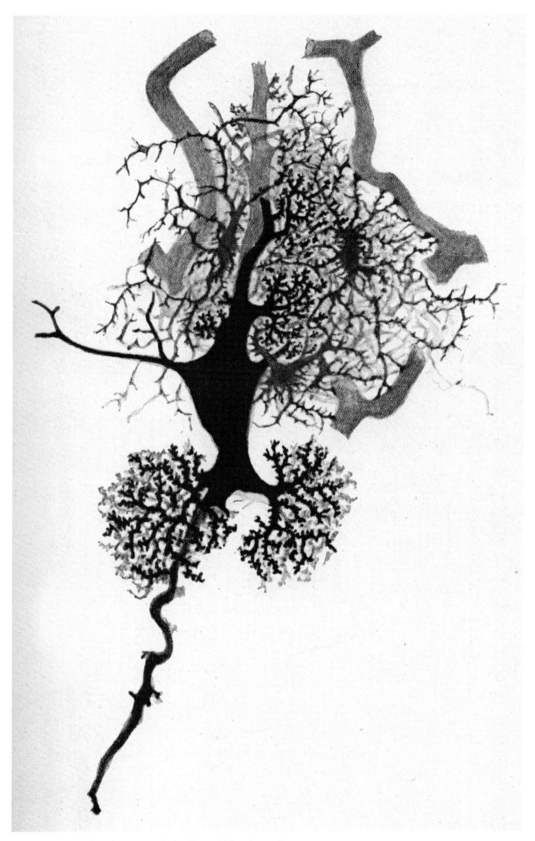

FIGURE 118. Berlucchi, 1923. Glial cells and blood vessels.

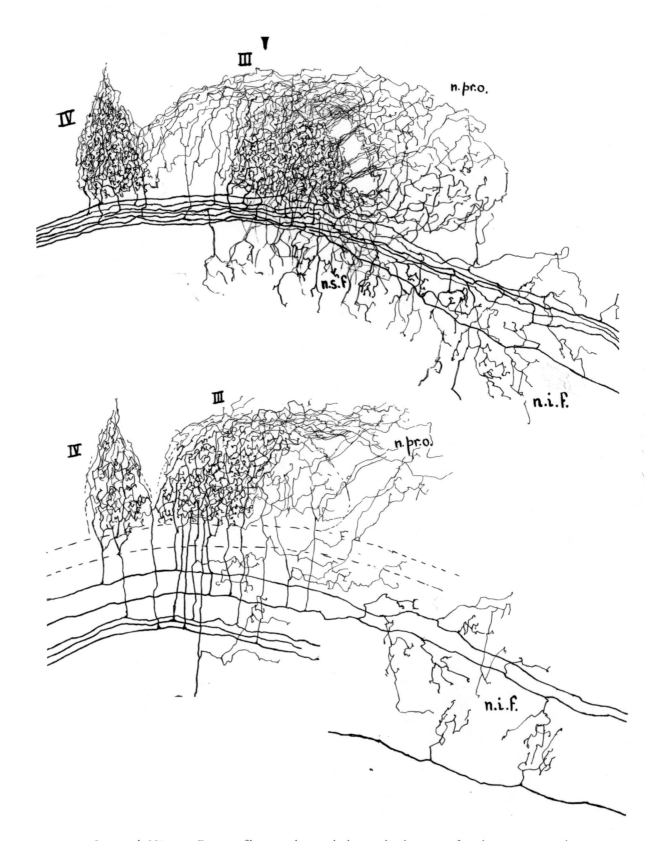

**FIGURE 119.** Lorente de Nó, 1924. Extrinsic fibers traveling in the longitudinal posterior fascicle to acoustic nuclei.

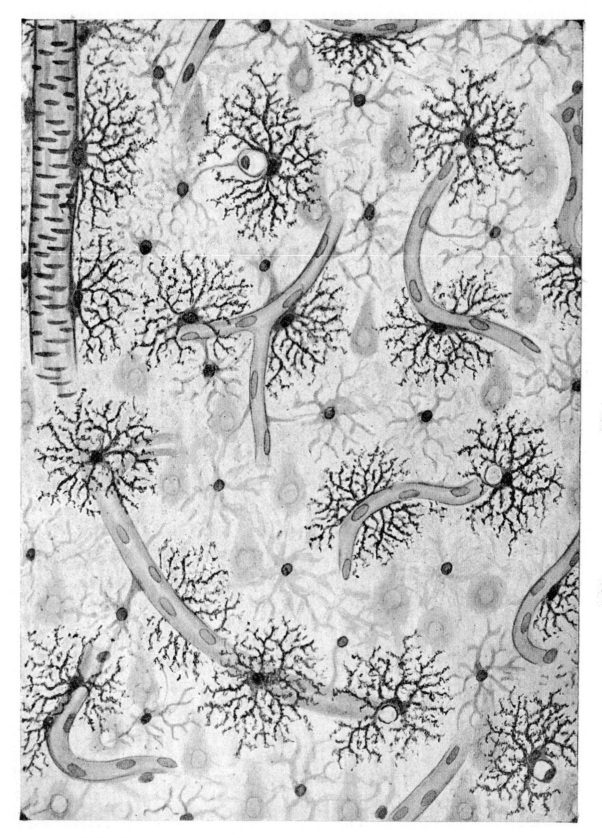

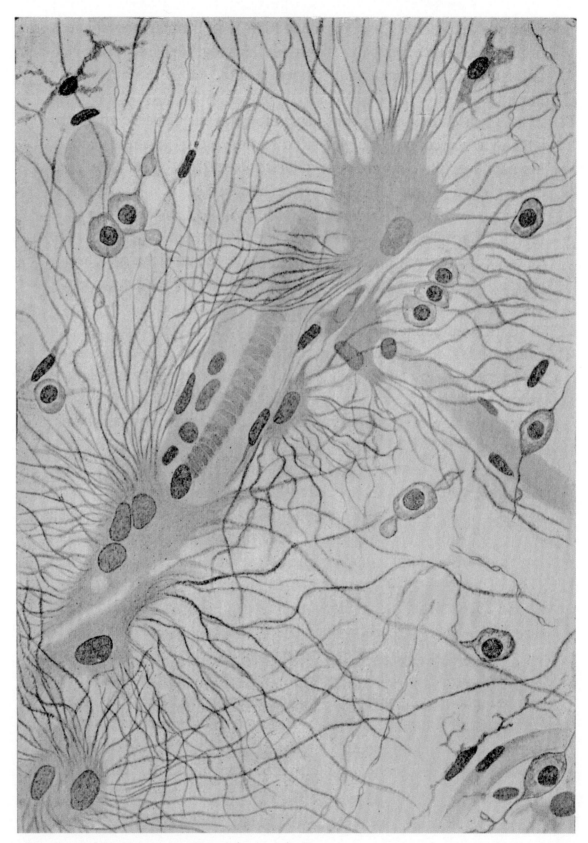

**FIGURE 121.** Del Río-Hortega, 1925. Perivascular neuroglia, II.

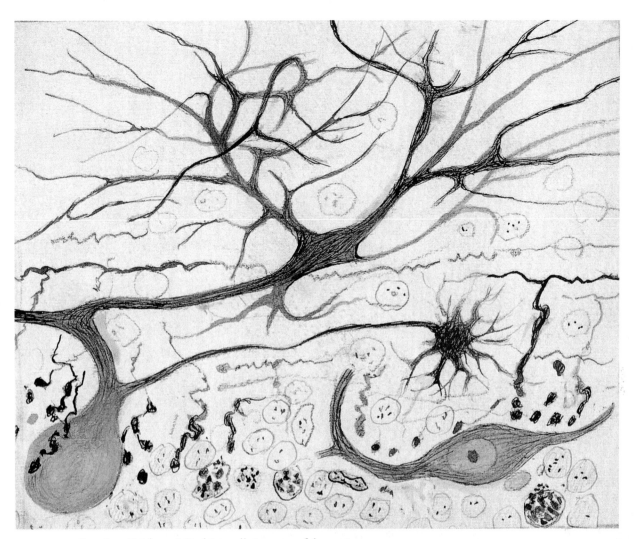

FIGURE 122. Ramón y Cajal, 1926. Purkinje cells in a case of dementia precox.

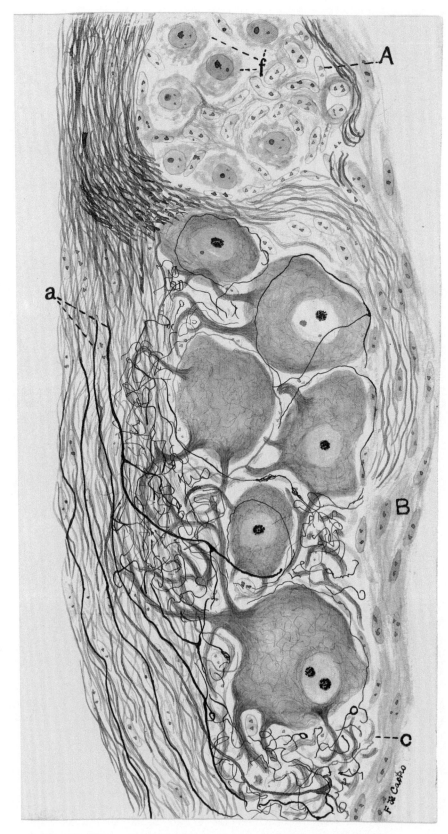

**FIGURE 123.** De Castro, 1926. Structure and innervation of the carotid body, I.

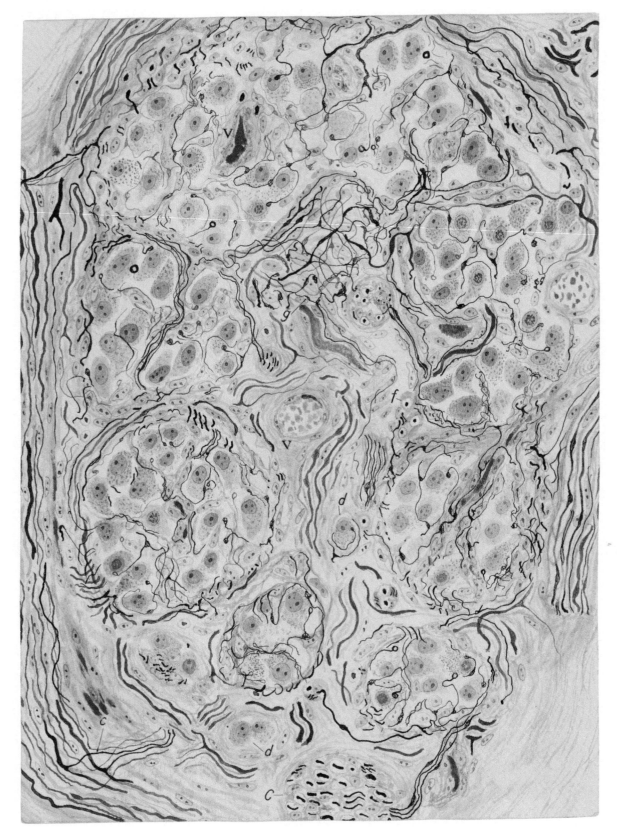

**FIGURE 124.** De Castro, 1926. Structure and innervation of the carotid body, II.

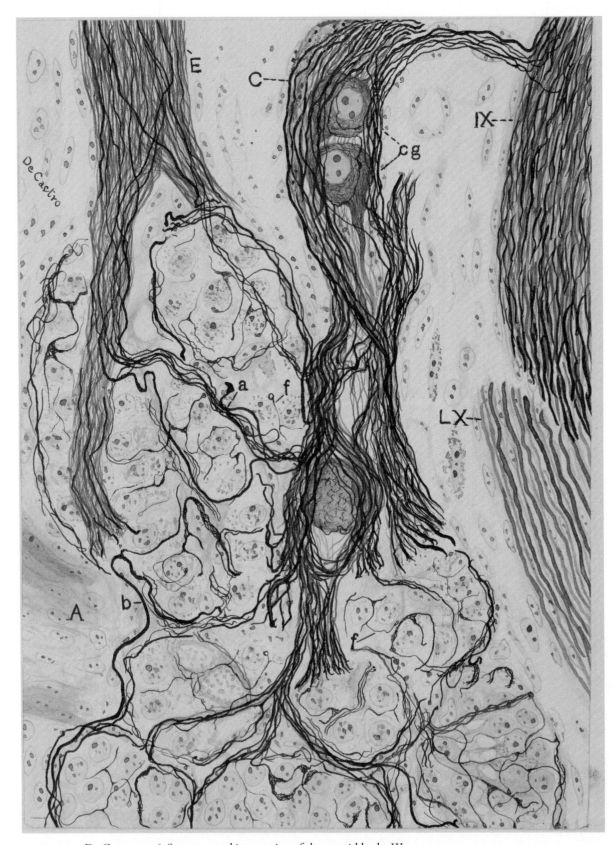

**FIGURE 125.** De Castro, 1926. Structure and innervation of the carotid body, III.

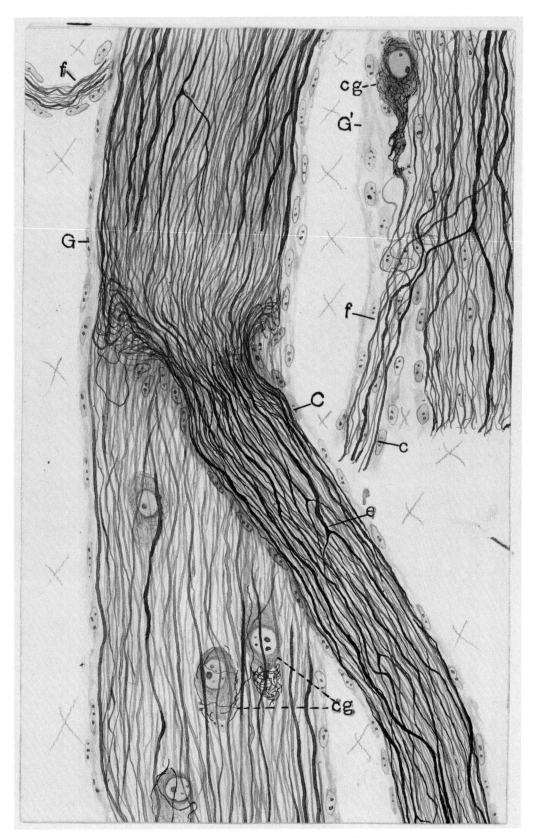

**FIGURE 126.** De Castro, 1926. Structure and innervation of the carotid body, IV.

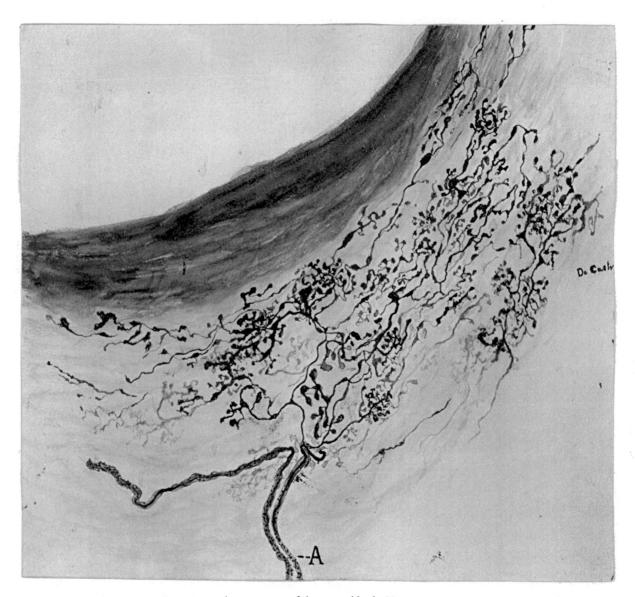

**FIGURE 127.** De Castro, 1926. Structure and innervation of the carotid body, V.

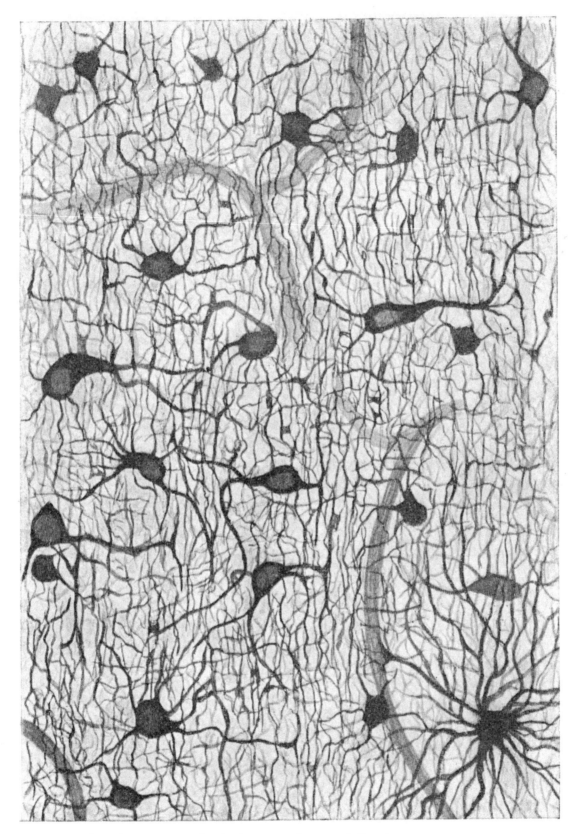

FIGURE 128. Del Río-Hortega, 1928. Oligodendrocytes in the cat cerebellar white matter.

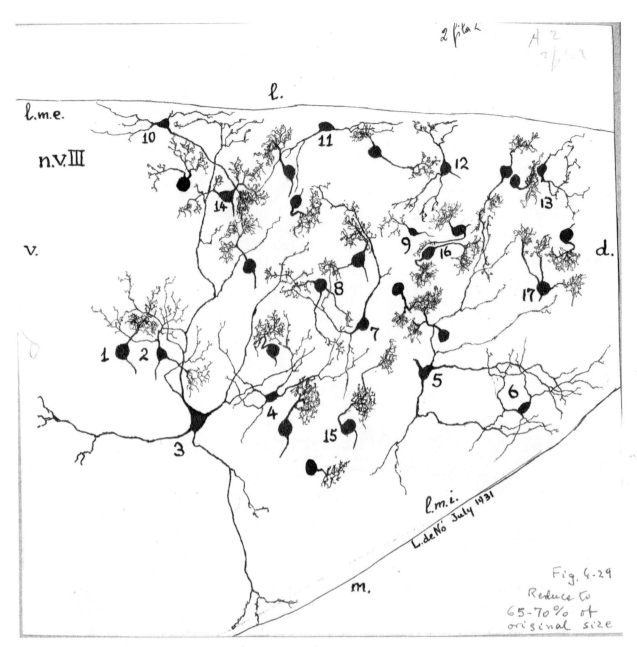

**FIGURE 133.** Lorente de Nó, 1931. Neurons in the acoustic nucleus.

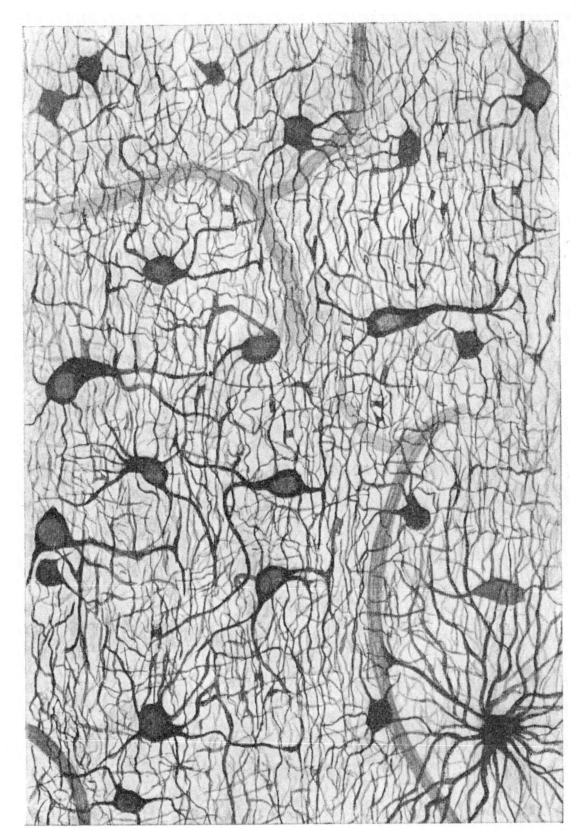

FIGURE 128. Del Río-Hortega, 1928. Oligodendrocytes in the cat cerebellar white matter.

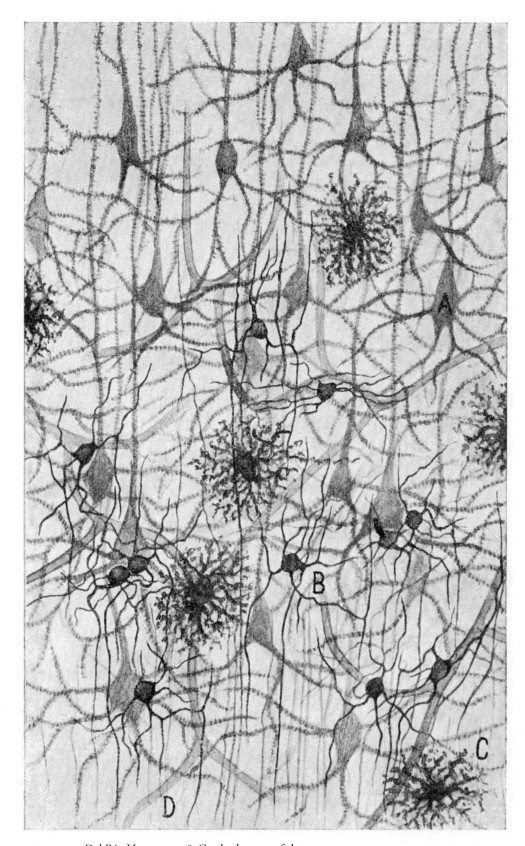

**FIGURE 129.** Del Río-Hortega, 1928. Cerebral cortex of the cat.

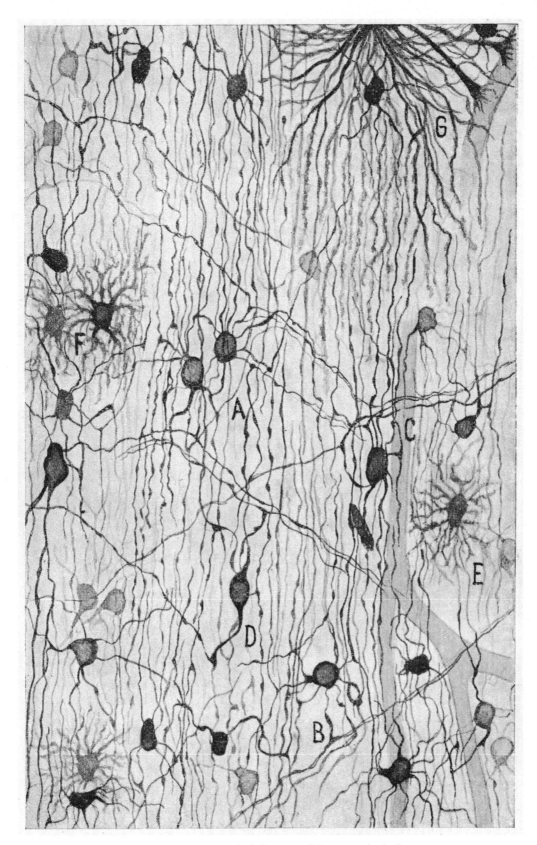

**FIGURE 130.** Del Río-Hortega, 1928. Neuroglial elements of the cat cerebral white matter.

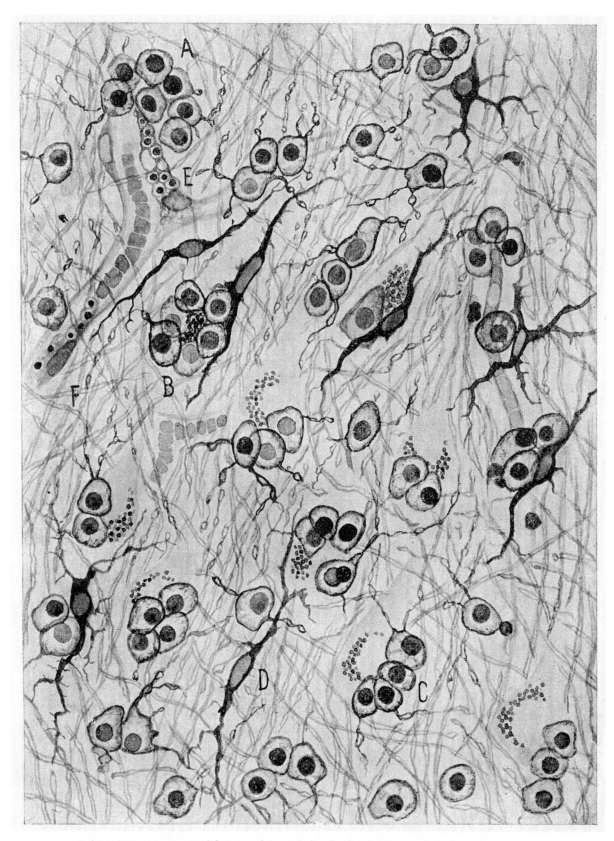

**FIGURE 131.** Del Río-Hortega, 1928. Proliferation of cortical oligodendrocytes in paralytic dementia.

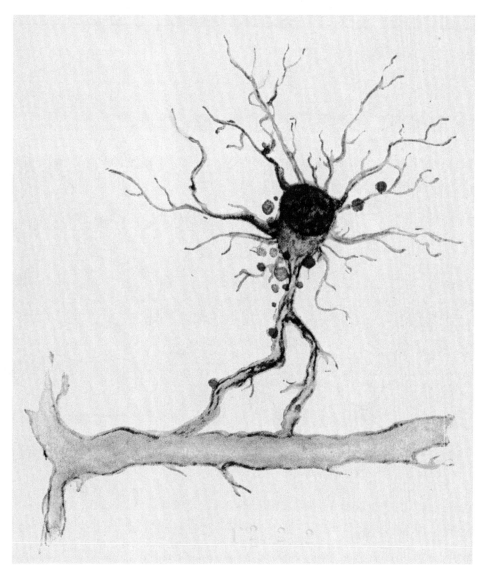

**FIGURE 132.** Berlucchi, 1930. Glial cell of the human white matter.

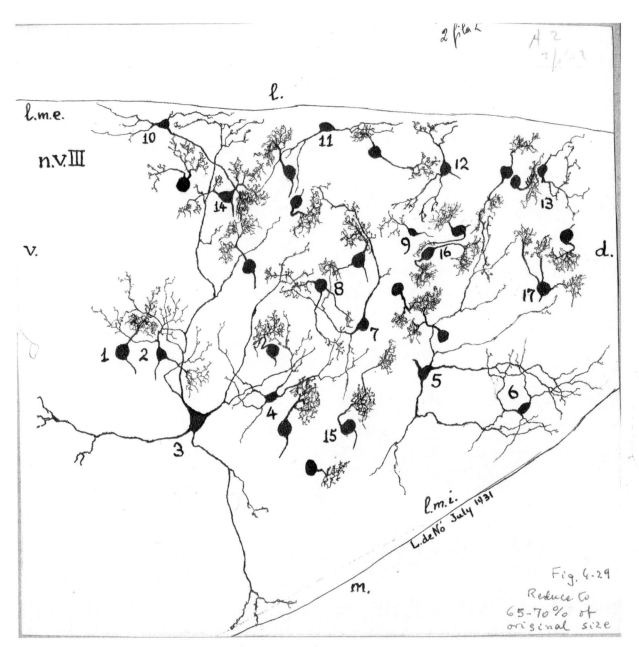

**FIGURE 133.** Lorente de Nó, 1931. Neurons in the acoustic nucleus.

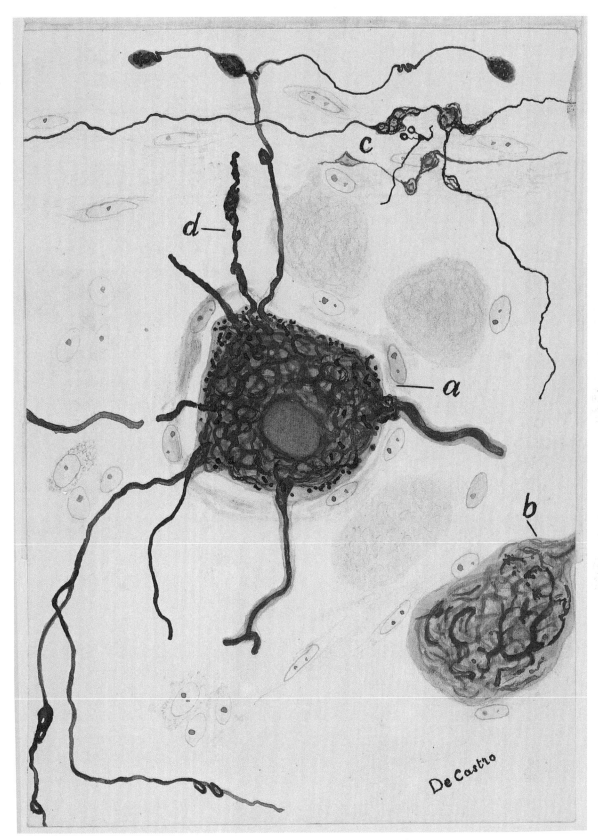

**FIGURE 134.** De Castro, 1932–1933. Section of a sympathetic ganglion.

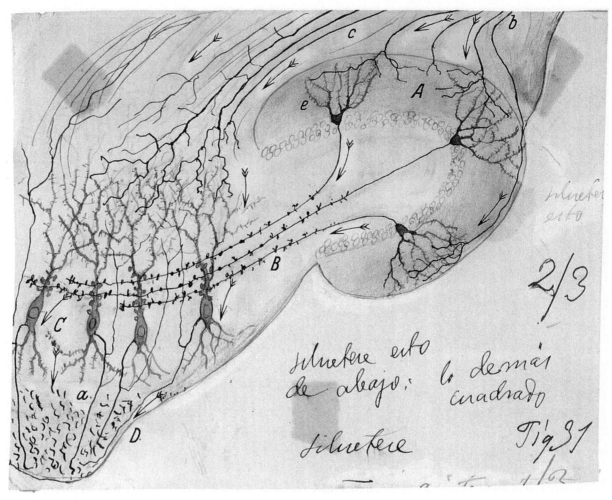

FIGURE 135. Ramón y Cajal, 1933. Diagram of the connections of the hippocampus.

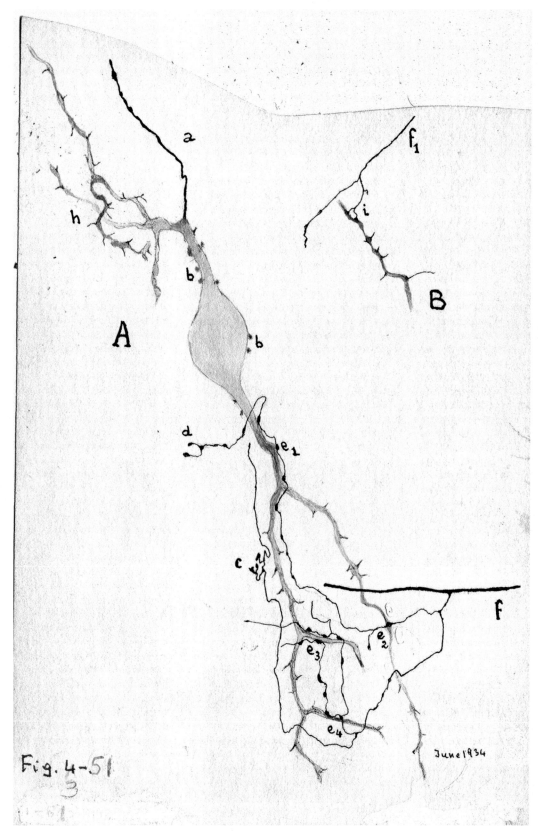

**FIGURE 136.** Lorente de Nó, 1934. Efferent neuron in the ventral acoustic nucleus.

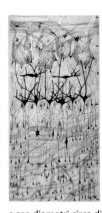

**FIGURE 13.**

Golgi, 1875. Olfactory bulb of a dog.

I singoli elementi riprodotti in questa tavola, vennero punto per punto con, esattezza scrupolosa disegnati coll' aiuto della camera chiara di Oberhauser. Il disegno rappresenta, semischematicamente, a 250 diametri circa di ingrandimento, un frammento di sezione verticale di un bulbo olfattorio di un cane. I tre diversi strati dell' organo sono indicati colle lettere A B C poste a lato. A, indica lo strato superficiale del bulbo, o strato delle fibre nervose periferiche. Esso vedesi essenzialmente costituito dai fasci di fibre nervose provenienti dalla mucosa olfattoria. Questi fasci, fra loro incrociandosi, si dirigono verso i glomeruli olfattori, entro i quali penetrano (in a a a), e si suddividono finamente. In mezzo agli stessi fasci si scorge anche un vaso sanguigno, che invia verticalmente verso l'interno dell' organo varie diramazioni. B, indica lo strato medio, o strato di sostanza grigia. Al confine periferico di questo stanno i glomeruli olfattori; al confine interno trovansi invece le grandi cellule nervose, disposte in regolare serie. Il prolungamento essenzialmente nervoso (b b b) (prolungamento-cilinder-axis) di queste ultime cellule, appare, con regola invariabile, verticalmente diretto verso gli strati interni del bulbo; i prolungamenti protoplasmatici (b' b' b') si portano invece verso i glomeruli nei quali penetrano e si ramificano complicatamente. Quest' ultimo andamento nel disegno vedesi riprodotto soltanto per uno dei prolungamenti (b"). Verso il mezzo di questo medesimo strato B vennero disegnate anche due grandi cellule nervose solitarie fusiformi, il cui prolungamento nervoso, colorato in azzurro, scende, ramificandosi, nello strato delle fibre nervose. All' ingiro dei glomeruli veggonsi alcune cellule nervose piccole. Di queste i prolungamenti rivolti verso i glomeruli hanno i caratteri dei protoplasmatici, mentre l' unico prolungamento che emana nell' opposta direzione (quello colorito in azzurro) ha i caratteri dei prolungamenti nervosi. C, finalmente indica lo strato interno o delle fibre nervose provenienti dal tractus. Nei vani lasciati dagli incrociantisi fasci stanno i piccoli elementi di forma prevalentemente piramidale, e di natura probabilmente nervosa. Nel mezzo dello strato veggonsi anche qui due cellule ben caratterizzate come nervose, sia per la forma e grandezza loro, sia per la presenza di

un prolungamento appartenente evidentemente al tipo dei nervosi (quello colorito in azzurro). Le fibrille risultanti dalle suddivisioni di questo prolungamento s' uniscono ai fasci provenienti dal tractus. Le complicate ramificazioni delle fibre nervose vennero omesse nel disegno, perchè non risultasse troppo complicato; il modo di decorrere e di ramificarsi delle medesime fibre per altro, può essere con approssimazione rilevato verso la periferia dello strato C. Ivi alcune di tali fibre staccansi dai fasci, e ramificandosi complicatamente oltrepassano con decorso tortuoso il confine della sostanza bianca, penetrano nello strato grigio, che parimenti atraversano, e molte di esse, ridotte a fibrille finissime, si ponno accompagnare fin entro i glomeroli. Lo stroma di cellule connettive venne riprodotto in modo possibilmente vicino al vero, per la quantità e pei suoi rapporti coi vasi, soltanto nelle parti profonde dello strato C, ove di fatto le cellule connettive raggiate sogliono essere assai numerose. Riguardo alle altre parti lo si vede soltanto accennato nella zona di confine tra la sostanza bianca e la grigia, nei glomeruli e nello strato delle fibre nervose periferiche. (Veggansi le parti del disegno colorate in rosso). [A, B, C have been added in the figure by author.] Golgi, C. (1875) Sulla fina struttura del bulbi olfattorii. Reggio-Emilia: Printer Stefano Calderini [Plate 7].

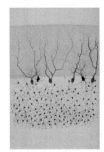

**FIGURE 14.**

Golgi, 1882. Cerebellum of a rabbit.

*Frammento di sezione verticale di una circonvoluzione cerebellare del coniglio.* Disegno fatto a particolare illustrazione dello *strato dei granuli.* Questi cosi detti granuli si presentano quali cellule nervose di forma globosa, piccolissime e fornite di 3, 4, 5 ed anche 6 prolungamenti, dei quali sempre uno solo offre i caratteri di prolungamento nervoso; siffatto prolungamento trovasi appena accennato (filo rosso). I prolungamenti, che pare si possano chiamare protoplasmatici, sebbene si presentino in modo un po' diverso dai prolungamenti protoplasmatici delle altre cellule gangliari, finiscono con un piccolo ammasso granuloso, al quale spesso veggonsi confluire le estremità dei corrispondenti prolungamenti dei circostanti granuli. Nella zona di passaggio tra lo strato molecolare e lo strato dei granuli sono pur disegnate altre due cellule, che dalle cellule di Purkinje, a lato delle quali sono poste, si differenziano oltrechè per la forma del corpo cellulare

e modo di ramificarsi dei prolungamenti protoplasmatici, anche, e soprattutto, pel contegno affatto diverso del prolungamento nervoso. Queste due cellule appartengono al tipo che già trovasi illustrato nelle Tavole XIV e XVII. Golgi, C. (1882–1883) Sulla fina anatomia degli organi centrali del sistema nervoso. *Riv. Sper. Freniat. Med. Leg.* Reprinted in *Opera Omnia*, vol I. *Istologia Normale*, Chapter 16. Milano: Ulrico Hoepli, 1903 [Plate 19].

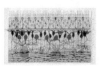

**FIGURE 15.**

Tartuferi, 1887. Structure of the retina.

Questa tavola serve a rappresentare l'immagine di una sezione verticale di retina *senza il suo apparato* di sostegno. 1 singoli elementi furono ad uno ad uno esattamente disegnati col prisma-carta del disegno all'altezza del piede del microscopio Hartnack, modello VIII, tubo chiuso, oc: 3, oggetto 9, immersione. Per chiarezza non furono designati che pochi elementi retinici, poichè altrimenti, essendo questi stipatissimi la figura sarebbe divenuta indecifrabile. Per la stessa ragione non furono designate le cellule le più superficiali del primo strato cerebrale *(cellule stellate).* Per la complicata tiratura della tavola non furono potute fare alcune piccole correzioni ; così alcune fibre dei bastoncini, come la prima a destra, sono state fatte dal litografo una piccola cosa troppo grosse; alcune fibrille terminali dei pennacchi sono state fatte un poco sottili, ma trattasi di piccolissime ed insignificanti differenze. La grossezza esatta delle fibre dei bastoncini è quella delle ultime quattro fibre a destra, a questa grossezza corrisponde quella delle fibrille terminali dei pennacchi. *1° Strato nevroepiteliale.* Alcune fibre dei bastoncini si vedono (come tal volta appariscono), tronche e terminanti con una varicosità. *2° Porzione fibrillare del primo strato cerebrale (rete sottoepiteliale).* Se molto fibrille dei pennacchi terminano senza connettersi con le fibre dei bastoncini, ciò dipende dall'essere state designate, per chiarezza della figura, solo poche cellule visive a bastoncino. *3° Porzione cellulare del primo strato cerebrale.* In nero sono rappresentate le *cellule a pennacchio;* le cellule colorate adiacenti alla rete sottoepiteliale sono le *grosse cellule superficiali.* Le cellule colorate adiacenti allo strato reticolare interno sono gli *spongioblasti. 4° Strato reticolare interno.* - Vi si vedono i processi verticali delle grosse cellule superficiali, i processi interni delle cellule a pennacchio e la rete di fiocchetti da questi formata; i prolungamenti degli spongioblasti ed i processi protoplasmatici delle cellule nervose dei due tipi descritti nel testo. Il fiocchetto dell'ultima cellula pennacchio a destra è veduto un poco obliquamente. Fu scelto per mostrare con evidenza come si origina dal processo interno della cellula a pennacchio. 5° *Strato delle cellule nervose e delle fibre nervose.* Tartuferi, F. (1887) Sull' anatomia della retina. *Arch. Scienze Mediche* 11, 425–441 [Plate 19].

### FIGURE 16.

Fusari, 1887. Structure of the central nervous system of teleosts, I.

Verschiedene Typen von Nervenzellen in hundertmaliger Vergrösserung. 1–3. Zellen des Thalamus opticus und der Vorderlappen. 4–8. Zellen des Opticusdaches. 9–14. Zellen der granulösen Schicht des Kleinhirnes (Granuli). 15–17. Zellen der moleculären Schicht des Kleinhirnes. 18–19. Zellen der Valvula cerebelli. 20. Zelle des Rückenmarkes. Fusari, R. (1887) Untersuchungen über die feinere Anatomie des Gehirnes des Teleostier. *Internat. Mschr. Anat. Physiol.* 4, 275–300 [Plate 9].

### FIGURE 17.

Fusari, 1887. Structure of the central nervous system of teleosts, II.

Paralcentraler Sagittalschnitt des Kleinhirnes von *Carassius* (50 fache Vergrösserung). A. Kleinhirn: I. Corticale Schicht; 2. Grenzschicht; 3. Körnerschicht; 4. Schicht der Centralfasern. B. Valvula cerebelli. C. Dach des Lobus opticus. D. Verlängertes Mark. Fusari, R. (1887) Untersuchungen über die feinere Anatomie des Gehirnes des Teleostier. *Internat. Mschr. Anat. Physiol.* 4, 275–300 [Plate 10].

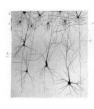

### FIGURE 18.

Martinotti, 1890. Cerebral cortex.

Stell ebenfalls den peripheren Teil der Gehirnrinde mit Silbernitrat (Argentum nitricum) behandelt dar. In der Schicht (a) bermerkt man characteristische Neurogliazellen, die als Schutz für die darunter liegende Schicht dienen (b). Die Protoplasmafortsätze der nervösen Zellen gelangen bis zur äussersten Grenze der Peripherie in die Schicht, welche sich unter der Pia befindet (a), wo sich keine markhaltigen Fasen vorfinden. In (c) shieht einen man nervösen Fortsatz, der von unten kommt und sich biegt, indem er sich in der Schicht

(b) zerteilt; in (d) einen nervösen Fortsatz, der von dem oberen Teil der Zelle ausgeht und sich hierau in der Schicht (b) zerteilt; in (e) einen Seitenfaden von einem nervösen Fortsatz des ersten Typus, der ebenfalls in die Schicht b übergeht; in (f) eine nervöse Faser, die von der Schicht (b) aus nach unten sich biegt und sich zerteilt. Martinotti, C. (1890) Beitrag zum Studium der Hirnrinde und dem Centralursprung der Nerven. *Int. Mschr. Anat. Physiol.* 7, 69–90 [Plate 4, Figure 2].

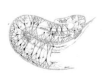

### FIGURE 19.

Schaffer, 1892. Structure of the hippocampus.

Schema des Ammonshornes. C- Stelle der Rindeneinrolhung, 1 - fusiforme, 2 - polymorphe, 3 – Golgi'sche Nervenzelle, 4 - Riesenpyramide, 5 – kleine Pyramide, 6 Nervenzelle der moleculären Schicht-, al - ascendirende Collateralen der Pyramiden, welche (theils auch jene der polymorphen Zellen) insgesammt in das Strat. lacunosum übergehen, 7- polygonale Nervenzelle der Fascia dentata, 8 – daselbst fusiforme Zelle. Sämmtliche Figuren sind mit Zeiss' Zeichenapparat bei einer Vergrösserung von 650 gezeichnet, mit Ausnahme der FIG. 6 und 12, welche mit Reichert's Oelimmersion 1/12 Ocul. III augefertigt wurden. Schaffer, K. 1892. Beitrag zur Histologie der Ammonshornformation. *Arch. Microsk. Anat.* 39, 611–632 [Plate 28, Figure 15].

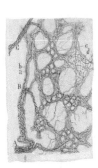

### FIGURE 20.

Ramón y Cajal, 1893. Auerbach plexus and ganglia of a mouse.

Corte paralelo á las túnicas musculares del intestino de la rata de pocos dias. Plexo de Auerbach visto de plano con los engrosamientos ganglionares cuyas células no se han teñido. A, nervio simpático que llegaba con una arteria del mesenterio; B, bifurcación del nervio simpático; C, otro nervio simpático aferente; *a*, fibras simpáticas gruesas; *b*, fibras finas; *c*, hueco para las células nerviosas; *d*, colaterales terminales dentro de los ganglios. Ramón y Cajal, S. (1893) *Los ganglios y plexos nerviosos del intestino de los mamíferos y pequeñas adiciones a nuestros trabajos sobre la médula y gran simpático general.* Madrid: Imprenta y Librería de Nicolás Moya [Figure 5].

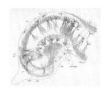

### FIGURE 21.

Kölliker, 1893. Hippocampus of a kitten.

Ammonshorn und *Fascia dentata* einer jungen Katze. Gez. b. Syst. II, Oc. I, k. Tub. *Golgi.* Buchstaben wie bei FIG. 777, ausserdem: *GA* Geflecht der Axonen der Körnerzellen; *Mf* Moosfasern, Hauptbündel; *Plic Plexus intercellularis* der Pyramidenzellen; *Pyr* Pyramidenzellen des dorsalen Blattes des Ammonshornes; *Str.z.S Stratum zonale* des *Subiculum* auf das obere Blatt des *Cornu Ammonis* übergehend; *grPyr* grosse Pyramidenzellen mit ihrer Fortsetzung in die Höhlung der *Fascia dentata*; *oMf* Moosfasern, oberfächliches Blatt; *pz* polymorphe Zellen des Ammonshornes; *tMf* Moosfasern, tiefes Blatt. Kölliker, A. von (1893) *Handbuch der Gewebelehre des Menschen*, vol. II. *Nervensystem des Menschen und der Thiere.* Leipzig: Engelmann [Figure 787].

### FIGURE 22.

Kölliker, 1893. Hippocampus of a human embryo.

Fascia dentata und angrenzende Theile des Ammonshornes von einem acht Monate alten menschlichen Embryo. Golgi. Gez. bei Syst. I. Oc. I, k. Tub. Naturgetreu nach mehreren Präparaten dargestellt. Buchstaben wie bei FIG. 777 und 789. Ausserdem: *Mf* Moosfasern, Hauptbündel; *Mf'* Moosfasern, Nebenbündel; a Zelle mit aufsteigendem Achsencylinder; *p* polymorphe Zelle der Fascia dentata. Kölliker, A. von (1893) *Handbuch der Gewebelehre des Menschen* Vol. II. *Nervensystem des Menschen und der Thiere.* Leipzig: Engelmann [Figure 789].

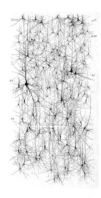

### FIGURE 23.

Kölliker, 1893. Human cerebral cortex.

Aus einer Centralwindung des Menschen, tiefer Theil. Golgi. Gez. bei Syst. III, Oc. III, 1g. Tub. *grP* Erste Lage der grossen Pyramiden; *klPII* Zweite Lage der kleinen Pyramiden; *PZ* Lage der polymorphen Zellen; *RP* Riesenpyramiden. Kölliker, A. von (1893) *Handbuch der Gewebelehre des Menschen* Vol. II. *Nervensystem des Menschen und der Thiere.* Leipzig: Engelmann [Figure 732].

**FIGURE 24.**

Retzius, 1894. Glial cells in the human cerebral cortex.

Die Neuroglia der Grosshirnrinde des Menschen. FIG. 4 und 5. Vertikalschnitte der Rinde von Windungen des Frontallappens von einem 45 *Cm. langen menschlichen Foetus.* Neurogliazellen sind in ihren verschiedenen foetalen Typen dargestellt. In der FIG. 5 sind ausserdem zwei Kleinpyramidenzellen und einige tangentiale Fasern (wahrscheinlich Fortsätze Cajal'scher Zellen), ebenso (unten rechts) ein von einer Gliazelle umstricktes Blutgefäss wiedergegeben. Sämmtliche Figuren der Tafel sind nach Golgi'schen Präparaten bei Vér. Obj. 6 und Ocul. 3 (eingeschob. Tubus) gezeichnet. Retzius, G. (1894) Die Neuroglia des Gehirns beim Menschen und bei Säugethieren. *Biol. Untersuch. Neue Folge* 6, 1–28 [Plate 2, Figure 5].

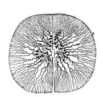

**FIGURE 25.**

Sala, 1894. Glial cells in the frog.

Células neuróglicas de la médula de rana adulta según Cl. A Sala. A, células ependimales; B, células neuróglicas del cordón lateral; C, células del cordón anterior; D, conos terminales constitutivos de la basal externa.
This drawing was used by Claudio Sala in his doctoral thesis titled "Neuroglia de los vertebrados. Estudios de histología comparada" (Faculty of Medicine, Madrid, 1894) (Figure 2). Cajal was a member of the committee that examined Sala's doctoral thesis, together with Professors Benito Hernando, Arturo Redondo, José Rivera and Emilio Loza y Collado. Ramón y Cajal, S. (1899–1904) *Textura del sistema nervioso del hombre y de los vertebrados.* Madrid: Moya [Figure 174].

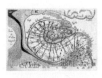

**FIGURE 26.**

Dejerine, 1895. Human hippocampal formation.

Schéma de la corne d'Ammon et de la circonvolution godronnée de l'homme vues sur une coupe vertico-transversale. La circonvolution godronnée est colorée en rouge; deux lignes interrompues - - - - -limitent les deux régions de la corne. Dejerine, J., and Dejerine-Klumpke, A. M. (1895) *Anatomie des Centres Nerveux,* vol 1. Paris: Rueff [Figura 351].

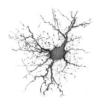

**FIGURE 27.**

Held, 1897. Cell of Deiters in the rabbit.

Zelle aus dem Deiters'schen Kern vom reifen Kaninchenfötus. Golgi-Präparat. Leitz' homogene Immersion $^1/_{12}$. Oc. 6. Schnittdicke 70 μ. Am Stück waren Nervenzellen und das Fasergeflecht der grauen Substanz zugleich gefärbt worden. Die schwarz gefärbte Zelle zeigt am Zellleib und deu zahlreichen Dendriten viele mit gefärbte und angefügte feinste Fäserchen *(x),* welche sicher keine Dendritenverzweigungen sind, sondern wegen ihrer Uebereinstimmung mit den vielen Nervenfasern der umgebenden grauen Substanz, aus denen sie auch zum Theil hervorgehen, als Nervenfäserchen anzusehen sind, welche an dieser Zelle zur Axencylinderendfläche znsammen gekommen sind. Einige sicher überkreuzende Fäserchen sind mit *xx* bebezeichnet. Da die mit *x* bezeichneten Nervenfäserchen, deren Uebergangsstellen vielfach kleine fussartige Verbreiterungen zeigen, mit den Dendriten zusammen imprägnirt sind, erscheinen sie bereits an diesem Silberpräparat nicht mehr als frei endende Axencylinder. Held, H. (1897) Beiträge zur Structur der Nervenzellen und ihrer Fortsätze. Dritte Abhandlung. *Arch. Anat. Phys. (Anat. Abt.)* 273–312 [Plate 14, Figure 4].

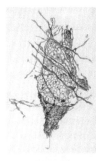

**FIGURE 28.**

Held, 1897. Pericellular axon terminals.

Nervöse pericelluläre Terminalnetze vom 20 Tage alten Kätzchen (Nuleus dendatus). Golgi - Präparat. Schnittdicke 70 μ. In FIG. 6 sind ausser einigen quer über das pericelluläre Terminalnetz hinweglaufenden uud an seiner Bildung unbetheiligten Nervenfasern die mit *a* bis *f* bezeichneten Axencylinder zu beobachten, welche zur Axencylinderendfläche der Zelle hier zusammenkommen. Die mit *a* bis c bemerkten Fasern sind am Präparat in ihrer netzartigen Verbindung deutlich zu verfolgen. Held, H. (1897) Beiträge zur Structur der Nervenzellen und ihrer Fortsätze. Dritte Abhandlung. *Arch. Anat. Phys. Anat. Abt.* 273–312 [Plate 14, Figure 6].

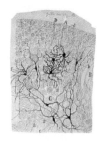

**FIGURE 29.**

Ramón y Cajal, 1897. Neurons in the lateral funiculus.

Corte transversal del cordón lateral de la médula cervical del gato recién nacido. A, foco especial del cordón lateral; B, substancia de Ronaldo del asta posterior; C, haces de la vía piramidal cruzada; *a,* axones de las células de la substancia reticular; *b, f,* células de la porción periférica de esta substancia; *e,* células de la porción interna de la misma; *d,* colaterales de la vía cerebelosa para el foco especial del cordón lateral. Ramón y Cajal, S. (1897) Nueva contribución al estudio del bulbo raquídeo. *Rev. Trim. Micrográf. Madrid* 2, 67–99 [Figure 3].

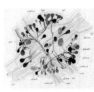

**FIGURE 30.**

Apáthy, 1897. Ganglion cells in the leech.

*Fig.* 1-4 etwas abgeplattete Mittelkörperganglien von Hirudo in Gsy nach Meth. 5 ebenfalls von Hirudo. 6 Lumbricus Nvg, Pa, Ca. 7 Anodonta Nvg, Ce, Ca [table legend]. FIG. 1. Das ganze Ganglion; vorwiegende, symmetrische Tinction von Ganglienzellen. Das Bild sucht die Farben des mikroskopischen Präparates wieder zu geben. 125 (pag. 561, 595–596, 600). Apáthy, S. (1897) Das leitende Element des Nervensystems und seine topographischen Beziehungen zu den Zellen. *Mitt. Zool. Stat. Neapel* 12, 495–748 [Plate 26, Figure 1].

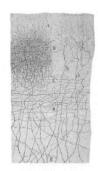

**FIGURE 31.**

Ramón y Cajal, 1899. Sensory plexus of the human cerebral cortex.

Plexo sensitivo de la corteza de la circunvolución frontal ascendente.- Feto humano de siete á ocho meses. A, ramas terminales para el límite superior de la zona tercera; B, plexo tupidísimo terminal de la zona de medianas pirámides; D, plexo medio de fibras horizontales; E, plexo profundo de tubos gruesos oblícuos; a, b, arborizaciones terminales. Ramón y Cajal, S. (1899) Estudios sobre la corteza cerebral humana. II. Estructura de la corteza motriz del hombre y mamíferos superiores. *Rev. Trim. Micrográf.* Madrid 4, 117–200 [Fig. 27].

**FIGURE 32.**

Ris, 1899. Optic lobe of the bird, I.

Taf. VI, Fig. 1–3 und Taf. VII, Fig. 1–2 sind mit Obj. 5, Oc. 2 von Leitz (Vergr. ca. 250) und einer Camera lucida nach Abbé gezeichnet. Bei der Vervielfältigung sind die Originalien dann zur bessern Raumausnützung in etwas verschiedenem Maassstabe verkleinert worden, so dass die Vergr. 250 auf die unten stehenden Zahlen reducirt wurde [table legend]. FIG. 3. Vgr. 150. Die Schichten 1–3 von der Spiegelmeise, aus verschiedenen Stellen und Schnitten des gleichen Organs zusammengestellt. 1. Verzweigungen der Opticusfasern; 2. Zellen, zweiten Typus der Schicht 2 mit annähernd sphärischer Ausbreitung der Protoplasmafortsätze; 3. desgl. mit tangentialer Ausbreitung; 4. eigenthümliche Zelle (1. Typus?) aus der Schicht 2a; 5. Zellen ersten Typus aus der Schicht 2a; 6. grosse Spindelzellen der Schicht 3; 6a und 6b desgl. mit vom tiefen Pol entspringendem Axenfortsatz; 7. kleine Spindelzellen der Schicht 3; 7a desgl. mit Verzweigung in den oberflächlichen Theilen der Schicht 2; 8. Zellen zweiten Typus der Schicht 3; 9. in Schicht 3 gelegene Zellen vom Typus der Schicht 4. Ris, F. (1899) Über den Bau des Lobus opticus der Vögel. *Arch. Mikros. Anat. Entwicklgsg.* 53, 106–130 [Plate 6, Figure 3].

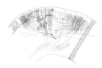

**FIGURE 33.**

Ris, 1899. Optic lobe of the bird, II.

Taf. VI, Fig. 1–3 und Taf. VII, Fig. 1–2 sind mit Obj. 5, Oc. 2 von Leitz (Vergr. ca. 250) und einer Camera lucida nach Abbé gezeichnet. Bei der Vervielfältigung sind die Originalien dann zur bessern Raumausnützung in etwas verschiedenem Maassstabe verkleinert worden, so dass die Vergr. 250 auf die unten stehenden Zahlen reducirt wurde [table legend]. FIG. 3. Vgr. 75. Halbschematische Zusammenstellung der verschiedenen Zell- und Fasertypen (Axenfortsätze roth). Ris, F. (1899) Ueber den Bau des Lobus opticus der Vögel. *Arch. Mikros. Anat. Entwicklgsg.* 53, 106–130 [Plate 7, Figure 3].

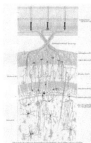

**FIGURE 34.**

Kopsch, 1899. Diagram of the retina of the squid.

*Schema vom Bau der Netzhaut und des Augenganglions von Loligo vulg.* Das Netzhautschema ist hergestellt unter Benutzung der durch v. Lenhossék gegebenen Figuren. Innerhalb der *Netzhaut* sind die zwei durch v. Lenhossék nachgewiesenen Zellenarten dargestellt. Jede derselben läuft aus in eine Stäbchenfaser, welche zwischen der Wand des Bulbus und der Netzhaut eine Strecke weit verläuft, dann die äussere Wand des Bulbus durchbricht und nun sich mit den aus der anderen Bulbushälfte kommenden Fasern kreuzt *(Stäbchenfaserbündelkreuzung)*, um sich auf das Ganglion opt. zu begeben, woselbst sie die äusserste Schicht *(Stäbchenfaserschicht)* bilden. Von dieser Schicht lösen sich unter bogenförmiger Umbiegung Gruppem von Stäbchenfasern ab, welche die *äussere Körnerschicht* durchsetzen und teils innerhalb der *reticulären Schicht (a, c)*, teils unterhalb der *Pallisadenzellenschicht* endigen *(b)*. An der Grenze der äusseren Körnerschicht und der Stäbchenfaserschicht liegen grosse Ganglienzellen *(D)*, deren Endigung nicht dargestellt ist. Die Zellen der äusseren Körnerschicht *(d)* verästeln sich dichotomisch innerhalb der reticulären Schicht. Innerhalb der *inneren* Körnerschicht sind zwei Arten von Zellen, eine reich verästelte *(e)*, die andere wenig verästelte *(f)*. Zwischen der inneren Körnerschicht und der Pallisadenzellenschicht liegen Riesenganglienzellen von horizontaler Verästelung *(g)*. Die Pallisadenzellen *(h)* sind eigenartige, den Spongioblasten der Wirbeltiere ähnliche Zellen. In der *Zone der regellos liegenden Ganglienzellen* unterhalb der Pallisadenzellen liegen eine Zellart *(k)*, welche ihre Fortsätze zu den letzteren sendet, und zweitens multipolare Ganglienzellen *(l)*. Das Aussehen der Zellen in den Zellnestern wird durch die Figuren *m* dargestellt. *i* sind grosse Ganglienzellen, wie sie überall im Mark vorkommen, und deren wahrscheinliche Dendritenbäume in *n* dargestellt sind. Durch die Strassen zwischen den Zellen der inneren Körnerschicht ziehen zahlreiche Fasern *(o)*, welche entweder directe Fasern aus den circumösophagealen Ganglienmassen sind oder von Zellen aus dem Mark stammen. Kopsch, Fr. (1899) Mitteilungen über das Ganglion opticum der Cephalopoden. *Internat. Mschr. Anat. Physiol.* 16, 33–54 [Plate, 5].

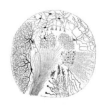

**FIGURE 35.**

Van Gehuchten, 1900. Neuronal components of the cerebellar cortex.

Les différents éléments constitutifs de la couche corticale grise du cervelet. Van Gehuchten, A. (1900) *Anatomie du système nerveux de l'homme.* Troisième édition. Imprimerie Des Trois Rois, Directeur A. Louvian: Uystpruyst [Figure 467].

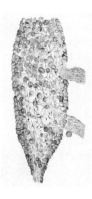

**FIGURE 36.**

Smirnow, 1900. Sympathetic ganglion cells in the frog.

Alle Figuren sind von den Präparaten, zum Teil mittelst der Camera lucida, bei entsprechender Vergrösserung abgenommen und die Zeichnungen darauf von meinem hochverehrten Kollegen, Herrn W. W. Saposchnikow, Professor der Botanik an der kaiserl. Universität zu Tomsk, photographisch hergestellt worden, für welche mühevolle Arbeit ich ihm hierdurch meinen verbindlichsten Dank sage. FIG. 6. Ein sympathischer Nervenknoten der Rana esculenta. Sichtbar sind zwei Rami communicantes. In dem Nervenknötchen ist eine sehr grosse Zahl sich abteilender, grösstenteils markhaltiger Nervenfasern enthalten, welche an den Czermak-Ranvierschen Einschnürungen in 2, 3, ja sogar 4 Zweige zerfallen. Diese Zweige sind bald von einer Myelinscheide umgeben, bald erscheinen einige von ihnen als marklose Fasern. Eine und dieselbe Nervenfaser verzweigt sich zuweilen in solcher Weise wiederholt in ihrem Verlaufe. Die Zweige einer und derselben Nervenfaser gehen in die spiraligen Nervenfasern zweier, dreier sympathischer Nervenzellen über, auf deren Protoplasma oberfläche sie eine Endausbreitung bilden. Auf solche Weise ist hier faktisch die Innervation einiger Zellen durch die Zweige einer und derselben Nervenfaser sichtbar. Das Präparat ist hergestellt, nachdem 3 Stunden zuvor Methylenblau in die Vena cutanea major injiziert worden war und durch pikrinsaures Ammonium fixiert Hartnacks Mikroskop Okul. 3, Obj. 4. Die Photographie ist in einem um 1/5 der Grösse der Zeichnung verkleinerten Massstabe aufgenommen. Smirnow, A. E. (1900) Zur kenntnis der morphologie der sympathischen ganglienzellen beim frosche. *Anat. Hefte* 14, 410–431 [Figure 6].

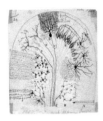

**FIGURE 37.**

Ramón y Cajal, 1904. Schema of the structure of the mammalian cerebellum.

Corte transversal semi-esquemático de una circunvolución cerebelosa de mamífero. A, zona molecular; B, zona de los granos; C, zona de substancia blanca; *a*, célula de Purkinje vista de plano; *b*, células estrelladas pequeñas de la zona molecular; *d*, arborizaciones finales descendentes que rodean las células de Purkinje; *e*, células estrelladas superficiales; *g*, granos con sus cilindros ejes ascendentes bifurcados en *i*; *h*, fibras musgosas; *j*, célula neuróglica en penacho; *n*, fibras trapadoras; *m*, célula neuróglica de la zona de los granos; *f*, células estrelladas grandes de la zona de los granos. Ramón y Cajal, S. (1899–1904) *Textura del sistema nervioso del hombre y de los vertebrados.* Madrid: Moya [Figura 369].

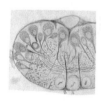

**FIGURE 38.**

Ramón y Cajal, 1904. Ventral chain ganglion of the earthworm.

Sección frontal de un ganglio del *Lumbricus.* Impregnación por el cloruro de oro. *a*, tubo colosal; *b*, columna neuróglica; *c*, corpúsculo multipolar; *d*, célula comisural; *e*, elementos monopolares. Ramón y Cajal, S. (1904) Neuroglia y neurofibrillas del Lumbricus. *Trab. Lab. Invest. Biol. Univ. Madrid* 3, 277–285 [Figure 3]. from the Royal Society, with permission.

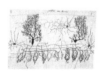

**FIGURE 39.**

Ramón y Cajal, 1904. Cerebellar cortex of a guinea pig.

Corte transversal de una lámina cerebelosa del cobaya de un mes. A, célula de cesta cuyo axon daba una revuelta; B, otra cuyo axon tenía una curva final; C, célula de axon horizontal que enviaba á las cestas una sola colateral descendente delgada; E, D, células de Purkinje dislocadas; *e*, punta de las cestas. Ramón y Cajal, S. (1899–1904) *Textura del sistema nervioso del hombre y de los vertebrados.* Madrid: Moya [Figure 372].

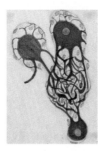

**FIGURE 40.**

Ramón y Cajal, 1905. Tricellular glomerulus from a man.

Glomérulo formado por dendritas pertenecientes á tres neuronas: *a*, axon (hombre de sesenta años). Ramón y Cajal, S. (1905) Las células del gran simpático del hombre adulto. *Trab. Lab. Invest. Biol. Univ. Madrid* 4, 79–104 [Figure 6].

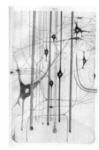

**FIGURE 41.**

Kolmer, 1905. Structure of the spinal cord of ammocoetes.

Schema der Lagerungs und Formverhältnisse im Rückenmark, nach verschiedenen Präparaten kombiniert. In der Mitte a der Centralkanal mit dem Centralfaden auf dem Querschnitt. *b*. Daneben die Querschnitte der Kolossalfasern. *c*. Gekreuzte Kolossalfaser. *d*. Grosse seitliche Zellen verschiedener Typen. *e*. Kleine seitliche Zellen. *f*. Randzellen. *g*. Verbindung mit den Bogenfasern. *h*. Hinterzellen. *i*. Hinterzelle in Verbindung mit hinterer Wurzelfaser. *k*. Übergangszelle. *l*. Spinalganglienzelle. *m*. Kleine Zellen der Mitte. *n*. Seitliche Kolossalzelle. *o*. Hintere Wurzelfaser. *p*. Vordere Wurzelfaser. *q*. Faser mit mäandrischem Verlauf längs der Müllerschen Fasern. *r*. H-förmig sich teilende Faser. *s*. Das wahrscheinlich anzunehmende Netz a der Oberflache. Kolmer, W. (1905) Zur kenntnis des rückenmarks von ammocoetes. *Anat. Hefte* 29, 163–214 [Figure 26].

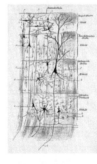

**FIGURE 42.**

Monakow, 1905. Diagram of the human cerebral cortex.

Schematischer Querschnitt durch die Großhirnrinde (vordere Zentralwindung) des Menschen, zum Teil nach Ramon y Cajal. Erste Schicht: *a* Fusiforme Zelle von Ramon y Cajal. *a*, Achsenzylinder derselben. *b* Dreieckige Zelle von Ramon y Cajal. *c* Polygonale Zelle. *c₁* Achsenzylinder derselben. Zweite Schicht: *d* Kleine Pyramidenzelle. *d₁* Achsenzylinder derselben. *e* Martinottische

Zelle. *e₁* Achsenzylinder derselben. Dritte Schicht: *f* Riesenpyramidenzelle. *f₁* Achsenzylinder derselben. *g* Golgische Zelle. *g₁* Achsenzylinder derselben. *K* Körner. Vierte Schicht: *e* Martinottische Zelle. *g* Polygonale Zelle (Golgische Zelle). *h* Polymorphe Zelle mit absteigend sich gabelndem Achsenzylinder (*h₁*). Monakow, C. von (1905) *Gehirnpathologie,* 2d. edition. Wien: Alfred Holder [Figure 112].

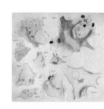

**FIGURE 43.**

Economo, 1906. Normal structure of ganglion cells.

FIG. 40. 2 Zellen mit Golginetz und Füllnetz aus dem Vorderhorn des RM. eines älteren Rindsembryo, Bethe's Methode, Zeiss' Apochr. 1,5, C. - Oc. 6, Abbé-Z.-A.; a, b, c, d Gliakerne. FIG. 41. Zelle mit Golgi- und Füllnetz aus dem hinteren Abschnitt des Vorderhorns eines älteren Rindsembryo, Bethe's Methode, Zeiss' Apochr.1 ,5, C.-Oc.8, Abbé-Z.-A.; A B Zelldendriten, C Capillare, SR. Schnürring, ax ax, Axencylinder, a, b, c, d, e Gliakerne. Verkleinert 2 : 3. FIG. 42. Zelle mit Golginetz aus dem RM. eines Kalbes, Bethe's Methode, Zeiss' Apochr.1,5, C.-Oc.8, bloss die Umrisse sind mit dem Zeichenapparat ausgeführt. FIG 43. Vorderhornzelle aus dem RM. eines jüngeren Rindsembryo, Cajal's Methode am Gelatineschnitte, Zeiss' Apochr. 1,5, C.-Oc. 6, Abbé-Z-A. FIG. 44, 45. Zwei Zelle aus dem RM. eines jüngeren Rindsembryo, Bethe's Methode, stark diff., Zeiss Apochr. 1,5, C.-Oc. 6, Abbé-Z.-A., g Gliakerne. FIG. 46. Vorderhornzelle aus dem RM. eines älteren Rindsembryo, Bethe's Methode, Zeiss' Apochr. 1,5, C.-Oc. 6, Abbé-Z.-A. FIG. 47. Zelle aus dem hinteren Abschnitt des Vorderhorns eines älteren Rindsembryo, Bethe's Methode, Zeiss' Apochr. 1,5, C.-Oc. 6, Abbé-Z.-A.; C₁ C₂ Capillaren, g,g₂ Gliakerne. FIG. 48. A und B dieselbe Vorderhornzelle aus dem RM. eines Rindsembryo bei verschiedener Einstellung, Bethe's Methode, Zeiss' Apochr. 1,5, C.-Oc. 8, Abbé-Z.-A.; g Gliakerne. Verkleinert 2: 3. Economo, C. J. (1906) Beiträge zur normalen Anatomie der Ganglienzelle. *Arch. Psychiat. Nervenk.* 41, 158–201 [Figures 40–48].

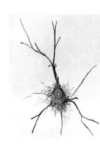

**FIGURE 44.**

Bielschowsky and Gallus, 1913. Atypical ganglion cell in tuberous sclerosis.

Atypische Ganglienzelle mit zarten

Fadenfortsätzen. (Silberimprägnation nach Bielschowsky.) Bielschowsky, M. and Gallus, K. (1913) Über tuberöse Sklerose. *J. Psychol. Neurol.* 20, 1–88 [Plate 2, Figure 5].

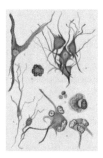

### FIGURE 45.

Bielschowsky and Gallus, 1913. Atypical cells in tuberous sclerosis, I.

(bezieht sich auf Fall III und außerdem auf einen Fall von Recklinghausenscher Krankheit). FIG. 1 und 2. Atypische Ganglienzellen, bei 2 in eigenartiger Gruppierung. (Silberimprägnation nach Bielschowsky.) FIG. 3. Riesenzellenähnliche Gliazelle. (Kernfärbung.) FIG. 4. Atypische "große" Zellen mit langen Fortsätzen. (Heldsche Färbung.) FIG. 5. "Große" Zelle mit riesigen Kernen aus einem kleinen Rindenherde von Recklinghausenscher Krankheit; links daneben zum Vergleich normale Gliakerne. (Heldsche Färbung.) FIG. 6. Links "große" Zelle aus einem Herde von tub. Sklerose; rechts "große" Zelle aus einem Rindenherde von Recklinghausenscher Krankheit. (Heldsche Färbung.) Vergr. übera Leitz Imm. 1/12. Oc. 1 und 3. Bielschowsky, M. and Gallus, K. (1913) Über tuberöse Sklerose. *J. Psychol. Neurol.* 20, 1–88 [Plate 3, Figures 1–6]

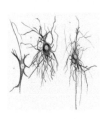

### FIGURE 46.

Bielschowsky and Gallus, 1913. Atypical cells in tuberous sclerosis, II.

(bezieht sich auf Fall VI). FIG. 1, 2, 4. Atypische sehr große und fortsatzreiche Ganglienzellen aus Rindenherden. (Silberimprägnation nach Bielschowsky.) Bielschowsky, M. and Gallus, K. (1913) Über tuberöse Sklerose. *J. Psychol. Neurol.* 20, 1–88 [Plate 5, Figures 1, 2, 4].

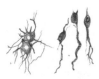

### FIGURE 47.

Bielschowsky and Gallus, 1913. Atypical cells in tuberous sclerosis, III.

(bezieht sich auf Fall IV und V). FIG. 4. "Große" fortsatzreiche Zellen mit Quellungserscheinungen. (Heldsche Färbung.) FIG. 5. Atypische Ganglienzellen. (Silberimprägnation nach Bielschowsky.) Vergr. bei ıa Leitz System 6, Oc. 3, sonst Leitz Immers. 1/12. Oc. 3. Bielschowsky, M. and Gallus, K (1913) Über tuberöse Sklerose. *J. Psychol. Neurol.* 20, 1–88 [Plate 4, Figures 4, 5].

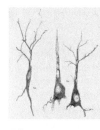

### FIGURE 48.

Bielschowsky and Gallus, 1913. Atypical cells in tuberous sclerosis, IV.

(bezieht sich auf Fall IV und V). FIG. 4a. Atypische Ganglienzelle. (Silberimprägnation nach Bielschowsky.) FIG. 5a. Wabig veränderte Ganglienzellen. (Kresylviolett.) Vergr. bei ıa Leitz System 6, Oc. 3, sonst Leitz Immers. 1/12. Oc. 3. Bielschowsky, M. and Gallus, K. (1913) Über tuberöse Sklerose. *J. Psychol. Neurol.* 20, 1–88 [Plate 4, Figures 4a, 5a].

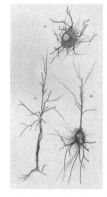

### FIGURE 49.

Bielschowsky and Gallus, 1913. Atypical cells in tuberous sclerosis, V.

(bezieht sich auf Fall VI). FIG. 6, 7, [9]. "Große" Zellen mit atypisch langen Fortsätzen. FIG. 10 und 12. Ganglienzellen mit fadenförmigen Fortsätzen. (Silberimprägnation.) Bielschowsky, M. and Gallus, K. (1913) Über tuberöse Sklerose. *J. Psychol. Neurol.* 20, 1–88 [Plate 5, Figures 9, 10, 12].

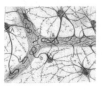

### FIGURE 50.

Ramón y Cajal, 1913. Cells of the cat Ammon's horn.

Células de la corteza gris del asta de Ammon del gato adulto. A, astrocitos; a, b, c, d, remolinos de ramas extendidas sobre la adventicia y procedentes de los pedículos vasculares. (La glia es de tipo fibroso y por tanto analoga á la de la substancia blanca). Ramón y Cajal, S. (1913) Contribución al conocimiento de la neuroglia del cerebro humano. *Trab. Lab. Invest. Biol. Univ. Madrid* 11, 255–315 [Figure 17].

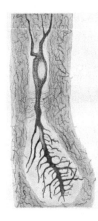

### FIGURE 51.

Lafora, 1914. Pyramidal cell dendritic neoformations in the senile dog.

Neoformaciones dendríticas en una célula piramidal del asta de Ammon de un perro senil. Obsérvese el espacio que rodea á la porción donde se producen las neoformaciones y la substancia homogénea que rellena el mismo (método de Bielschowsky). Lafora, G. (1914) Neoformaciones dendríticas en las neuronas y alteraciones de la neuroglia en el perro senil. *Trab. Lab. Invest. Biol. Univ. Madrid* 12, 39–53 [Figure 1].

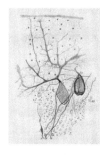

### FIGURE 52.

Schaffer, 1914. Structure of the cerebellar cortex.

Zwei Purkinjesche Zellen; zur Zelle *a* gehört der Axon A, zur *b* der Axon A'. Nähere Schilderung s. im Text. A" ist ein offenbar rückläufiger Axonseitenast, der an der *Stelle eine lokale Schwellung erlitt. AG = amöboide Gliazellen. Schaffer, K. (1914) Zum normalen und pathologischen Fibrillenbau der Kleinhirnrinde. *Z. Gesamte Neurol. Psychiatr.* 21, 1–48; 49–76 [Figure 19].

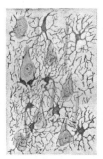

### FIGURE 53.

Achúcarro, 1914. Human *stratum lucidum*.

*Stratum lucidum* del hombre. Método áurico de Cajal. Abundante ramificación y estructura reticulada de los astrocitos. Achúcarro, N. (1914) Contribución al estudio gliotectónico de la corteza cerebral. El asta de Ammon y la fascia dentata. *Trab. Lab. Invest. Biol. Univ. Madrid* 12, 229–272 [Figure 4].

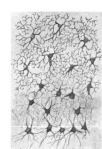

### FIGURE 54.

Achúcarro, 1914. Human *fascia dentata*.

*Fascia dentata* del hombre. Método áurico de Cajal. En la parte superior de la figura la capa molecular poblada de numerosas células enanas de ramificaciones profusas y de carácter protoplásmico. Cada capa granulosa los astrocitos son fibrosos. Las células de la capa polimorfa forman una barrera limitante con la capa granulosa. Achúcarro, N. (1914) Contribución al estudio gliotectónico de la corteza cerebral. El asta de Ammon y la fascia dentata. *Trab. Lab. Invest. Biol. Univ. Madrid* 12, 229–272 [Figure 7].

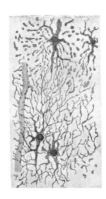

**FIGURE 55.**

Achúcarro, 1914. Human *stratum radiatum.*

*Stratum radiatum* en el hombre. Método áurico de Cajal. Los astrocitos son eminentemente protoplásmicos y su estructura esponjosa es manifiesta. El cuerpo de las células se alarga en la dirección perpendicular á la superficie. En las células de la parte superior de la figura se ve la fragmentación de las prolongaciones ó klasmatodendrosis. Achúcarro, N. (1914) Contribución al estudio gliotectónico de la corteza cerebral. El asta de Ammon y la fascia dentata. *Trab. Lab. Invest. Biol. Univ. Madrid* 12, 229–272 [Figure 5].

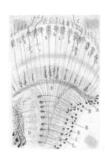

**FIGURE 56.**

Ramón y Cajal and Sánchez y Sánchez, 1915. Retina and optic lobe of the horsefly.

Sección horizontal de la retina profunda y lóbulo óptico del tábano.A, acúmulo de neuronas generadoras de fibras centrífugas arborizadas en el epióptico *(a, c);* B, corteza granular del lóbulo óptico donde residen los somas de centrífugas acabadas en el plexo primero difuso de1a zona plexiforme interna *(b);* C, centrífugas largas ó perforantes para la retina intermediaria y cuyo soma reside en el ganglio angular A; D, ganglio ovoideo del lóbulo óptico; L, foco laminar; K, kiasma profundo. Ramón y Cajal, S., and Sánchez y Sánchez, D. (1915) Contribución al conocimiento de los centros nerviosos de los insectos. *Trab. Lab. Invest. Biol. Univ. Madrid* 13, 1–164 [Figure 40].

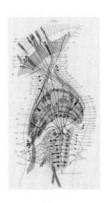

**FIGURE 57.**

Ramón y Cajal and Sánchez y Sánchez, 1915. Schema of the retina and visual centers of the fly.

Esquema de la retina y centros ópticos de la mosca azul. *Acg':* Arborizaciones de una célula gangliónica colosal en la retina profunda; *Apc:* Amacrina de arborización terminal localizada en el plexo difuso cuarto; *App:* Amacrina de arborización terminal localizada en el plexo difuso primero; *Apr:* Amacrina de penacho recurrente periférico; *Aps:* Amacrina de arborización terminal localizada en el plexo difuso segundo; *Apt:* Amacrina de arborización terminal localizada en el plexo difuso tercero; *Arp:* Amacrina de arborización terminal retrógrada profunda; *Asp:* Amacrina de arborización terminal localizada en el plexo difuso primero; *Cai:* Células de asociación interfocal; *Cc:* Célula centrífuga corta; *Cg, Cg', C'g", Cg"':* Células gangliónicas con dos ramas terminales, una para el lóbulo óptico y otra para el segmento laminar del mismo; *Cg$^{IV}$:* Células gangliónicas con una sola rama terminal destinada al primer plexo difuso del lóbulo óptico; *Cmp, Cmp', Cmp":* Células monopolares pequeñas; *Cpa, Cpa':* Centrífugas profundas arciformes; *Crp:* Célula centrífuga para la retina profunda; *Fcl:* Fibra centrífuga larga que termina en la frontera externa de la retina intermediaria; *Fph:* Fibra centrípeta terminada por amplio penacho horizontal en el segundo plexo difuso de la retina profunda; *Lsp:* Lámina serpenteante primera del epióptico; *Lss:* Lámina serpenteante segunda del epióptico; *Lst:* Lámina serpenteante tercera del epióptico; *Pdc:* Plexo difuso cuarto del epióptico; *Pdp:* Plexo difuso primero del epióptico; *Pds:* Plexo difuso segundo del epióptico: *Pdt:* Plexo difuso tercero del epióptico; *Tcd:* Terminación centrípeta difusa en la retina profunda; *Tcg$^{IV}$:* Terminación en el primer plexo difuso del lóbulo óptico de la expansión no bifurcada de ciertas células gangliónicas (Cg$^{IV}$); *Tcm, Tcm':* Terminaciones de monopolares gigantes; *Tfl, Tfl', Tfl":* Terminaciones de fibras ópticas largas; *Tgl:* Terminaciones de células gangliónicas en el foco laminar del lóbulo óptico; *Tpr:* Terminación en la retina intermediaria de la expansión periférica de una célula de mango retrógrado de la corteza ganglionar anterior; *Tpr':* Terminación en la retina intermediaria de la expansión periférica de una célula de mango retrógrado de la corteza ganglionar posterior. Ramón y Cajal, S., and Sánchez y Sánchez, D. (1915) Contribución al conocimiento de los centros nerviosos de los insectos. *Trab. Lab. Invest. Biol. Univ. Madrid* 13, 1–164 [Plate 2].

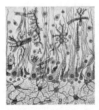

**FIGURE 58.**

Ramón y Fañanás, 1916. Neuroglia in the rabbit cerebellum.

Neuroglia protoplásmica de la zona molecular del cerebelo del conejo. A, capa molecular; B, capa de los granos. (Método del oro-sublimado). Ramón y Fañanás, J. (1916) Contribución al estudio de la neuroglia del cerebro *Trab. Lab. Invest. Biol. Univ. Madrid* 14, 161–179 [Figure 2].

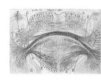

**FIGURE 59.**

Ramón y Cajal, 1917. Cerebroid ganglion of the cuttlefish.

Corte horizontal del centro cerebroide de la sepia de algunas semanas. Figura semiesquemática. A, cordón óptico cruzado; B, terminación de este cordón en el foco peduncular contrapuesto; C, vía óptica refleja nacida en el núcleo peduncular; D, manojo de la corona óptica radiante destinada al lóbulo anterior del foco cerebroide; E, cordón destinado al lóbulo medio; F, corteza del núcleo peduncular. Ramón y Cajal, S. (1917) Contribución al conocimiento de la retina y centros ópticos de los cefalópodos. *Trab. Lab. Invest. Biol. Univ. Madrid* 15, 1–82 [Figure 38].

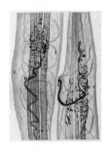

**FIGURE 60.**

Tello, 1917. Human neuromuscular spindle.

Huso neuromuscular de feto humano de seis meses. Aumento, 570 diámetros. A, fibra gruesa de la ramificación en garra G; B, fibra gruesa de la ramificación hederiforme E y F; C, vaina conectiva; H, fibras motrices; I, fibras finísimas. Tello, J. F. (1917) Génesis de las terminaciones nerviosas motrices y sensitivas. En el sistema locomotor de los vertebrados superiores. *Trab. Lab. Invest. Biol. Univ. Madrid* 15, 101–199 [Figure 32].

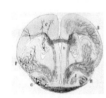

**FIGURE 61.**

Ramón y Cajal [Pedro], 1918. Forebrain of the lizard, I.

Representación esquemática del cerebro de la lacerta en su tercio posterior. A, comisura posterior; B, terminación de las fibras más externas de la comisura intercortical posterior; C, origen de estas fibras; D, fornix; E, thenia trasversalis; F, origen de las fibras de la thenia; G, células situadas debajo del fascículo basal; H, fascículo basal; I, fascículo córtico-medial; L, fascículo septo-cortical. Ramón y Cajal, P. (1918) Nuevo estudio del encéfalo de los reptiles. *Trab. Lab. Invest. Biol. Univ. Madrid* 16, 309–333 [Figure 2].

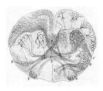

**FIGURE 62.**

Ramón y Cajal [Pedro], 1918. Forebrain of the lizard, II.

*Representación esquemática de un corte del cerebro al nivel de la comisura anterior.* A, fascículos córtico-basilares (decusados); B, comisura de los núcleos esféricos (no decusada); C, comisura interestriada (decusada); D, comisura olfatoria (no decusada); E, ramificaciones de las fibras del fascículo córtico-basilar; FF, fascículos basales; I, thenia transversalis; J, fascículo bulbo-olfativo para el núcleo esférico (raíz externa olfatoria); L, radiación ondulada del fascículo interestriado en el interior del cuerpo estriado y origen de fibras; M, fascículos septo-corticalis; P, *commisura pallii* anterior. Ramón y Cajal, P. (1918) Nuevo estudio del encéfalo de los reptiles. *Trab. Lab. Invest. Biol. Univ. Madrid* 16, 309–333 [Figure 6].

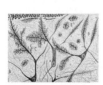

**FIGURE 63.**

Del Río-Hortega, 1918. Cells in the dog *fascia dentata.*

Células con apéndices penniformes pertenecientes a la fascia dentata del perro adulto. A, capa de los granos; B, región de los corpúsculos polimorfos; C, D, prolongaciones en forma de pluma y de ramillete; E, dendritas seccionadas transversalmente. Método de Cajal. Del Río-Hortega, P. (1918) Particularidades histológicas de la Fascia dentata en algunos mamíferos. *Trab. Lab. Invest. Biol. Univ. Madrid* 16, 291–308 [Figure 1].

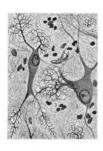

**FIGURE 64.**

Del Río-Hortega, 1918. Cells in the horse *fascia dentata.*

Dos corpúsculos de la fascia dentata del caballo viejo. A, célula que posee por arriba dendritas arborescentes (C) y por abajo apéndices penniformes (E); B, célula provista de gran penacho dendrítico (D) próximo al soma; F, prolongación seccionada transversalmente. Método del carbonato argéntico. Particularidades histológicas de la Fascia dentata en algunos mamíferos. *Trab. Lab. Invest. Biol. Univ. Madrid* 16, 291–308 [Figure 2].

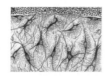

**FIGURE 65.**

Del Río-Hortega, 1918. Cells in the ram *fascia dentata.*

Aspecto de la fascia dentata del carnero, coloreada por el método de Cajal. A, granos; B, zona de corpúsculos polimorfos, de los que irradian abundantísimos apéndices ramificados, que, en C, F, G, H, nacen principalmente del soma, y en D, E del soma y prolongaciones polares; I, célula que sólo emite dendritas por su parte inferior; J, K, corpúscnlos de tipo fusiforme. Del Río-Hortega, P. (1918) Particularidades histológicas de la Fascia dentata en algunos mamíferos. *Trab. Lab. Invest. Biol. Univ. Madrid* 16, 291–308 [Figure 5].

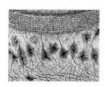

**FIGURE 66.**

Del Río-Hortega, 1918. Cells in the bull *fascia dentata.*

Fascia dentata del toro. A, capa de los granos; B, zona de los corpúsculos polimorfos; D, E, F, G, diversos tipos celulares, de los que nacen infinitos apéndices dicotomizados y entrelazados. Método de Cajal. Del Río-Hortega, P. (1918) Particularidades histológicas de la Fascia dentata en algunos mamíferos. *Trab. Lab. Invest. Biol. Univ. Madrid* 16, 291–308 [Figure 7].

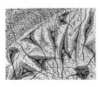

**FIGURE 67.**

Del Río-Hortega, 1918. Cells in the ox *fascia dentata.*

Fascia dentata del buey senil. A, granos; B, región de los corpúsculos polimorfos; C, D, E, F, G, diferentes tipos de células vellosas. Obsérvese el número infinito de apéndices somáticos y el apretado plexo pericelular que forman. Método de Cajal. Particularidades histológicas de la Fascia dentata en algunos mamíferos. *Trab. Lab. Invest. Biol. Univ. Madrid* 16, 291–308 [Figure 8].

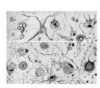

**FIGURE 68.**

Del Río-Hortega, 1918–1919. Neuroglial cells of the aging human cerebral cortex.

Restos de las células neuróglicas en algunas regiones corticales del cerebro senil. A, G, mechones y anillos gliofibrilares correspondientes a células desaparecidas; D, F, gliocitos que sólo conservan el núcleo y las madejas gliofibrilares; B, C, E, amiboides cuyas fibrillas intrasomáticas se prolongan por las expansiones; I, M, espesos glomérulos perinucleares; H, J, L, células quísticas con restos de glomérulos fibrilares; K, célula fibrosa, no amiboide, con atrofia fibrilar de sus prolongaciones. Del Río-Hortega, P. (1918–1919) Sobre la verdadera significación de las células neuróglicas llamadas amiboides. *Bol. Soc. Esp. Biol.* Año 8, 229–243 [Figure 6].

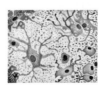

**FIGURE 69.**

Del Río-Hortega, 1918–1919. Human cerebral cortex in a case of tuberculous meningo-encephalitis.

Corteza cerebral humana en un caso de meningo-encefalitis tuberculosa subaguda. A, célula protoplásmica en tumefacción y clasmatodendrosis; B, células preamiboides; C, D, amiboides típicas. Coloración: carbonato argéntico amoniacal. Del Río-Hortega, P. (1918–1919) Sobre la verdadera significación de las células neuróglicas llamadas amiboides. *Bol. Soc. Esp. Biol.* Año 8, 229–243 [Figure 1].

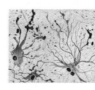

**FIGURE 70.**

Del Río-Hortega, 1918–1919. Cerebral white substance in a case of paralytic dementia.

Substancia blanca cerebral en un caso de demencia paralítica. A y C, células fibrosas preamiboides; B, célula con tumefacción poco acentuada. Obsérvese la existencia de fibrillas intraprotoplásmicas. Del Río-Hortega, P. (1918–1919) Sobre la verdadera significación de las células neuróglicas llamadas amiboides. *Bol. Soc. Esp. Biol.* Año 8, 229–243 [Figure 2].

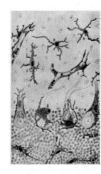

**FIGURE 71.**

Collado, 1919. Cerebellar microglia of the rabbit with rabies.

Microglía cerebelosa en el conejo rábico: A, E, células que abrazan a los vasos; B, D, células de la capa molecular, con toscos apéndices; C, célula con protoplasma ensanchado; F, G, H, I, microglía que envuelve al cuerpo de las células de Purkinje; J, K, corpúsculos laminares próximos a los vasos de la capa granulosa. (Método de Río-Hortega.) Collado, C. (1919) Participación de la microglía en el substratum patológico de la rabia. *Bol. Soc. Esp. Biol.* 9, 175–191 [Figure 4].

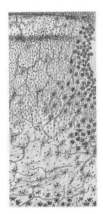

### FIGURE 72.

Del Río-Hortega, 1919. Migration and transformation of microglia in the vicinity of a cerebral injury.

**Emigración y transformación de la microglía en la proximidad de una herida cerebral de veinticuatro horas (gato de dos dias): A, microglía globulosa de la substancia blanca; B, microglía ramificada emigrante; C, microglía globulosa de los bordes de la herida.** Del Río-Hortega, P. (1919) El tercer elemento de los centros nerviosos. Poder fagocitario y movilidad de la microglía. *Bol. Soc. Esp. Biol.* Año 9, 154–166 [Figure 2 ].

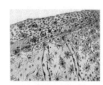

### FIGURE 73.

Del Río-Hortega, 1919. Migration of microglia in the vicinity of a cerebral injury.

**Emigración de la microglía a los espacios meníngeos en la herida cerebral de cuarenta y ocho horas.** Del Río-Hortega, P. (1919) El tercer elemento de los centros nerviosos. Poder fagocitario y movilidad de la microglía. *Bol. Soc. Esp. Biol.* Año 9, 154–166 [Figure 5].

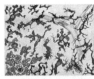

### FIGURE 74.

Del Río-Hortega, 1919. Transformation of microglia in the normal rabbit.

**Evolución morfológica de la microglía en el conejo normal de cuatro dias.Véase la transición de las formas redondeadas (A) en mamelonadas (B), pseudopódicas (C, D, E) y ramificadas (F).** Del Río-Hortega, P. (1919) El tercer elemento de los centros nerviosos. Poder fagocitario y movilidad de la microglía. *Bol. Soc. Esp. Biol.* Año 9, 154–166 [Figure 6].

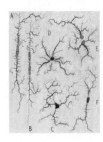

### FIGURE 75.

Del Río-Hortega, 1920. Human microglia.

**Principales tipos existentes en la microglía humana en estado normal. A, célula**

bipolar, en forma de bastoncito; B, célula alargada, provista de dos núcleos; C, célula multipolar, con expansiones ramificadas; D, célula multipolar, con apéndices espinosos; E, pareja isogénica; F, corpúsculo bipolar, con apéndices bifurcados. Del Río-Hortega, P. (1920) Estudios sobre la neuroglia. La microglía y su transformación en células en bastoncito y cuerpos gránulo-adiposos. *Trab. Lab. Invest. Biol. Univ. Madrid* 18, 37–82 [Figure 1].

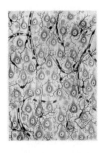

### FIGURE 76.

Del Río-Hortega, 1920. Microglia in the Ammon's horn of the normal rabbit.

**Distribución de la microglía en el asta de Ammon** *(stratum radiatum)* **del conejo normal. Obsérvese la variada morfología de los corpúsculos microgliales y sus relaciones con los vasos. (Coloración: técnica II).** Del Río-Hortega, P. (1920) Estudios sobre la neuroglia. La microglía y su transformación en células en bastoncito y cuerpos gránulo-adiposos. *Trab. Lab. Invest. Biol. Univ. Madrid* 18, 37–82 [Figure 3].

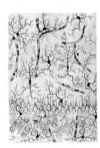

### FIGURE 77.

Del Río-Hortega, 1920. Distribution of microglia in the rabbit cerebral cortex.

**Distribución de la microglía en la corteza cerebral del conejo. Véase la forma variada de los corpúsculos microgliales y, sobre todo, las relaciones que tienen con los vasos (satélites vasculares) y con las células nerviosas (satélites neuronales). (Coloración: técnica II).** Del Río-Hortega, P. (1920) Estudios sobre la neuroglia. La microglía y su transformación en células en bastoncito y cuerpos gránulo-adiposos. *Trab. Lab. Invest. Biol. Univ. Madrid* 18, 37–82 [Figure 4].

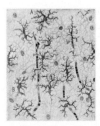

### FIGURE 78.

Del Río-Hortega, 1920. Microglia in the Ammon's horn of a rabbit that died from an infectious disease.

**Caracteres de la microglía en el asta de Ammon** *(stratum radiatum)* **de un conejo muerto de enfermedad infecciosa. Nótese el engrosamiento y aspecto espinoso de las expansiones**

celulares. A, corpúsculo provisto de abundantes ramas; B, célula con prolongaciones cortas y reticuladas; C, D, células alargadas verticalmente que tienden a transformarse en *Stäbchenzellen*. La neuroglia protoplásmica aparece débilmente teñida. (Coloración: técnica 1). Del Río-Hortega, P. (1920) Estudios sobre la neuroglia. La microglía y su transformación en células en bastoncito y cuerpos gránulo-adiposos. *Trab. Lab. Invest. Biol. Univ. Madrid* 18, 37–82 [Figure 5].

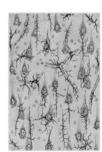

### FIGURE 79.

Del Río-Hortega, 1920. Microglia of the human cerebral cortex from a case of acute meningitis.

**Caracteres de la microglía de la corteza cerebral humana, en un caso de meningitis subaguda. Obsérvese la formación de células en bastoncito. A, célula de forma estrellada; B, C, satélites neuronales; D, corpúsculo alargado; E, F, G, H, diferentes tipos de** *Stäbchenzellen;* **I, J, K, L, satélites vasculares íntimamente adosadas a los vasos. (Coloración: técnica I).** Del Río-Hortega, P. (1920) Estudios sobre la neuroglia. La microglía y su transformación en células en bastoncito y cuerpos gránulo-adiposos. *Trab. Lab. Invest. Biol. Univ. Madrid* 18, 37–82 [Figure 6].

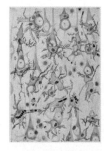

### FIGURE 80.

Del Río-Hortega, 1920. Microglia of the rabbit cerebral cortex in the vicinity of a wound.

**Microglía de la corteza cerebral del conejo en la proximidad de una herida producida dos días antes con un punzón candente. Obsérvese el aspecto monstruoso de los corpúsculos microgliales, que ofrecen la más variada forma globulosa y laminar. A, B, C, satélites neuronales; D, satélite apical, de aspecto laminar; E, G, satélites vasculares; F, célula aplanada íntimamente adosada a un vaso; H, I, J, pequeños corpúsculos redondeados; K, L, núcleos neuróglicos. (Coloración: técnica I).** Del Río-Hortega, P. (1920) Estudios sobre la neuroglia. La microglía y su transformación en células en bastoncito y cuerpos gránulo-adiposos. *Trab. Lab. Invest. Biol. Univ. Madrid* 18, 37–82 [Figure 9].

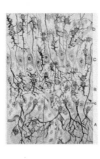

**FIGURE 81.**

De Castro, 1920. Olfactory bulb of the cat.

Corte transversal del bulbo olfatorio del gato de ocho días. Método áurico de Caja1. A, zona glomerular; B, capa molecular; C, capa de las células mitrales; D, porción inferior de la zona de los granos; *a,* tallo radial de una célula epitelial dislocada implantado en un vaso; *c,* otra expansión radial que termina libremente; *b,* astrocito con núcleo en forma de bizcocho. De Castro, F. (1920) Algunas observaciones sobre la histogénesis de la neuroglia en el bulbo olfativo. *Trab. Lab. Invest. Biol. Univ. Madrid* 18, 83–108 [Figure 1].

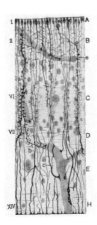

**FIGURE 82.**

De Castro, 1920. Optic lobe of the lizard.

Lóbulo óptico del lagarto. Método del oro-sublimado de Cajal. A la derecha se indican las capas según la disposición neuróglica y a la izquierda la correspondiente en la arquitectura nerviosa según P. Ramón. A, capa epitelial; B, capa de las fibras radiales; C, zona fasciculada; E, capa de las trompas y colaterales; H, zona de los pies terminales; *a,* tallo exuberantemente erizado por vellosidades; *c,* tallo con una colateral implantada en un vaso e hipertrofiada; *e,* célula epitelial desplazada; *f,* trompa de paso en una de las ramas terminales del tallo. De Castro, F. (1920) Algunas observaciones sobre la histogénesis de la neuroglia en el bulbo olfativo. *Trab. Lab. Invest. Biol. Univ. Madrid* 18, 83–108 [Figure 9].

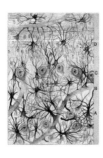

**FIGURE 83.**

De Castro, 1920. Human olfactory bulb.

Bulbo olfativo humano. Método áurico de Cajal, previa fijación en nitrato de urea. A, subestrato superficial de la zona molecular, con numerosas células de forma *cefalopódica;* B, subestrato profundo; C, capa de las células mitrales; D, zona de los granos. De Castro, F. (1920) Estudios sobre la neuroglia de la corteza cerebral del hombre y de los animales. I. La arquitectonia neuróglica y vascular del bulbo olfativo. *Trab. Lab. Invest. Biol. Univ. Madrid* 18, 1–35 [Figure 2].

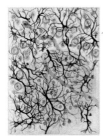

**FIGURE 84.**

De Castro, 1920. Olfactory glomerulus of the adult dog.

Glomérulo olfativo del perro adulto. *g,* elementos fibrosos *intraglomerulares; a,* corpúsculos *radioglomerulares; f,* células fibrosas más superficiales de la zona molecular, exhibiendo el máximo de sus prolongaciones orientadas hacia la profundidad. Adviértanse los numerosos núcleos que pueblan esta zona, pertenecientes todos a la glía adendrítica de Cajal. De Castro, F. (1920) Estudios sobre la neuroglia de la corteza cerebral del hombre y de los animales. I. La arquitectonia neuróglica y vascular del bulbo olfativo. *Trab. Lab. Invest. Biol. Univ. Madrid* 18, 1–35 [Figure 5].

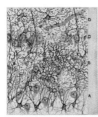

**FIGURE 85.**

De Castro, 1920. Plexiform layer and mitral cells of the adult cat.

Corte de las capas plexiforme y de las células mitrales del gato adulto. Método del oro-sublimado. A, subestrato superficial con robustos elementos fibrosos; B, subzona profunda de la molecular dotada de numerosos astrocitos de tipo mixto; C, capa de las células mitrales; D, zona de las colaterales de Cajal o segmento más superficial de la capa de los granos; *g,* terminación del tallo radial de las células epiteliales dislocadas. Nótese la riqueza en apéndices penniformes vacuolados que cubren las dendritas de la glía de las zonas centrales. En el centro de la capa B se ven dos astrocitos de apariencia protoplásmica. De Castro, F. (1920) Estudios sobre la neuroglia de la corteza cerebral del hombre y de los animales. I. La arquitectonia neuróglica y vascular del bulbo olfativo. *Trab. Lab. Invest. Biol. Univ. Madrid* 18, 1–35 [Figure 7].

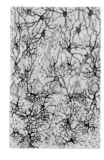

**FIGURE 86.**

De Castro, 1920. Olfactory bulb of adult dog.

Corte del bulbo olfativo del perro adulto, comprendiendo las capas molecular (A), de las células mitrales (B), y de los granos (C, D). Los astrocitos de las zonas A, B y C pertenecen al tipo mixto de Cajal. En la glía del estrato granuloso C, D, el polo profundo es singularmente rico en prolongaciones, las cuales, después de larga excursión, terminan por insertarse en capilares. El último piso del estrato D, encierra elementos muy esclerosos. Son muy numerosos los pies chupadores implantados sobre los vasos de estas regiones. De Castro, F. (1920) Estudios sobre la neuroglia de la corteza cerebral del hombre y de los animales. I. La arquitectonia neuróglica y vascular del bulbo olfativo. *Trab. Lab. Invest. Biol. Univ. Madrid* 18, 1–35 [Figure 8].

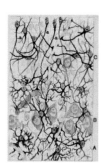

**FIGURE 87.**

De Castro, 1920. Structure of neuroglia in the human cerebral cortex.

Capa molecular (A), de los elementos mitrales (B), y de los granos (C), del conejo adulto. Método áurico de Cajal. Los corpúsculos de las zonas A, B, son muy granulosos, con protoplasma polarizado y parecen pertenecer a una variedad poco diferenciada del tipo mixto. En C los elementos son fibrosos; *a,* células epiteliales dislocadas; en una de ellas se ve el tallo radial en su larga exploración, acabar insertándose en un vaso de esta misma zona. Los pies vasculares abundan menos que en el gato y perro. De Castro, F. (1920) Estudios sobre la neuroglia de la corteza cerebral del hombre y de los animales. I. La arquitectonia neuróglica y vascular del bulbo olfativo. *Trab. Lab. Invest. Biol. Univ. Madrid* 18, 1–35 [Figure 9].

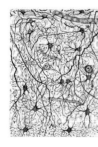

**FIGURE 88.**

De Castro, 1920. Olfactory bulb of the cat.

Corte horizontal del bulbo olfatorio del gato de un año, comprendiendo sólo la capa de los granos. Método del oro-sublimado. Los astrocitos de los distintos pisos son del tipo mixto. *a,* células epiteliales dislocadas; *f,* vasos capilares con numerosos pies implantados en su superficie. De Castro, F. (1920) Estudios sobre la neuroglia de la corteza cerebral del hombre y de los animales. I. La arquitectonia neuróglica y vascular del bulbo olfativo. *Trab. Lab. Invest. Biol. Univ. Madrid* 18, 1–35 [Figure 10].

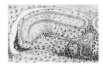

**FIGURE 89.**

Del Río-Hortega, 1921. Cross-section of the rabbit brain.

Corte transversal del cerebro de conejo de cuatro días: A, cuerpo calloso; B, comisura interammónica, con microglía globulosa; C, microglía emigrante al asta de Ammon; D, hipocampo; E, plexo coroideo; F, ventrículo lateral; G, fimbria; H, I, tálamo óptico; J, tela coroidea superior; K, ganglio habenular. Del Río-Hortega, P. (1921) El tercer elemento de los centros nerviosos. Histogénesis y evolución normal; éxodo y distribución regional de la microglia. *Mem. Real Soc. Esp. Hist. Nat.* 11, 213–268 [Figure 1].

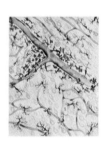

**FIGURE 90.**

Del Río-Hortega, 1921. Perivascular microglia.

Sección vertical de la protuberancia de conejo de cuatro días: A, vaso; B, F, microglía perivascular, con tuberosidades y pseudópodos; C, célula ramificada; D, célula cuyas ramas siguen la dirección de las fibras nerviosas; E, satélites vasculares. Del Río-Hortega, P. (1921) El tercer elemento de los centros nerviosos. Histogénesis y evolución normal; éxodo y distribución regional de la microglia. *Mem. Real Soc. Esp. Hist. Nat.* 11, 213–268 [Figure 5].

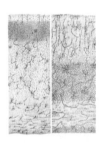

**FIGURE 91.**

Del Río-Hortega, 1921. Microglia in the cerebral and cerebellar cortex.

(*Left*) FIG. 14. Circunvolución cerebral de conejo de un dia: E, epéndimo; D, substancia blanca, desde donde asciende la microglía a los planos inferiores y medios de la corteza (A, B); A, capa molecular. (*Right*) FIG. 19. Microglía cerebelosa en el conejo adulto: A, zona plexiforme; B, células de Purkinje; C, capa granulosa; D, substancia blanca de las laminillas. Del Río-Hortega, P. (1921) El tercer elemento de los centros nerviosos. Histogénesis y evolución normal; éxodo y distribución regional de la microglia. *Mem. Real Soc. Esp. Hist. Nat.* 11, 213–268 [Figures 14, 19].

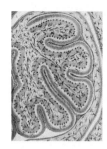

**FIGURE 92.**

Del Río-Hortega, 1921. Cerebellar microglia.

Microglía cerebelosa en el conejo de cuatro días: A, cuarto ventrículo; B, velo medular; C, laminilla cerebelosa; D, microglía que emigra por la substancia blanca; E, célula microglial llegada a la substancia gris. Del Río-Hortega, P. (1921) El tercer elemento de los centros nerviosos. Histogénesis y evolución normal; éxodo y distribución regional de la microglia. *Mem. Real Soc. Esp. Hist. Nat.* 11, 213–268 [Figure 18].

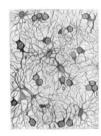

**FIGURE 93.**

Del Río-Hortega, 1921. Glial cells with few processes.

Glía de escasas radiaciones en la substancia blanca cerebelosa del mono adulto: A, células con prolongaciones dicotomizadas; B,C, células con gruesos brazos protoplásmicos; D, células con apéndices nudosos; E, tres células muy juntas; F, neuroglia fibrosa; G, microglía. Del Río-Hortega, P (1921) Estudios sobre la neuroglia. La glia de escasas radiaciones. (Oligodendroglia). *Bol. Soc. Esp. Hist. Nat.* 21, 63–92 [Figure 5].

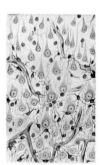

**FIGURE 94.**

Del Río-Hortega, 1921. Oligodendroglia in the monkey cerebral cortex.

Disposición de la oligodendroglía en la substancia gris cerebral del mono: A, capa de pequeñas pirámides casi exenta de células enanas: B, piramidales grandes con satélites de escasas radiaciones; C, vaso; D, microglía; E, núcleo de un gliocito protoplásmico; F, plexo de fibrillas nudosas. Del Río-Hortega, P. (1921) Estudios sobre la neuroglia. La glia de escasas radiaciones. (Oligodendroglia). *Bol. Soc. Esp. Hist. Nat.* 21, 63–92 [Figure 15].

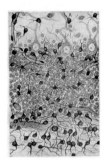

**FIGURE 95.**

Del Río-Hortega, 1921. Oligodendroglia in the monkey cerebellar cortex.

Disposición de la oligodendroglía en el cerebelo del mono: A, zona molecular; B, célula de Purkinje; C, capa de los granos con gliocitos de escasas radiaciones; D, gliocito con caracteres indecisos; E, gliocito de largas radiaciones; F, vaso con abundantes satélites; G, substancia blanca; H, gliocito voluminoso. Del Río-Hortega, P. (1921) Estudios sobre la neuroglia. La glia de escasas radiaciones. (Oligodendroglia). *Bol. Soc. Esp. Hist. Nat.* 21, 63–92 [Figure 16].

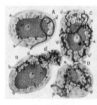

**FIGURE 96.**

De Castro, 1921. Sensory ganglion neurons.

Diversos elementos irritados, mostrando algunos momentos de su evolución. *A,* corpúsculo irritado con puntas o espinas sobre el soma; *B,* otro más adelantado, con numerosas excrescencias en el axón y en la robusta asa de fenestramiento; *C,* célula irritada con crecidas dendritas subcapsulares, gruesas y finas, todas armadas de apéndices lanciformes; *D,* glomérulo axónico de un elemento irritado exhibiendo gran diversidad de apéndices implantados en su superficie, mientras está cobijado por la cápsula. En esta figura puede reconocerse que el número de satélites es proporcional al desarrollo de los brotes dendríticos. De Castro, F. (1921) Estudio sobre los ganglios sensitivos del hombre en estado normal y patológico. Formas celulares típicas y atípicas. *Trab. Lab. Invest. Biol. Univ. Madrid* 19, 241–340 [Figure 24].

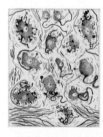

**FIGURE 97.**

De Castro, 1921. Gasser ganglion in a case of osteomalacia, I.

Corte del ganglio de Gasser de un caso de osteomalacia muy avanzado. (En la construcción de la figura se han reunido tres campos microscópicos contiguos). *o* y *e,* células mono polares con puntas de irritación; *n* y *c,* corpúsculos irritados de gran volumen;

f, otra con numerosísimos apéndices y excrecencias en el soma y axón; g, elemento irritado, dotado a su vez de apéndice armado de bola; a, célula ganglónica con expansión fibrosa de extraordinaria longitud. De Castro, F. (1921) Estudio sobre los ganglios sensitivos del hombre en estado normal y patológico. Formas celulares típicas y atípicas. *Trab. Lab. Invest. Biol. Univ. Madrid* 19, 241–340 [Figure 25].

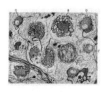

**FIGURE 98.**

De Castro, 1921. Alteration of the Gasser ganglion.

Corte del ganglio de Gasser atacado de un proceso supurativo, exhibiendo diversas variedades de fenestramientos en los corpúsculos residentes. c y b, formas sencillas con evolución del aparato fenestrado; a, e y g, corpúsculos fenestrados complejos; d, célula lobulada y fenestrada; n, nódulo residual, con restos de neurona muerta; o, f e i, apéndices o fibras orientadas al nódulo residual inervado, central. Repárese en a, cuán parecido es el corpúsculo, salvo diferencias de volumen, con los del *Orthagoriscus mola*. En el corte, hállanse numerosos acúmulos granulosos, restos procedentes de neuronas y axones demolidos. De Castro, F. (1921) Estudio sobre los ganglios sensitivos del hombre en estado normal y patológico. Formas celulares típicas y atípicas. *Trab. Lab. Invest. Biol. Univ. Madrid* 19, 241–340 [Figure 13].

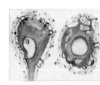

**FIGURE 99.**

De Castro, 1921. Sensory ganglion neurons.

A y B, células de tamaño mediano del *Orthagoriscus mola*, exhibiendo la doble formación de los fenestramientos; c, canales impresos en la superficie celular; I, perforaciones en el protoplasma, ocupadas por tejido conjuntivo; a, asas finísimas brotando de la superficie; b, otras robustas; g, núcleos del tejido conjuntivo envolvente. (Tomadas de una preparación de G. Levi.) De Castro, F. (1921) Estudio sobre los ganglios sensitivos del hombre en estado normal y patológico. Formas celulares típicas y atípicas. *Trab. Lab. Invest. Biol. Univ. Madrid* 19, 241–340 [Figure 17].

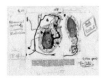

**FIGURE 100.**

De Castro, 1921. Gasser ganglion in a case of osteomalacia, II.

Células del ganglio de Gasser de una mujer con osteomalacia muy avanzada. c, elemento monopolar normal, con el *glomérulo situado a distancia,* formando la cápsula un zurrón o pedículo sesil; A, corpúsculo irritado, de configuración somática normal, brotan del soma apéndices, c, c', erizados de puntas en su extremo libre. Repárese en el axón durante su porción intracapsular, la abundancia de apéndices diversos retoñados, g, a, que cesan bruscamente, en cuanto éste traspasa su envoltura; b, colateral ramifcada de tipo regenerativo; o, bifurcación del axón. De Castro, F. (1921) Estudio sobre los ganglios sensitivos del hombre en estado normal y patológico. Formas celulares típicas y atípicas. *Trab. Lab. Invest. Biol. Univ. Madrid* 19, 241–340 [Figure 23].

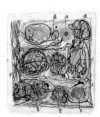

**FIGURE 101.**

De Castro, 1921. Plexiform ganglion of the vagus nerve, I.

Corte del ganglio plexiforme del vago de un alcohólico (caso 10) reunidas tres porciones del mismo corte. E, corpúsculo monopolar dotado de complicado glomérulo axónico y una fibra brotada de éste terminada en anillo; F, célula ganglónica, en torno de la cual fibras aferentes forman ovillo; C, otra con expansiones muy gruesas; D, nódulo residual neurotizado; B, gruesa maza extracapsular; A, otra capsulada monstruosa con degeneración hialínica periférica. Notese en F que, alguna fibra que contribuye en la formación del nido, llega a la cápsula arrollándose helicoidalmente en torno a la neurita. De Castro, F. (1921) Estudio sobre los ganglios sensitivos del hombre en estado normal y patológico. Formas celulares típicas y atípicas. *Trab. Lab. Invest. Biol. Univ. Madrid* 19, 241–340 [Figure 29].

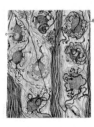

**FIGURE 102.**

De Castro, 1921. Plexiform ganglion of the vagus nerve, II.

Corte del ganglio plexiforme del vago, *cuya raiz periférica habíase seccionado seis días antes* durante la intervención operatoria (caso 50). Todos los corpúsculos son multipolares, en algunos, la semejanza con los simpátiros es extraordinaria. o, a, g e i, elementos con numerosas prolongaciones cortas, largas y finas o gruesas, terminadas por pequeñas tumefacciones; c, célula ganglónica con expansiones cortas coronadas por macitas y con asas u ojales fibrosos sobre la superficie; f, otra desgarrada propiamente dicha, con puntas de irritación y satélites cargadas de granos argentófilos; b, pelotón fibroso distinto de los nódulos residuales asentando en el conjuntivo intersticial. De Castro, F. (1921) Estudio sobre los ganglios sensitivos del hombre en estado normal y patológico. Formas celulares típicas y atípicas. *Trab. Lab. Invest. Biol. Univ. Madrid* 19, 241–340 [Figure 34].

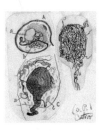

**FIGURE 103.**

De Castro, 1921. Changes of sensory ganglion cells.

Elementos nerviosos del plexo gangliforme del vago de un alcohólico. A, célula con vacuolas pequeñas b, y colosales a; C, corpúsculo nervioso de gran tamaño, con retículo neurofibrillar bien aparente y apéndices rosariformes subcapsulares con vacuolas a; B, nódulo residual inervado por fibras de excursión laberíntica. De Castro, F. (1921) Estudio sobre los ganglios sensitivos del hombre en estado normal y patológico. Formas celulares típicas y atípicas. *Trab. Lab. Invest. Biol. Univ. Madrid* 19, 241–340 [Figure 28].

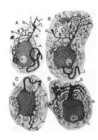

**FIGURE 104.**

De Castro, 1921. Sensory ganglion cells: multipolar elements.

Varios elementos multipolares. A, célula con fenestramiento del ganglio de Gaserio del niño recién nacido, con un tallo g, brotado del soma que, produce, a modo de *surtidor,* numerosos apéndices terminados en mazas d; A, otro del plexo gangliforme del vago del niño normal recién nacido, todos sus apéndices poseen mazas; C corpúsculo ganglónico del plexiforme del vago de un niño (8 años) con tuberculosis pulmonar, irradiando del cuerpo celular gran cantidad de apéndices e; D, célula ganglónica de un sujeto adulto normal. De Castro, F. (1921) Estudio sobre los ganglios sensitivos del hombre en estado normal y patológico. Formas celulares típicas y atípicas. *Trab. Lab. Invest. Biol. Univ. Madrid* 19, 241–340 [Figure 26].

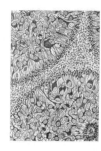

**FIGURE 105.**

Del Río-Hortega, 1922. Structure of the pineal gland, I.

Pineal de mujer joven: A, células parenquimatosas; B, radiaciones marginales claviformes; *C*, espacio interlobulillar sembrado de mazas; *D*, vaso con abundantes mazas apoyadas en la adventicia. Del Río-Hortega, P. (1922) Constitución histológica de la glándula pineal. I. Células Parenquimatosas. In *Libro en honor de D. Santiago Ramón y Cajal*, vol 1, 315–359. Madrid: Jiménez y Molina [Figure 2].

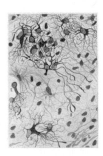

### FIGURE 106.

Del Río-Hortega, 1922. Structure of the pineal gland, II.

Agrupaciones celulares envueltas por neuroglia en la región superficial de la epífisis: *A, C, D, E*, células con penachos de apéndices, algunos claviformes; *B*, prolongaciones largas con ensanchamientos terminales; *F*, célula neuróglica; *G*, fibras neuróglicas abultadas en maza. Del Río-Hortega, P. (1922) Constitución histológica de la glándula pineal. I. Células Parenquimatosas. In *Libro en honor de D. Santiago Ramón y Cajal*, vol 1, 315–359. Madrid: Jiménez y Molina [Figure 6].

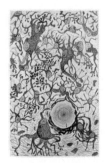

### FIGURE 107.

Del Río-Hortega, 1922. Structure of the pineal gland, III.

Células parenquimatosas hipertróficas en una pineal con marcados signos de regresión: *A, C, E*, corpúsculos gigantes con numerosos brazos tortuosos *F, H*, células profundamente alteradas por la proximidad de un acervulus (*I*); *B*, agrupación de expansiones abultadas; *D*, células de tipo más pequeño; *G*, neuroglia pálidamente teñida. Del Río-Hortega, P (1922) Constitución histológica de la glándula pineal. I. Células Parenquimatosas. In *Libro en honor de D. Santiago Ramón y Cajal*, vol 1, 315–359. Madrid: Jiménez y Molina [Figure 7].

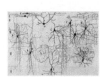

### FIGURE 108.

Lorente de Nó, 1922. Mouse cortical interneurons.

Células de axon corto de las capas I, II, III y IV. *A* y *B*, células cuyo axon genera un plexo vertical; *C*, célula de axon bipenachado; *D, F, H*, células de axon ascendente; *E*, células de axon corto, rudimentarias, de la capa I; *G*, célula cuyo axon da un plexo horizontal en la capa III; *I*, célula de axon corto glomerular (capa IV); *K*, célula de axon glomerular (capa V). Del Río-Hortega, P. (1922). La corteza cerebral del ratón. (Primera contribución.-La corteza acústica). *Trab. Lab. Invest. Biol. Univ. Madrid* 20, 41–78 [Figure 7].

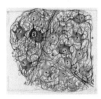

### FIGURE 109.

De Castro, 1922–1923. Semilunar ganglion.

Corte del ganglio semilunar del feto de término. Las células son estrelladas, sus dendritas, todavía delgadas, contienen numerosos retoños de ramillas; por el entrecruzamiento de unas prolongaciones con otras fórmase un intrincado plexo protoplásmico intercelular. *A*, fascículos de fibras de Remak y pregangliónicas; *d, e*, fibras aferentes ramificadas por el plexo protoplásmico; *a*, axon de una célula simpática. (Piridina alcohol.) De Castro, F. (1922–1923) Evolución de los ganglios simpáticos vertebrales y prevertebrales. Conexiones y citoarquitectonia de algunos grupos de ganglios, en el niño y hombre adulto. *Trab. Lab. Invest. Biol. Univ. Madrid* 20, 113–208 [Figure 42].

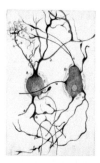

### FIGURE 110.

De Castro, 1922–1923. Human superior cervical ganglion cells, I.

Células grandes del ganglio cervical superior. Hombre de cuarenta y cinco años. *B*, célula cuyas dendritas se hacen filiformes y muestran en su trayecto ensanchamientos protoplásmicos reticulados, singularmente en los puntos de asiento de dicotomías (*f*); *A*, otra con iguales caracteres, aunque algo menos aparentes; *J*, dendrita que daba origen a una rama de colosal diámetro; *e*, arborización final de una dendrita formando una placa receptora; *a*, axon. De Castro, F. (1922–1923) Evolución de los ganglios simpáticos vertebrales y prevertebrales. Conexiones y citoarquitectonia de algunos grupos de ganglios, en el niño y hombre adulto. *Trab. Lab. Invest. Biol. Univ. Madrid* 20, 113–208 [Figure 17].

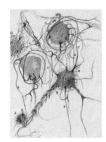

### FIGURE III.

De Castro, 1922–1923. Human superior cervical ganglion cells, II.

Células ganglionares del cervical superior. Hombre de cuarenta años. *A, D*, elementos con dendritas largas; *C, B*, otras con expansiones primordiales y accesorias; *b*, prolongación protoplásmica que lejos del soma formaba un complicado receptor *F*, al que llegaban dendritas de otros elementos vecinos; *e*, dendrita con dos receptores, en el trayecto y extremo *o, o'; g*, dendrita que constituía en toda su extensión un receptor y termina formando un nido pericelular *J*. y, en parte, en un fascículo; *f*. prolongación que acaba ramificándose en un fascículo; *a*, neuritas. De Castro, F. (1922–1923) Evolución de los ganglios simpáticos vertebrales y prevertebrales. Conexiones y citoarquitectonia de algunos grupos de ganglios, en el niño y hombre adulto. *Trab. Lab. Invest. Biol. Univ. Madrid* 20, 113–208 [Figure 18].

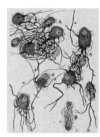

### FIGURE 112.

De Castro, 1922–1923. Human superior cervical ganglion cells, III.

Diversas modalidades de congregaciones neuronales en el cervical superior. Hombre de veinticinco años. *A*, glomérulo pluricelular; *B, C*, otros bicelulares; *I, e*, dendritas arborizadas en los zurrones dendríticos de otros elementos; *f*, dendrita arribada a un glomérulo; *a*, cilindro-eje. De Castro, F. (1922–1923) Evolución de los ganglios simpáticos vertebrales y prevertebrales. Conexiones y citoarquitectonia de algunos grupos de ganglios, en el niño y hombre adulto. *Trab. Lab. Invest. Biol. Univ. Madrid* 20, 113–208 [Figure 24].

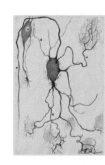

### FIGURE 113.

De Castro, 1922–1923. Human lumbar ganglion, I.

Ganglio lumbar de una mujer de treinta años. *A*, grueso elemento simpático, cuyas dendritas se ramificaban por la zona de dispersión de las dendritas accesorias de otros elementos (*e, f, g, d*); *b, c*, extremos de expansiones terminadas en tractos protoplásmicos; *a*, axon. De Castro, F. (1922–1923) Evolución de los ganglios simpáticos vertebrales y prevertebrales. Conexiones y citoarquitectonia de algunos grupos de ganglios, en el niño y hombre adulto. *Trab. Lab. Invest. Biol. Univ. Madrid* 20, 113–208 [Figure 38].

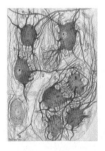

### FIGURE 114.

De Castro, 1922–1923. Human lumbar ganglion, II.

Corte de un ganglio lumbar. Hombre de treinta y ocho años. *f*, nido dendrítico pericelular; *d*, expansión protoplásmica larga que remata entre las dendritas accesorias de otro elemento; *b, g*, matorrales de dendritas accesorias; *e*, prolongaciones protoplásmicas con tallos colaterales; *c*, dendrita rematada en maza; *a*, fibra aferente ramificada, en parte, por el matorral dendrítico, *g*. De Castro, F. (1922–1923) Evolución de los ganglios simpáticos vertebrales y prevertebrales. Conexiones y citoarquitectonia de algunos grupos de ganglios, en el niño y hombre adulto. *Trab. Lab. Invest. Biol. Univ. Madrid* 20, 113–208 [Figure 39].

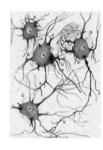

### FIGURE 115.

De Castro, 1922–1923. Cells of the human semilunar ganglion, I.

Células del ganglio semilunar del niño. *A*, célula con dendritas primordiales y accesorias; *D*, otra cuyas expansiones accesorias o cortas se esparcen en finas ramillas por un paraje ocupado por elementos satélites (glomérulo). *C*, elemento con dendritas primordiales o largas sólo. (*A, D, C*, del niño de once años); *B*, otra neurona simpática cuyas dendritas largas poseen numerosos tallos colaterales (niño de trece años); *d*, dendritas cortas o accesorias y tallos colaterales; *e. c*, terminación de unas dendritas largas; *a*, axon. De Castro, F. (1922–1923) Evolución de los ganglios simpáticos vertebrales y prevertebrales. Conexiones y citoarquitectonia de algunos grupos de ganglios, en el niño y hombre adulto. *Trab. Lab. Invest. Biol. Univ. Madrid* 20, 113–208 [Figure 45].

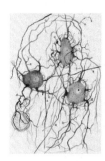

### FIGURE 116.

De Castro, 1922–1923. Cells of the human semilunar ganglion, II.

Células simpáticas del ganglio semilunar de una mujer de treinta años, muerta por precipitación. *d*, dendrita primordial con tallos colaterales y terminada en ovilıo o nido dendrítico pericelular; *b, g, f*, dendritas con numerosos tallos colaterales; *n*, terminación de una de estas dendritas; *d*, receptor en forma de cáliz; *e*, otra con pocos tallos colaterales; 1, prolongación protoplásmica cubierta de tallitos a modo de uñas en la primera porción; *m*, dendrita accesoria; *c*, otra terminada en bola; *a*, axon; *o*, rama colateral esparcida por el ganglio. De Castro, F. (1922–1923) Evolución de los ganglios simpáticos vertebrales y prevertebrales. Conexiones y citoarquitectonia de algunos grupos de ganglios, en el niño y hombre adulto. *Trab. Lab. Invest. Biol. Univ. Madrid* 20, 113–208 [Figure 46].

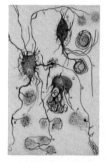

### FIGURE 117.

De Castro, 1922–1923. Cells of the human superior cervical ganglion.

Celulas del ganglio cervical superior del hombre de cuarenta años. *B*, elemento que forma dos nidos dendríticos pericelulares; *C*, otro cuyas expansiones robustas abrazaban el soma de una neurona simpática; *D*, placa receptora; *b, c, o, f.* prolongaciones largas terminadas entre las expansiones de otros ele· mentos; *a*, axon; *d*, neurita que emitía varias colaterales cortas cerca de otro elemento. De Castro, F. (1922–1923) Evolución de los ganglios simpáticos vertebrales y prevertebrales. Conexiones y citoarquitectonia de algunos grupos de ganglios, en el niño y hombre adulto. *Trab. Lab. Invest. Biol. Univ. Madrid* 20, 113–208 [Figure 23].

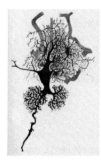

### FIGURE 118.

Berlucchi, 1923. Glial cells and blood vessels.

Rapporti tra ciuffi di proliferazione dendritica, cellule di glía e vasi sanguigni. Metodo della reazione nera. Oc. 4 comp., obb. apocr. 3 mm 0,96 Zeiss tubo 160 alt. tav. (ridotta a 2/3). Berlucchi, C. (1923) Le cellule polimorfe della fascia dentata in animali allo stato di senilità. *Riv. Patol. Nerv. Ment.* 28, 241–256 [Figure 5].

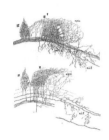

### FIGURE 119.

Lorente de Nó, 1924. Extrinsic fibers traveling in the longitudinal posterior fascicle to acoustic nuclei.

Indian ink drawing made by Lorente de Nó in Upsala, Sweden, when he was 22 years old. The drawing derives from a Golgi-impregnated, longitudinal section and it discloses extrinsic fibers traveling in the longitudinal posterior fascicle (f.l.p.). Axonal terminals resolve successively in the neuropil of the occulomotor (i.e., IV and III) and solitary tract (n.i.f.) nuclei. The bottom drawing depicts the mode of individual parent axons traveling in the postro-dorsal fascicle and a reticular core bundle (r.t.) resolving in the motor and solitary tract nuclei; the latter fibers were regarded by Lorente de Nó as the connectional substrate accounting for the role of reticular nuclei in influencing eye reflexes.

Rafael Lorente de Nó (1902–1990) was the last and best-known of Santiago Ramón y Cajal's disciples; he spent most of his active researcher life working at the Rockefeller Institute in the United States. Born in Zaragoza, Spain in 1902, Lorente de Nó worked first under Pedro Ramón y Cajal's supervision and, from 1919 to 1934, with Santiago Ramón y Cajal. In addition to Santiago Ramón y Cajal himself, Lorente de Nó worked with two of the most influential neuroscientists of the last century, namely, Rober Bárany in Sweden and Oskar Vogt in Germany. Lorente de Nó's most important contributions to neuroscience related to cytological organization of the brain and to nerve physiology. His early Lorente de Nó works, made when he was a teenager, involved classic silver impregnations combined with a variety of surgical and experimental approaches. Contributions of Lorente de Nó to basic neurocytology included the internal organization, neuron types, and local connectivity from the auditory, entorhinal, and somato-sensory isocortices, as well as to the Ammon´s horn. Still working in the Santiago Ramón y Cajal and Bárány laboratories, Lorente de Nó made a series of publications describing the neuronal circuitry of the primary brain stem and reticular nuclei. Lorente de Nó was a gifted scientist: a polyglot with an outstanding memory and a versatile intellect, which together with his strong, almost belligerent character, made him a rather controversial person. The strength of his scientific contributions is evidenced by their actual impact. Among these are the modular (i.e., columnar) organization, the synaptic delay, synaptic summation, nerve volume conduction, and cybernetic (negative feedback) neuron circuit. The three figures (119, 133, and 136) presented here belong to Lorente de Nó's extensive monograph on the primary acoustic nuclei. The text and figures are provided by Dr. Jorge Larriva-Sahd.  Lorente de Nó, R. (1976) Some unsolved problems concerning the cochlear nerve. *Ann. Otol. Rhinol. Laryngol.* (Suppl. 34) 85, 1–28.

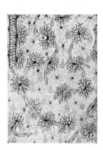

## FIGURE 120.

Del Río-Hortega, 1925. Perivascular neuroglia, I.

Distribución de la neuroglia perivascular en la corteza cerebral (Imagen compuesta con detalles observados en varias preparaciones).  Del Río-Hortega, P. (1925) Algunas observaciones acerca de la neuroglia perivascular. Boletin de la Sociedad Española de Historia Natural, abril de 1925. (Pág. 1–21 y 184–210) [Figure 1].

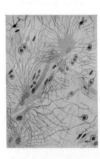

## FIGURE 121.

Del Río-Hortega, 1925. Perivascular neuroglia, II.

Gliocitos perivasculares muy aplanados, pertenecientes a la región ammónica del cerebro humano. En la figura existen, además, algunos corpúsculos microgliales y de oligodendroglía, caracterizados estos últimos por su forma redondeada y sus escasas expansiones varicosas. Técnica: carbonato argéntico.  Del Río-Hortega, P. (1925) Algunas observaciones acerca de la neuroglia perivascular. Boletin de la Sociedad Española de Historia Natural, abril de 1925. (Pág. 1–21 y 184–210) [Figure 9].

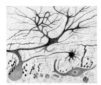

## FIGURE 122.

Ramón y Cajal, 1926. Purkinje cells in a case of dementia precox.

Morceau de la couche moléculaire du cervelet dans un cas de démence précoce compliquée; *A*, cellule de Purkinje pourvue de dendrites aberrantes; *a*, branche se terminant au moyen d'une étoile *(b)*; *B*, corpuscule de Purkinje en voie d'atrophie; *C*, renflement considérable d'une tige protoplasmique.  Ramón y Cajal, S. (1926) Sur quelques lésions du cervelet dans un cas de démence précoce. *Trav. Lab. Recherches. Biol. Univ. Madrid* 24, 181–190 [Figure 1].

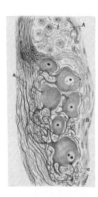

## FIGURE 123.

De Castro, 1926. Structure and innervation of the carotid body, I.

Segment d'une branche sympathique carotidienne du chat adulte douze jours après avoir sectionné le nerf glossopharyngien: *B*, microganglion sympathique avec ses fibres préganglionnaires a arrivées de la moelle épinière; *c*, glomérule dendritique avec des fibrilles préganglionnaires terminées en anneau; *A*, petit glomérule glandulaire dénervé enchâssé dans le trajet du nerf sympathique; *f*, cellules glandulaires sans terminaison dans lesquelles celle-ci a dégénéré. Pyridine, nitrate d'argent réduit.  De Castro, F. (1926) Sur la structure et l'innervation de la glande intercarotidienne (glomus caroticum) de l'homme et des mammifères, et sur un nouveau système d'innervation autonome du nerf glosopharyngien. *Trav. Lab. Rech. Biol.* 24, 365–432 [Figure 11].

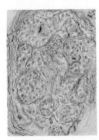

## FIGURE 124.

De Castro, 1926. Structure and innervation of the carotid body, II.

Coupe de la glande intercarotidienne humaine (Femme de vingt ans, morte subitement par accident et dont l'autopsie a été faite trois heures après la mort). Hydrate de chloral, nitrate d'argent réduit; coloration nucléaire à l'hématoxyline. *c*, fascicule à fibres médullées et amédullées; *g*, plexus périglomérulaire; *f*, fibres médullées coupées

de travers; *c*, collatérales à axones myéliniques; *d*, cellules glandulaires isolées; *v*, vaisseaux sanguins. Dans le plexus intraglomérulaire les fibres terminent à l'aide d'anneaux ou de petites massues sur les cellules (terminaisons épilemmales).  De Castro, F. (1926) Sur la structure et l'innervation de la glande intercarotidienne (glomus caroticum) de l'homme et des mammifères, et sur un nouveau système d'innervation autonome du nerf glosopharyngien. *Trav. Lab. Rech. Biol.* 24, 365–432. [Figure 8].

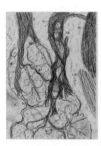

## FIGURE 125.

De Castro, 1926. Structure and innervation of the carotid body, III.

Fragment d'une coupe de la glande intercarotidienne de la souris d'un mois el demi; IX^e paire; *LX*, branche pharyngienne de la X^e paire; *C, nerf intercarotidien; c, g*. cellules sympathiques sur le trajet de ce nerf ; *f*, terminaisons des fibres du plexus intraglomérulaire; *a*, axones du *nerf intercarotidien* qui pénètrent dans la branche sympathique carotidienne *E; A*, artère. Fixation en sommiphène azotique. Coupe horizontale et légèrement oblique de la tête.  De Castro, F. (1926) Sur la structure et l'innervation de la glande intercarotidienne (glomus caroticum) de l'homme et des mammifères, et sur un nouveau système d'innervation autonome du nerf glosopharyngien. *Trav. Lab. Rech. Biol.* 24, 365–432. [Figure 10].

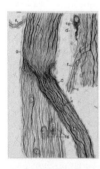

## FIGURE 126.

De Castro, 1926. Structure and innervation of the carotid body, IV.

Coupe longitudinale du nerf glossopharyngien *G, G'*, du rat de deux mois: *C, nerf intercarotidien; g,ce*, éléments sympathiques; *e*, division d'une fibre médullée; *c*, collatérale d'un *gros* axone destiné à une branche sympathique; *f*, branche pour un nerf sympathique. Somniphène azotique.  De Castro, F. (1926) Sur la structure et l'innervation de la glande intercarotidienne (glomus caroticum) de l'homme et des mammifères, et sur un nouveau système d'innervation autonome du nerf glosopharyngien. *Trav. Lab. Rech. Biol.* 24, 365–432 [Figure 16].

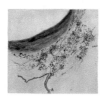

**FIGURE 127.**

De Castro, 1926. Structure and innervation of the carotid body, V.

Vaste arborisation terminale sensitive (type I) du sinus carotidien du chat adulte. Méthode d'Ehrlich-Dogiel modifiée : A, tube nerveux médullé qui donne naissance à la terminaison. Gr. 450 diamètres. De Castro, F. (1926) Sur la structure et l'innervation de la glande intercarotidienne (glomus caroticum) de l'homme et des mammifères, et sur un nouveau système d'innervation autonome du nerf glosopharyngien. *Trav. Lab. Rech. Biol.* 24, 365–432 [Figure 8].

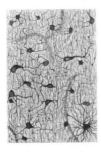

**FIGURE 128.**

Del Río-Hortega, 1928. Oligodendrocytes in the cat cerebellar white matter.

Conjunto de oligodendrocitos en la substancia blanca cerebelosa de gato. Las expansiones protoplásmicas forman rico plexo envolviendo a fibras nerviosas y vasos. Del Río-Hortega, P. (1928) Tercera aportacion al conocimiento morfologico e interpretacion funcional de la oligodendroglia. *Mem. R. Soc. Esp. Hist. Nat.* 14, 5–122 [Figure 12].

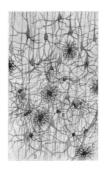

**FIGURE 129.**

Del Río-Hortega, 1928. Cerebral cortex of the cat.

Aspecto de la corteza cerebral de gato con neuronas (*A*); oligodendroglía (*B*); glía protoplásmica (*C*), y vasos (*D*). Del Río-Hortega, P. (1928) Tercera aportacion al conocimiento morfologico e interpretacion funcional de la oligodendroglia. *Mem. R. Soc. Esp. Hist. Nat.* 14, 5–122 [Figure 24].

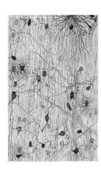

**FIGURE 130.**

Del Río-Hortega, 1928. Neuroglial elements of the cat cerebral white matter.

Elementos neuróglicos de la substancia blanca cerebral de gato. *A,* oligodendrocitos con largas expansiones que siguen a fibras nerviosas; *B, C, D,* oligodendrocitos con numerosos apéndices divididos en *T; E, F,* astrocitos enanos; *G,* astrocito fibroso. Del Río-Hortega, P. (1928) Tercera aportacion al conocimiento morfologico e interpretacion funcional de la oligodendroglia. *Mem. R. Soc. Esp. Hist. Nat.* 14, 5–122 [Figure 28].

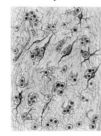

**FIGURE 131.**

Del Río-Hortega, 1928. Proliferation of cortical oligodendrocytes in paralytic dementia.

Tumefacción transparente y proliferación de los oligodendrocitos de la corteza cerebral en la demencia paralítica. *A,* pléyade vascular; *B,C,* grupos perineuronales (pseudoneuronofagía); *D,* microglía; *E,* célula endotelial con inclusiones; *F,* fibras nerviosas recubiertas por expansiones de oligodendrocitos. (Carbonato argéntico.) Del Río-Hortega, P. (1928) Tercera aportacion al conocimiento morfologico e interpretacion funcional de la oligodendroglia. *Mem. R. Soc. Esp. Hist. Nat.* 14, 5–122 [Figure 61].

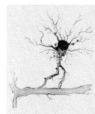

**FIGURE 132.**

Berlucchi, 1930. Glial cell of the human white matter.

Cellula gliale come nella figura precedente osservata a più forte ingrandimento. Berlucchi, C. (1930) Ricerche intorno ad alcuni reperti istologici nel sistema nervoso centrale dei feti e dei neonati. *Riv. Patol. Nerv. Ment.* 35, 69–182 [Figure 2].

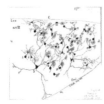

**FIGURE 133.**

Lorente de Nó, 1931. Neurons in the acoustic nucleus.

This figure shows cells impregnated with the Golgi-Cox method as observed in a transverse section through the oral end of the ventral acoustic nucleus. Although brush cells are the most numerous, other distinct neuron-types may also be seen. Cells 2, 7, 8, 12, and 14 correspond to basket, projecting cells. Neurons 4 to 6, 9 to 11, and 13 correspond to medium-sized short axon cells. Cell 3 is a giant short axon neuron having two long dendrites piercing the external marginal (*left*) and internal marginal (l.m.i.) laminae. (The text and figure are provided by Dr. Jorge Larriva-Sahd. See legend of Figure 119 for further details.) Drawing published in: Lorente de Nó, R. (1976) Some unsolved problems concerning the cochlear nerve. *Ann. Otol. Rhinol. Laryngol.* (Suppl. 34) 85, 1–28.

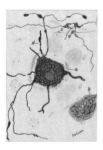

**FIGURE 134.**

De Castro, 1932–1933. Section of sympathetic ganglion.

Coupe de ganglion sympathique de chat, greffé depuis 6 jours dans un muscle du même animal: *a, b,* cellules ganglionnaires avec dégénération hydropique; la substance neurofibrillaire est coagulée et ressemble à un squelette spongieux; *d,* dendrite altérée et avec rétraction longitudinale; *c,* processus d'altération dans une plaque réceptrice. De Castro, F. (1932–1933) Quelques recherches sur la transplantation de ganglions nerveux (cérebro-spinaux et sympathiques) chez les mammifères. Etudes comparatives sur la capacité réactionnelle et la résistance vitale des neurones survivants dans les greffes. *Trav. Lab. Rech. Biol.* 28, 237–302 [Figure 14].

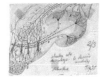

**FIGURE 135.**

Ramón y Cajal, 1933. Diagram of the connections of the hippocampus.

Esquema encaminado a presentar la conexión establecida entre el axón de los granos de la *fascia dentata* y las gruesas pirámides del Asta de Ammon (región inferior de ésta). *A,* capa moñecular de la *fascia dentata*; *B,* axón de los granos; *C,* pirámides grandes; *D,* fimbria; *c, b,* fibras aferentes llegadas de los centros olfativos secundarios; *a,* axón. Las flechas señalan la dirección de las corrientes. Ramón y Cajal, S. (1933) ¿Neuronismo o reticularismo? Las pruebas objetivas de la unidad anatómica de las células nerviosas. *Arch. Neurobiol.* 13, 1–144 [Figure 39].

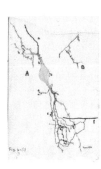

**FIGURE 136.**

Lorente de Nó, 1934. Efferent neuron in the ventral acoustic nucleus.

Axons were drawn with India ink and a neuron cytoplasm (i.e., soma plus dendrites) with watercolors.

A. Branches of a cochlear fiber (f) provide multiple contacts (e1–e4) with dendrites of a putative efferent neuron (shaded). Presynaptic boutons (b) without identifiable stem axons. B. Another cochlear fiber (f1) originating terminal boutons (i) terminating in a dendritic shaft (shaded). (The text and figure are provided by Dr. Jorge Larriva-Sahd. See legend of Figure 119 for further details.) Lorente de Nó, R. (1976) Some unsolved problems concerning the cochlear nerve. *Ann. Otol. Rhinol.* Laryngol. (Suppl. 34) 85, 1–28.

# THE COLORFUL PERIOD: INTERNAL STRUCTURE AND CHEMISTRY OF THE CELLS

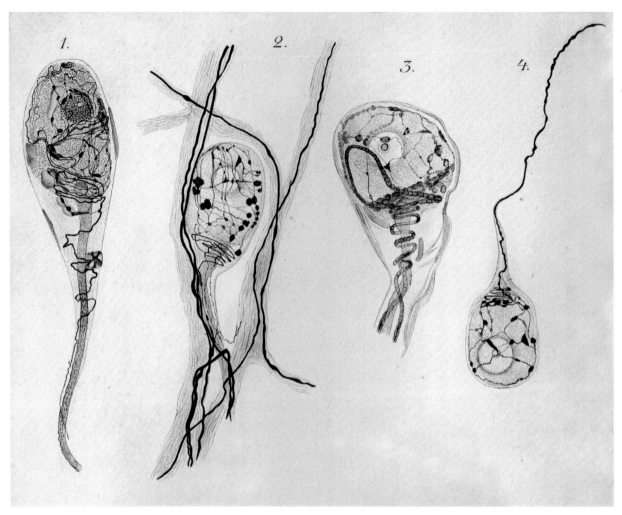

**FIGURE 137.** Smirnow, 1890. Structure of sympathetic nerve cells.

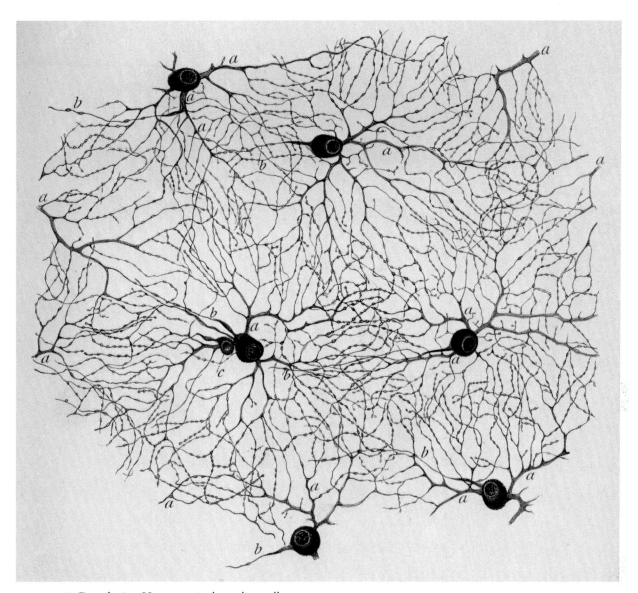

FIGURE 138. Dogiel, 1891. Human retinal ganglion cells.

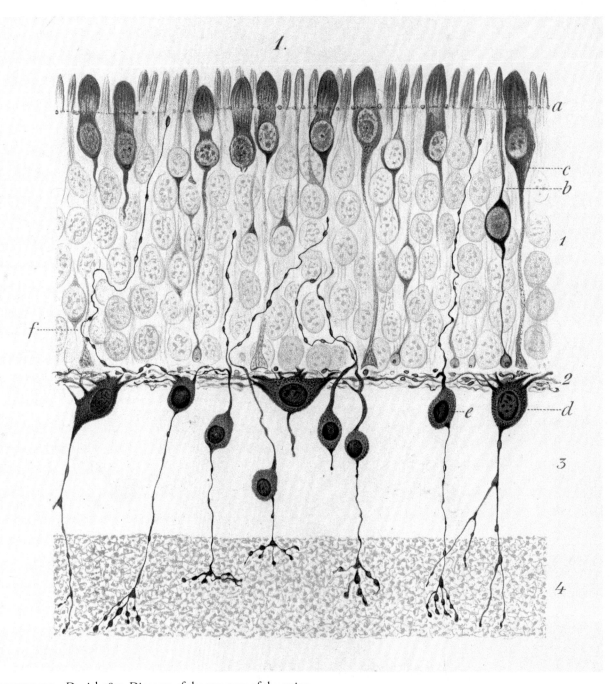

**FIGURE 139.** Dogiel, 1891. Diagram of the structure of the retina.

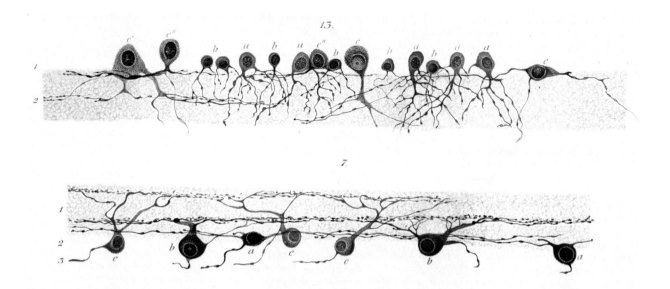

**FIGURE 140.** Dogiel, 1891. Nerve cells of the human retina.

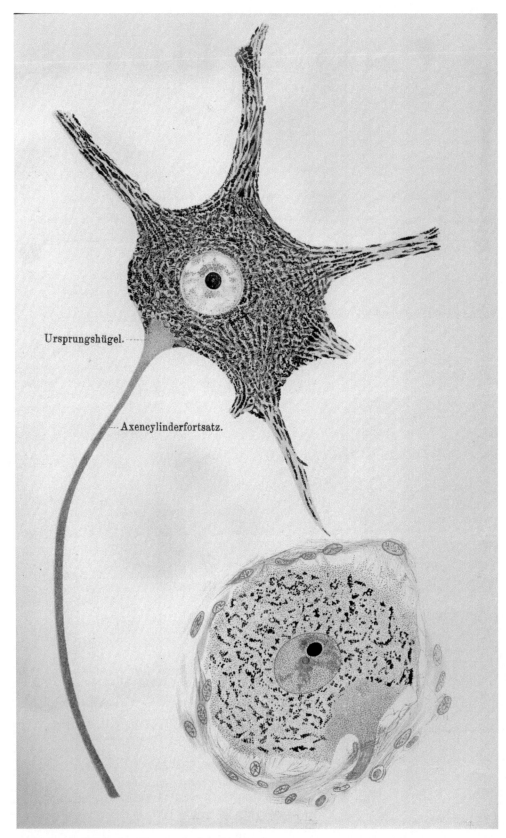

Ursprungshügel.

Axencylinderfortsatz.

**FIGURE 141.** Held, 1895. Neurons in the spinal cord.

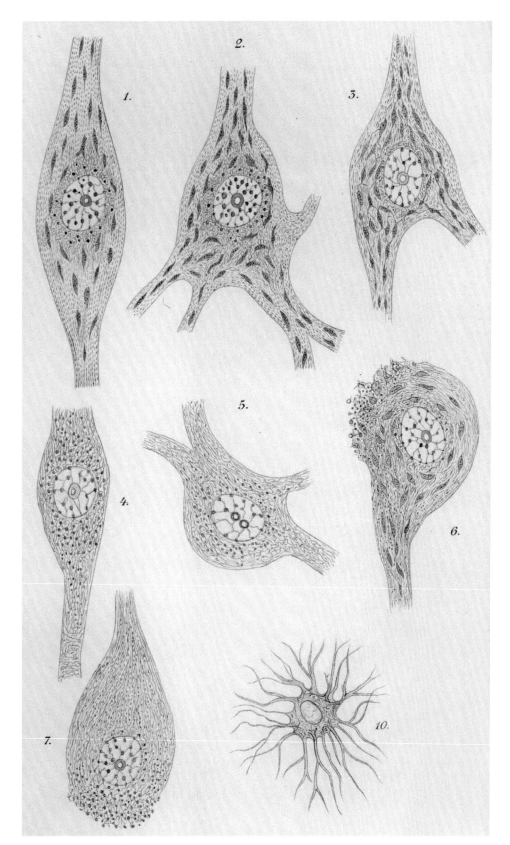

**FIGURE 142.** Arnold, 1898. Cells from the spinal cord of the cow.

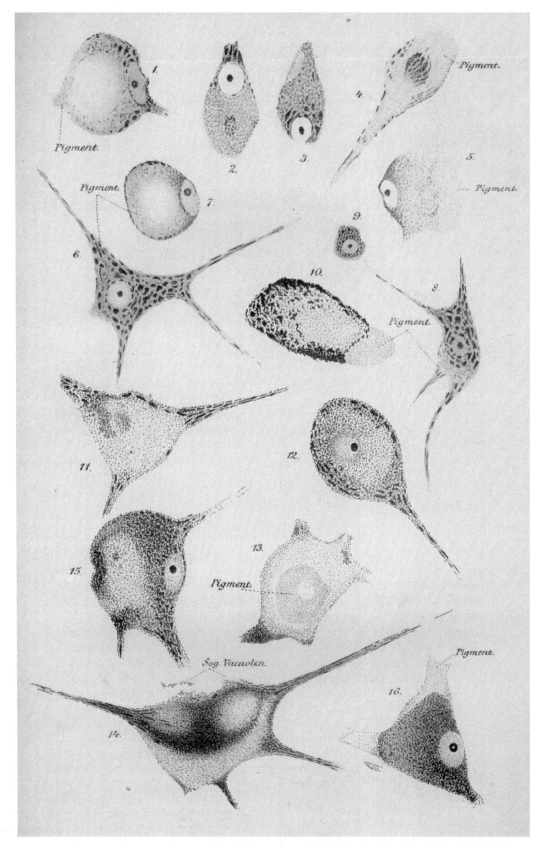

**FIGURE 143.** Juliusburger and Meyer, 1898. Ganglion cells of the spinal cord.

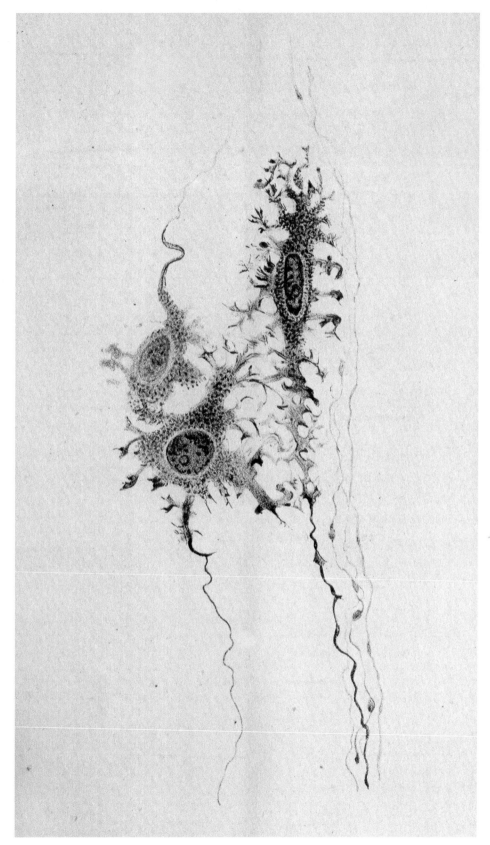

FIGURE 144. Dogiel, 1899. Cells of the Auerbach plexus.

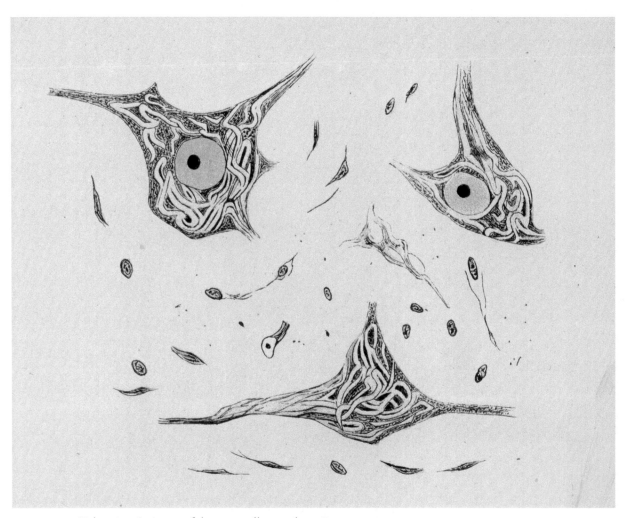

FIGURE 145. Nelis, 1899. Structure of the nerve cell protoplasm, I.

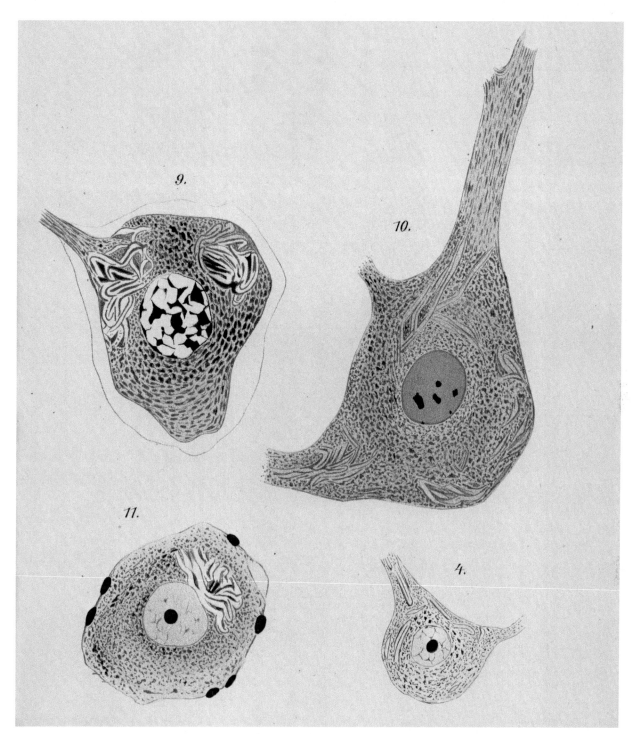

**FIGURE 146.** Nelis, 1899. Structure of the nerve cell protoplasm, II.

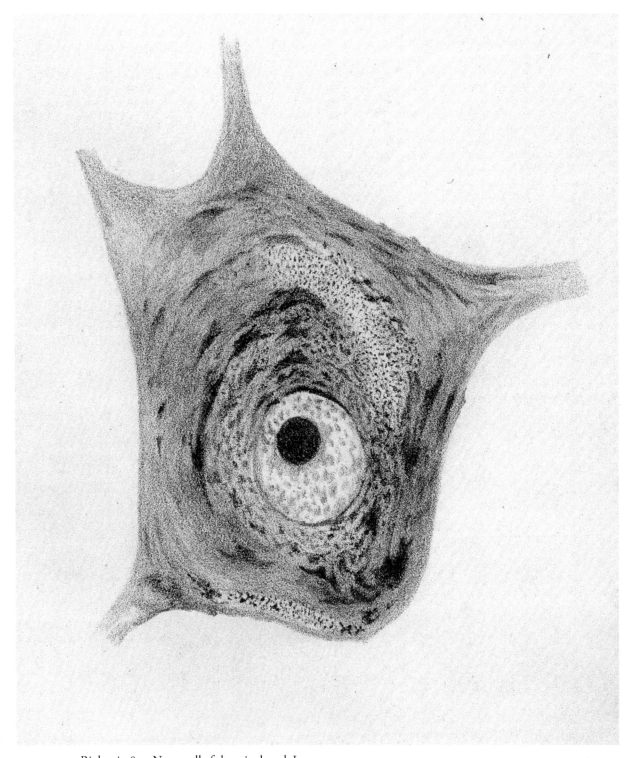

**FIGURE 147.** Righetti, 1899. Nerve cell of the spinal cord, I.

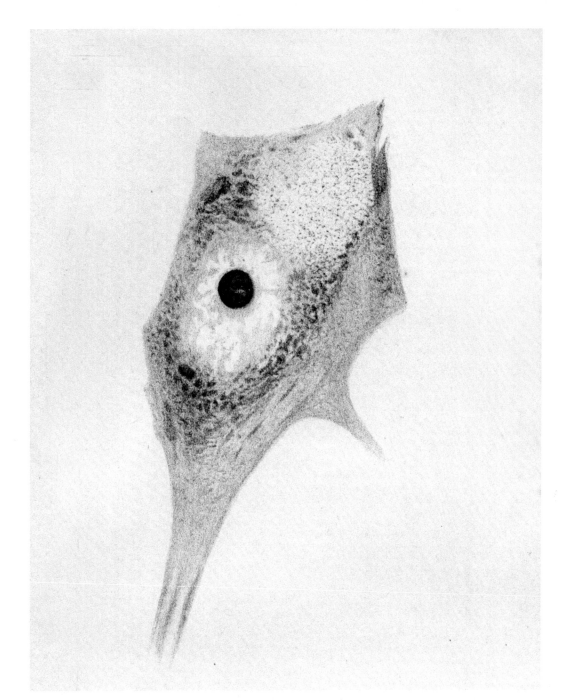

**FIGURE 148.** Righetti, 1899. Nerve cell of the spinal cord, II.

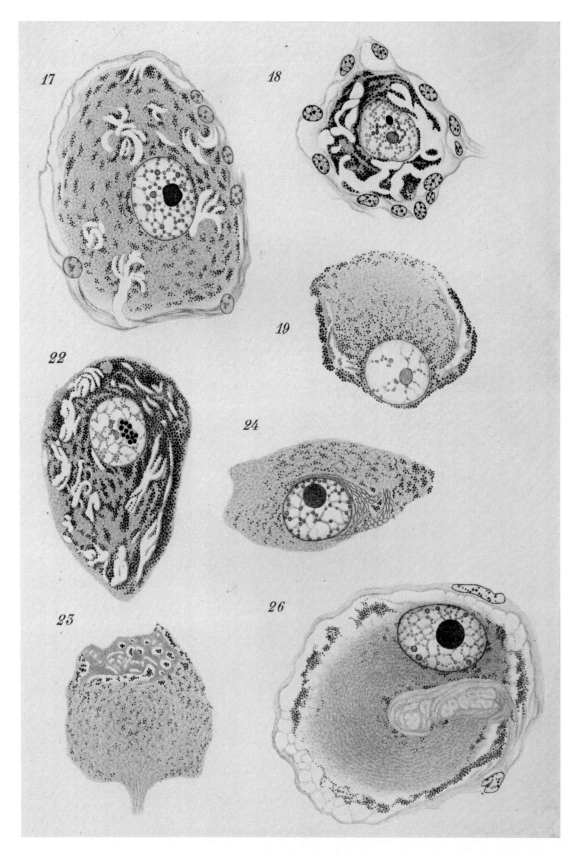

**FIGURE 149.** Holmgren, 1900. Fine structure of nerve cells, I.

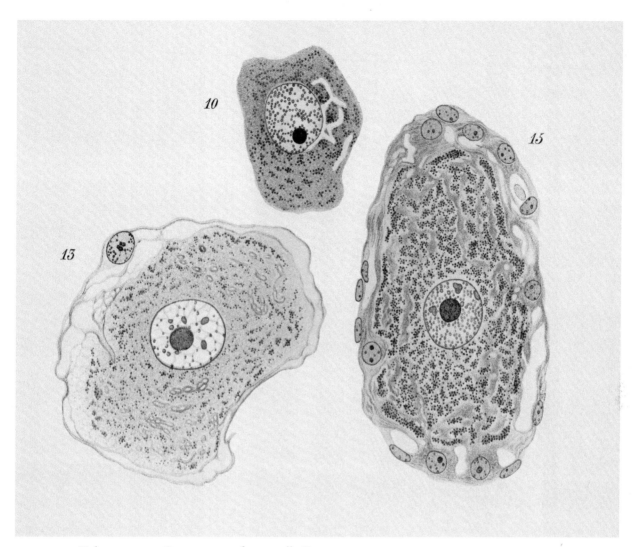

FIGURE 150. Holmgren, 1900. Fine structure of nerve cells, II.

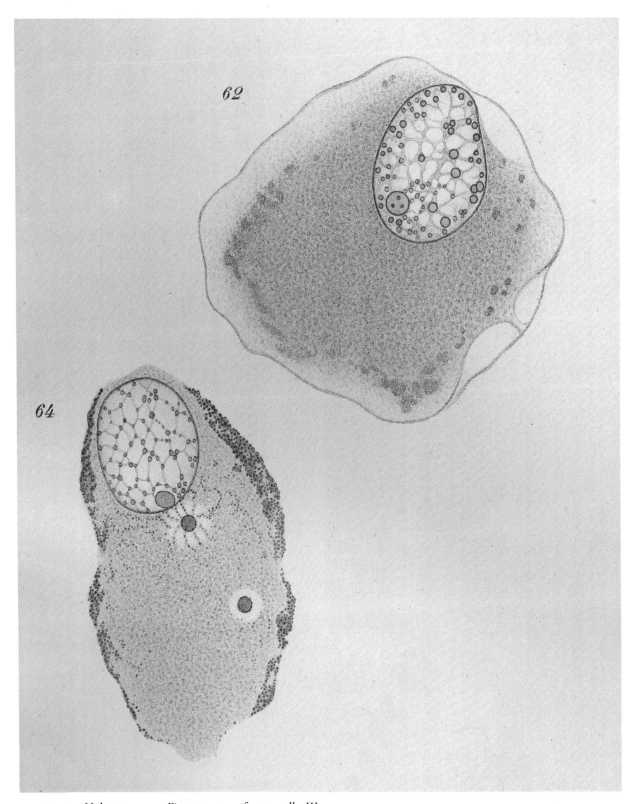

**FIGURE 151.** Holmgren, 1900. Fine structure of nerve cells, III.

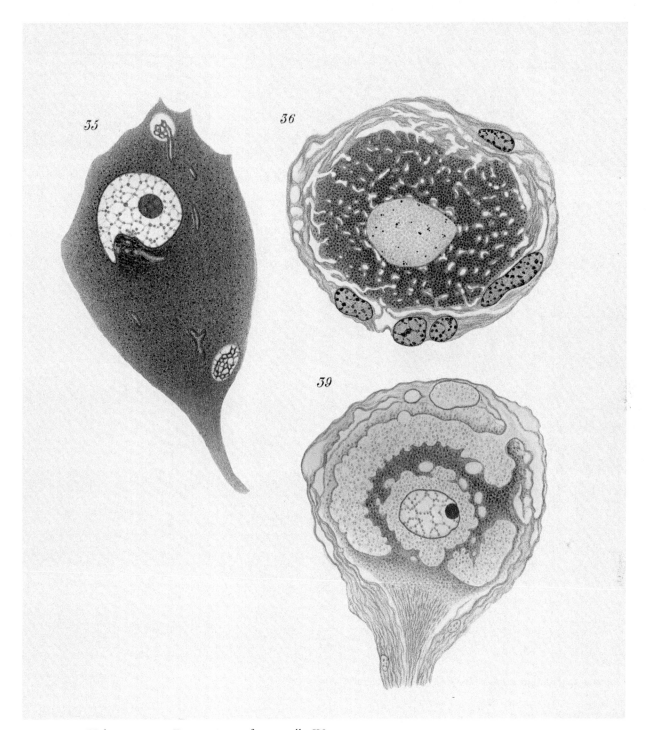

**FIGURE 152.** Holmgren, 1900. Fine structure of nerve cells, IV.

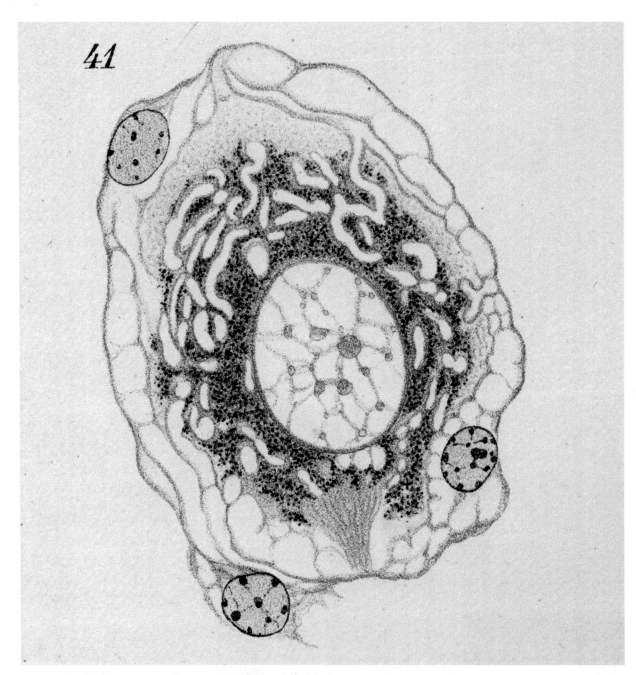

**FIGURE 153.** Holmgren, 1900. Fine structure of nerve cells, V.

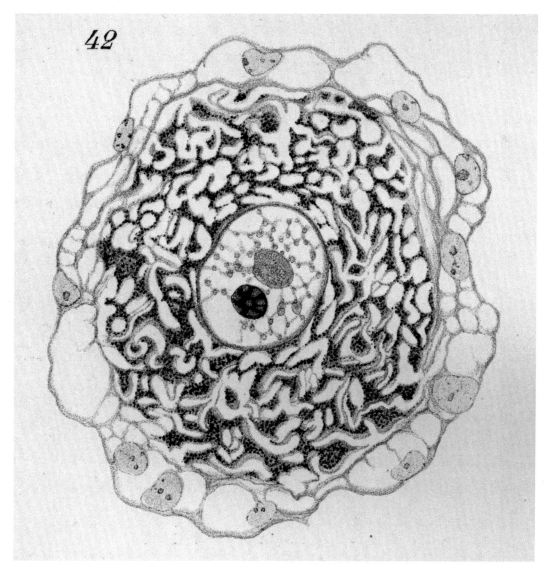

FIGURE 154. Holmgren, 1900. Fine structure of nerve cells, VI.

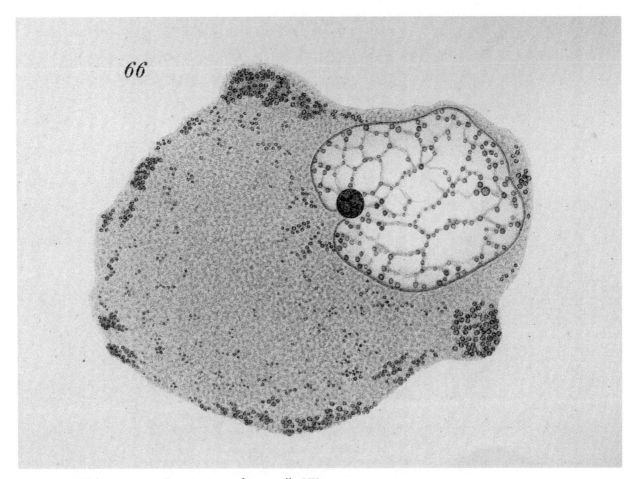

**FIGURE 155.** Holmgren, 1900. Fine structure of nerve cells, VII.

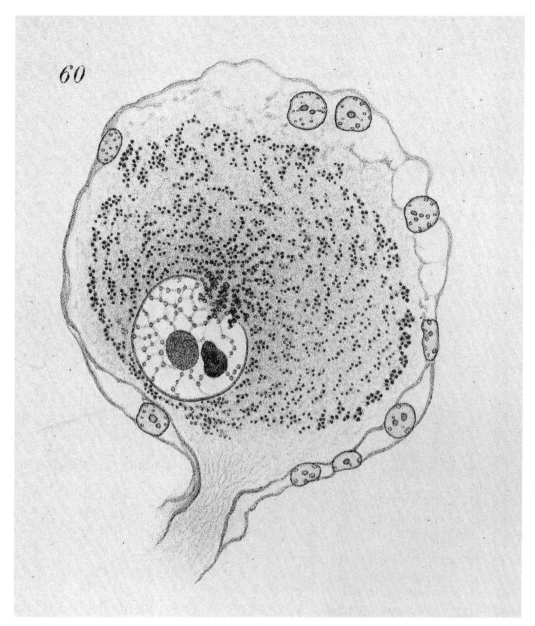

**FIGURE 156.** Holmgren, 1900. Fine structure of nerve cells, VIII.

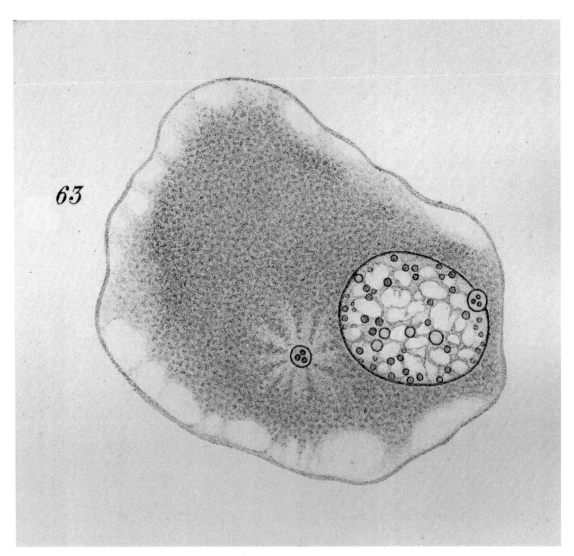

FIGURE 157. Holmgren, 1900. Fine structure of nerve cells, IX.

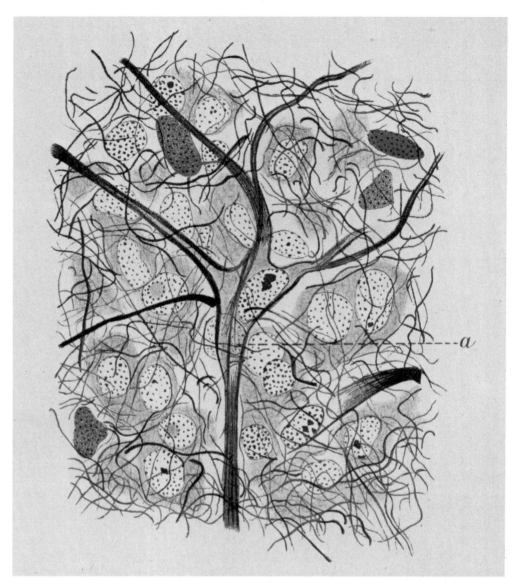

**FIGURE 158.** Dimitrova, 1901. Structure of the pineal gland.

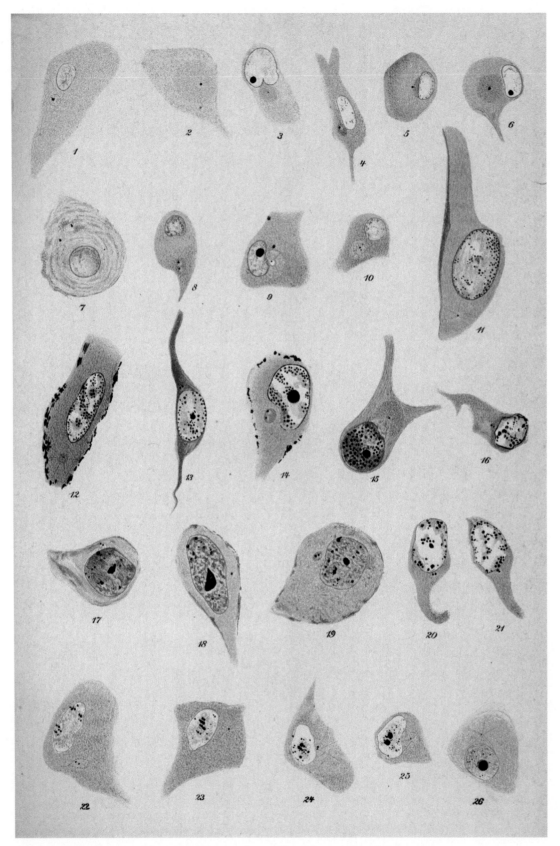

**FIGURE 159.** Kolster, 1901. Structure of anterior horn cells of the spinal cord, I.

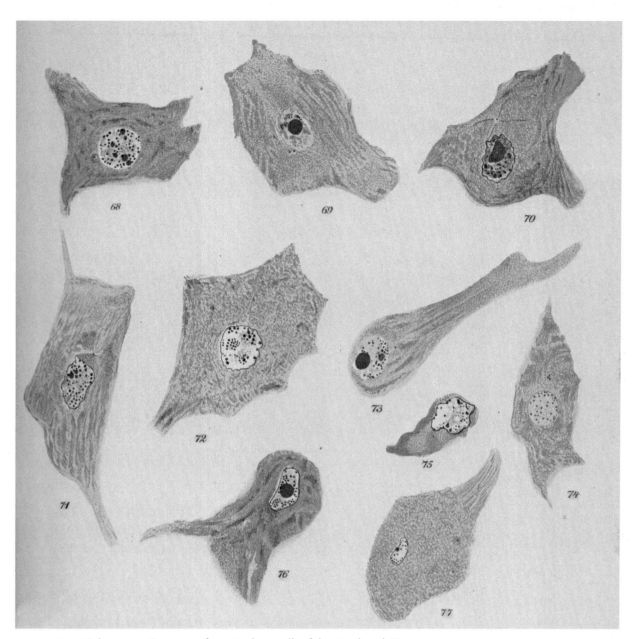

FIGURE 160. Kolster, 1901. Structure of anterior horn cells of the spinal cord, II.

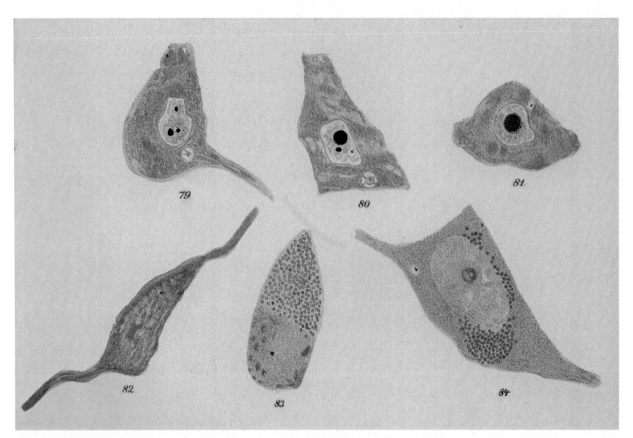

**FIGURE 161.** Kolster, 1901. Structure of anterior horn cells of the spinal cord, III.

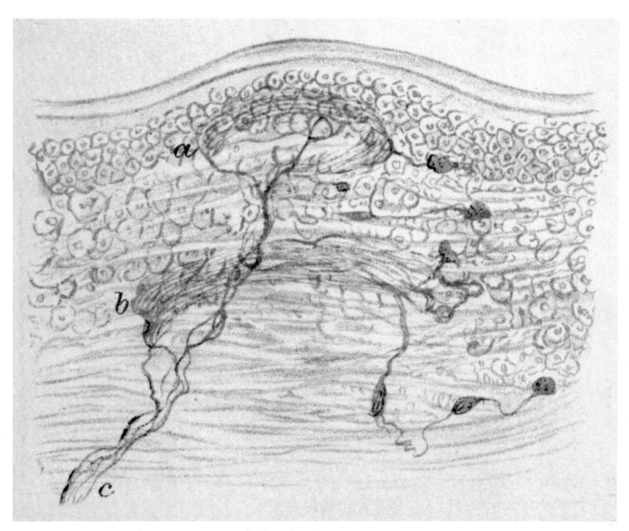

**FIGURE 162.** Leontowitsch, 1901. Innervation of human skin, I.

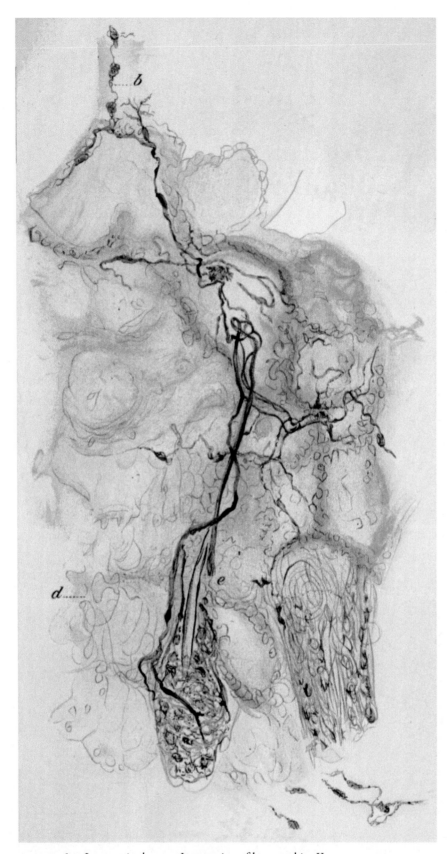

**FIGURE 163.** Leontowitsch, 1901. Innervation of human skin, II.

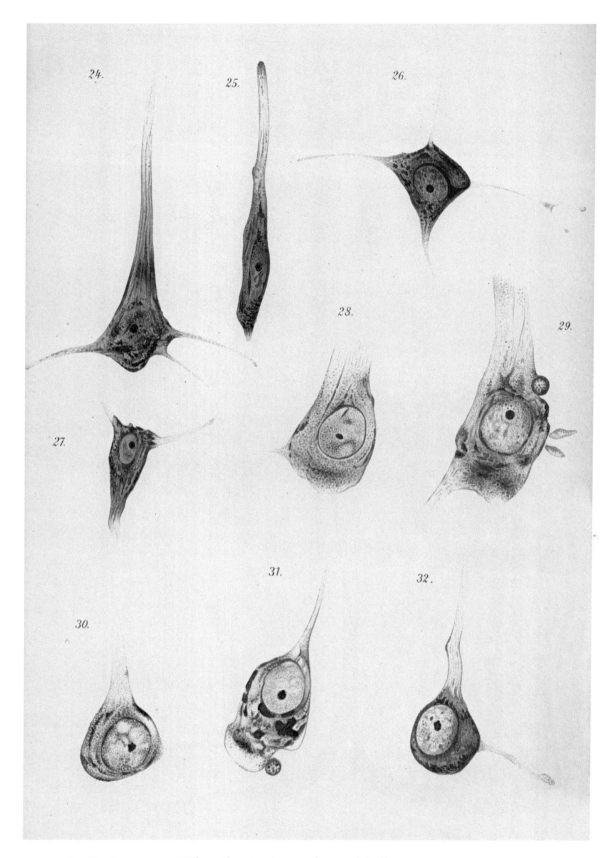

**FIGURE 164.** Van Durme, 1901. Different functional states of pyramidal cells.

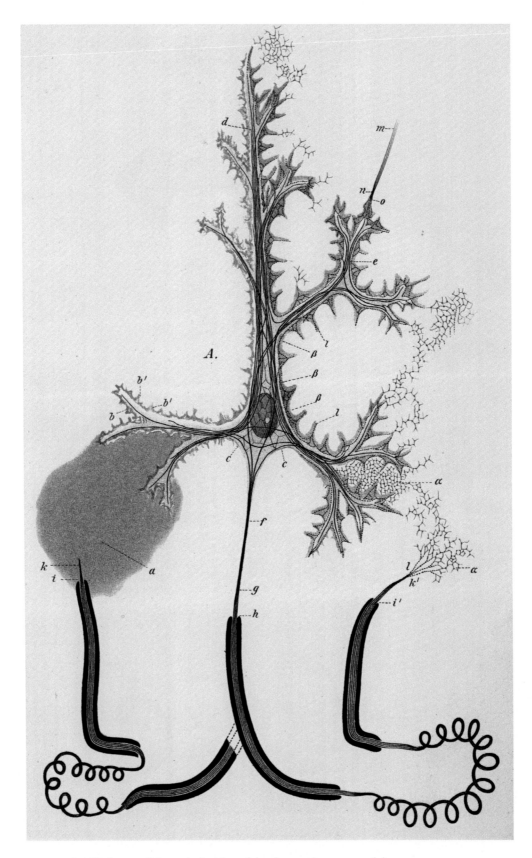

**FIGURE 165.** Nissl, 1903. Schematic drawing of the elemental structure of the nervous system.

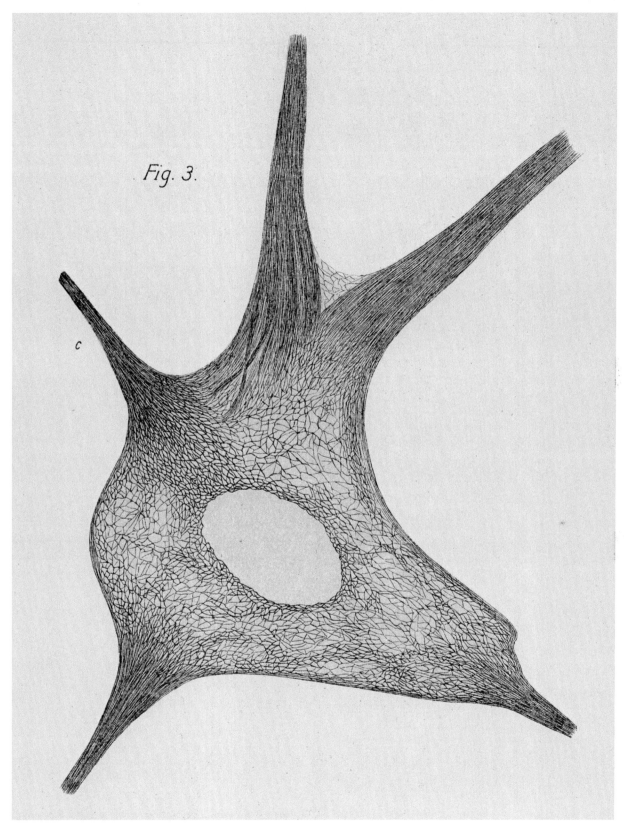

FIGURE 166. Donaggio, 1904. Endocellular fibrillary reticulum.

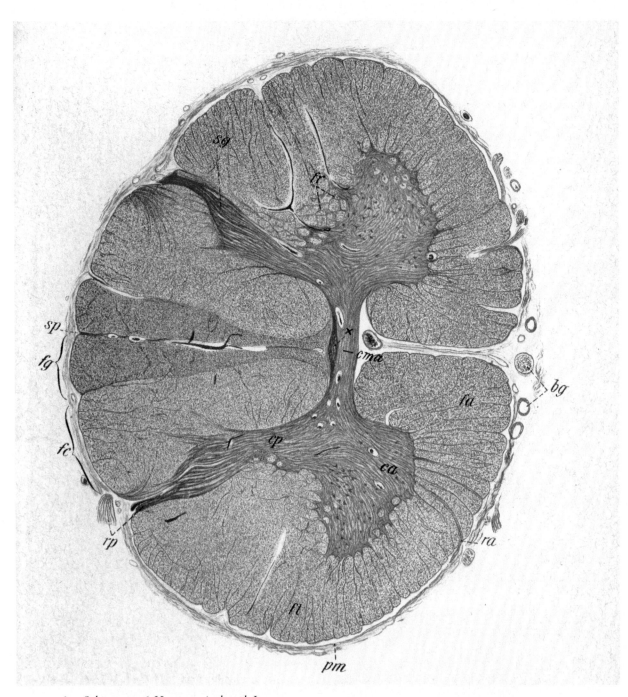

**FIGURE 167.** Sobotta, 1906. Human spinal cord, I.

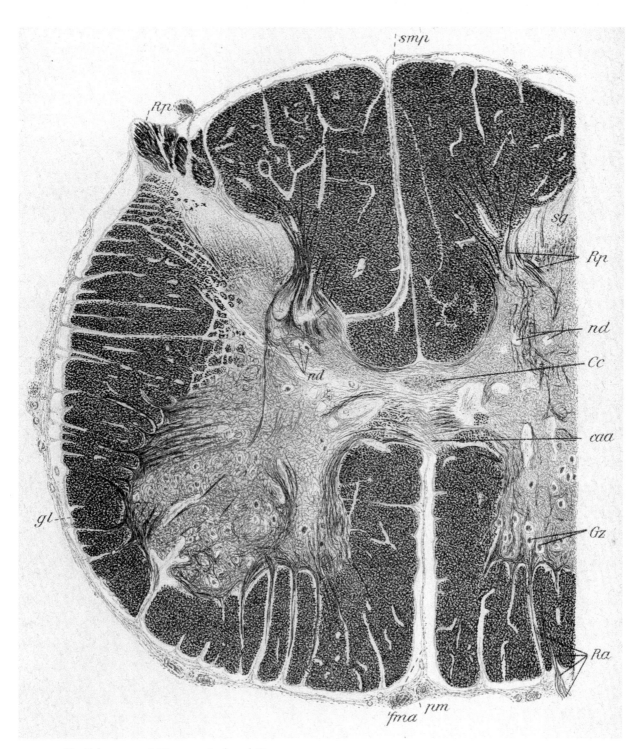

**FIGURE 168.** Sobotta, 1906. Human spinal cord, II.

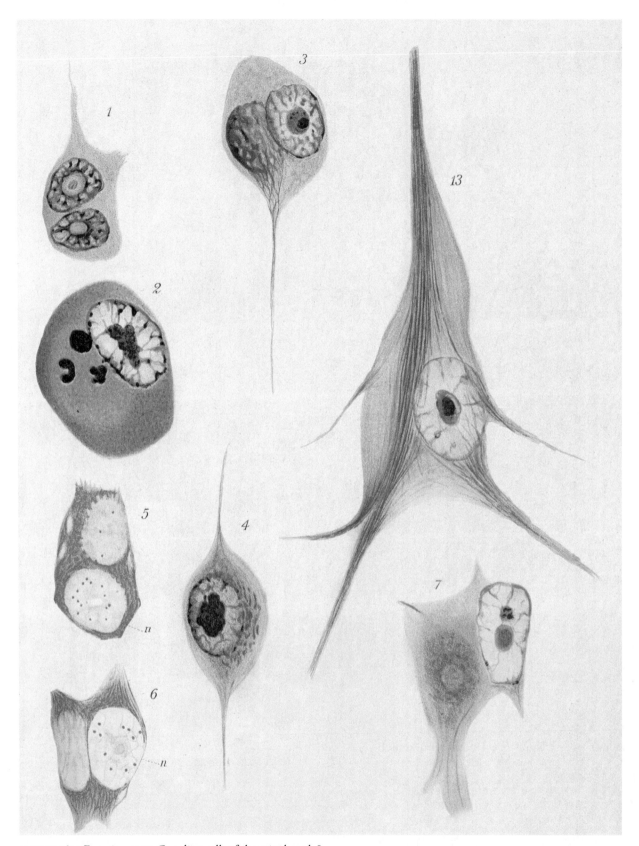

**FIGURE 169.** Fragnito, 1907. Ganglion cells of the spinal cord, I.

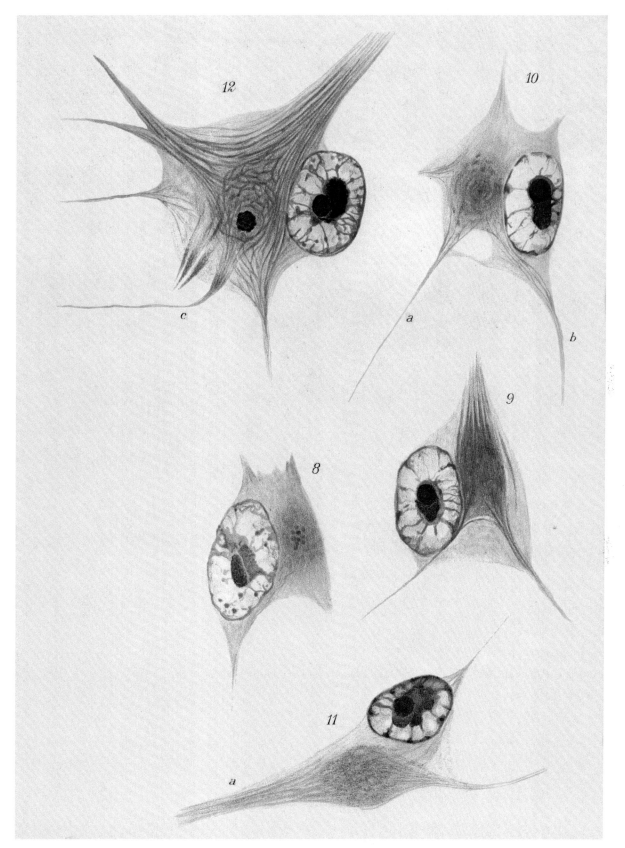

FIGURE 170. Fragnito, 1907. Ganglion cells of the spinal cord, II.

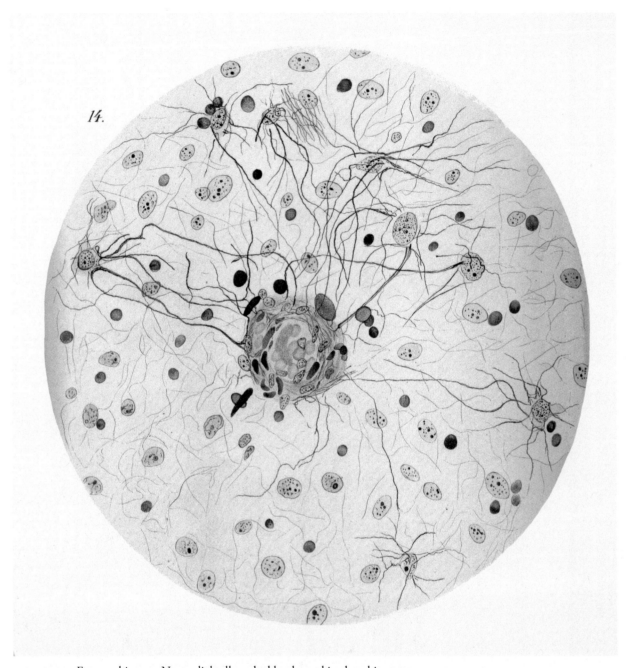

**FIGURE 171.** Franceschi, 1907. Neuroglial cells and a blood vessel in the white matter.

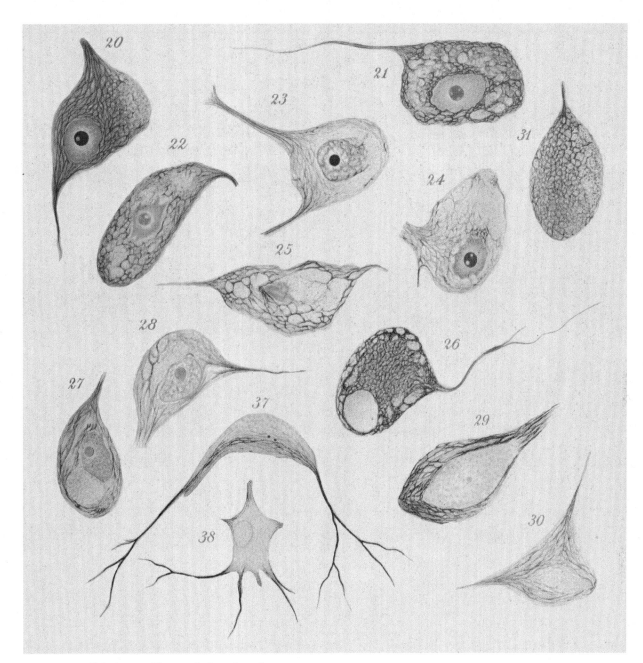

**FIGURE 172.** Sciuti, 1907. Nerve cell alterations, I.

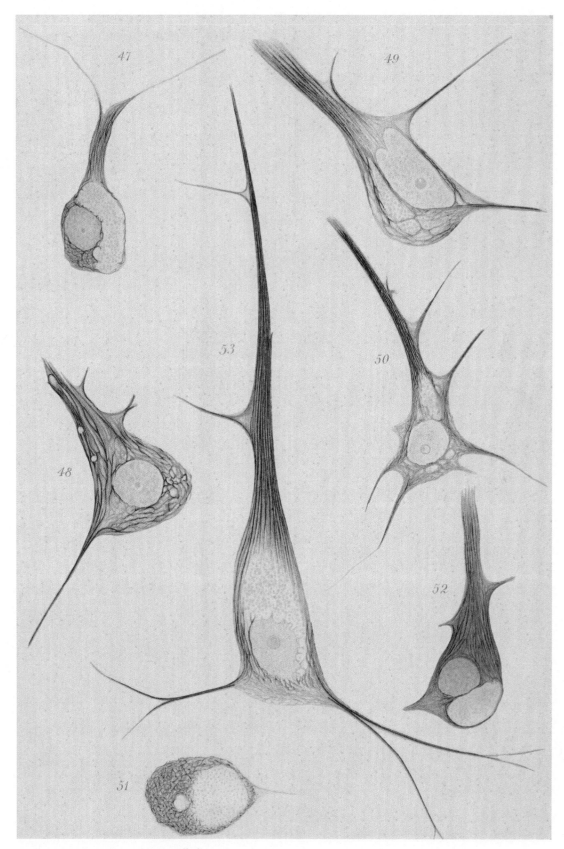

**FIGURE 173.** Sciuti, 1907. Nerve cell alterations, II.

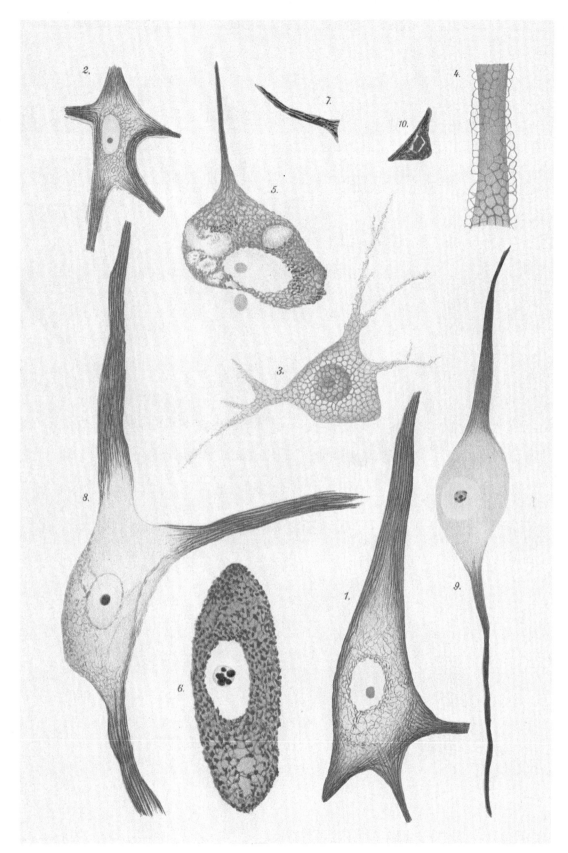

**FIGURE 174.** Gurewitsch, 1908. Internal structure of nerve cells.

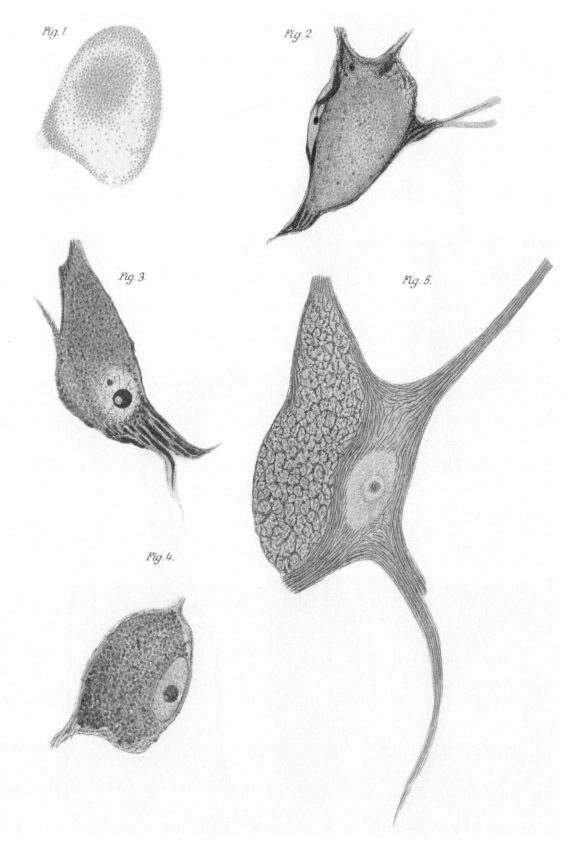

**FIGURE 175.** Calligaris, 1908. Cells of the locus coeruleus, I.

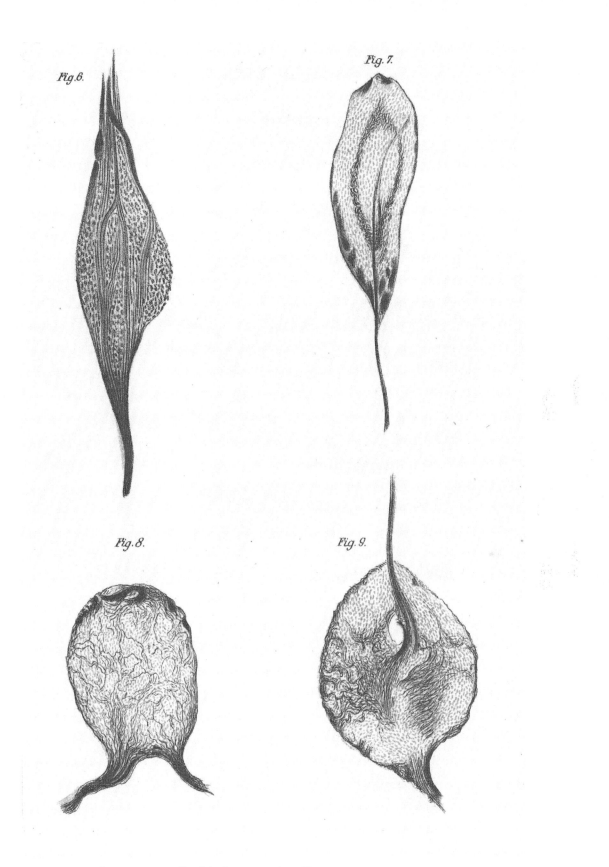

**FIGURE 176.** Calligaris, 1908. Cells of the locus coeruleus, II.

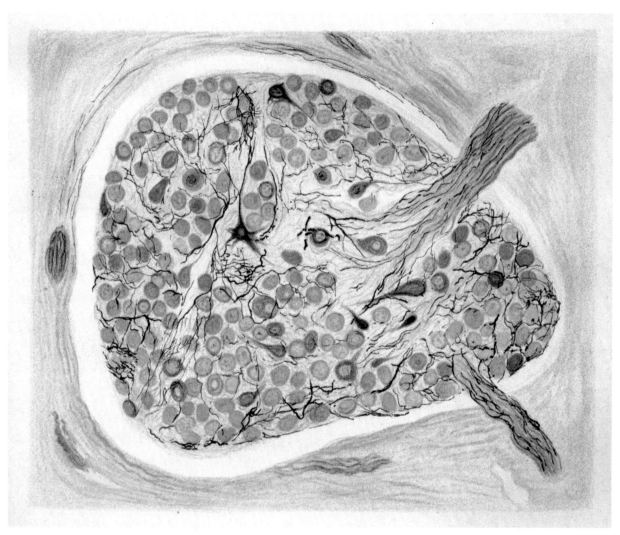

FIGURE 177. Luna, 1908. Sympathetic ganglion.

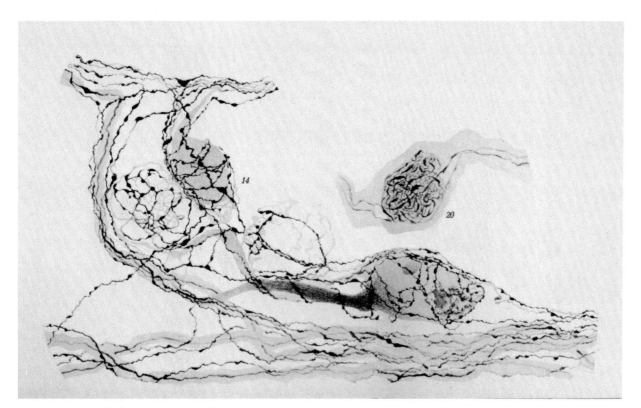

FIGURE 178. Michailow, 1908. Intracardiac nervous system.

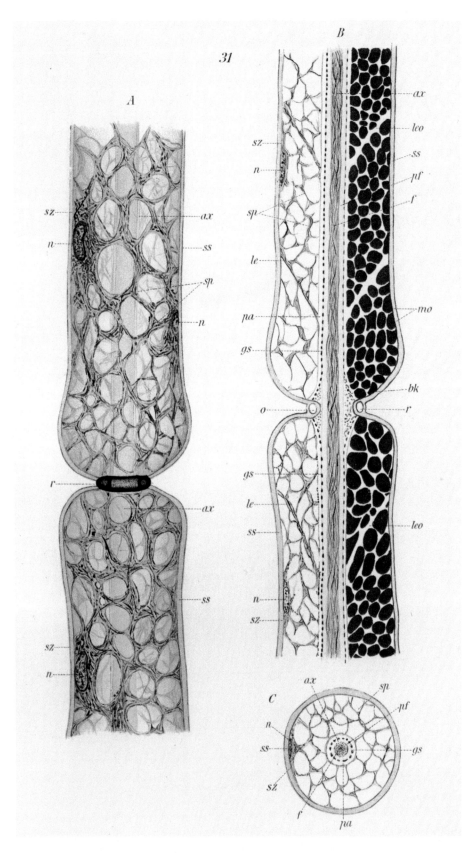

FIGURE 179. Nemiloff, 1908. Nerve fibers, I.

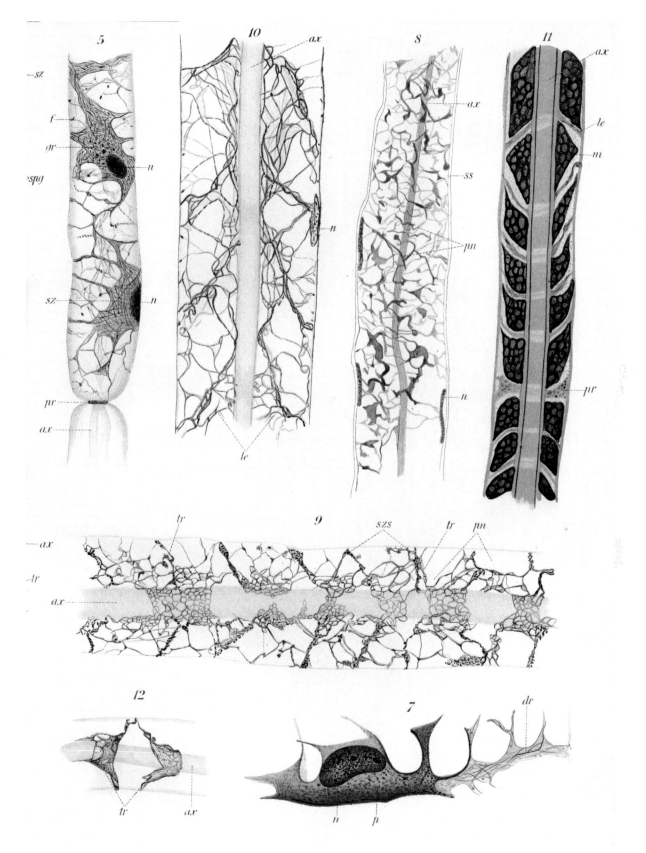

**FIGURE 180.** Nemiloff, 1908. Nerve fibers, II.

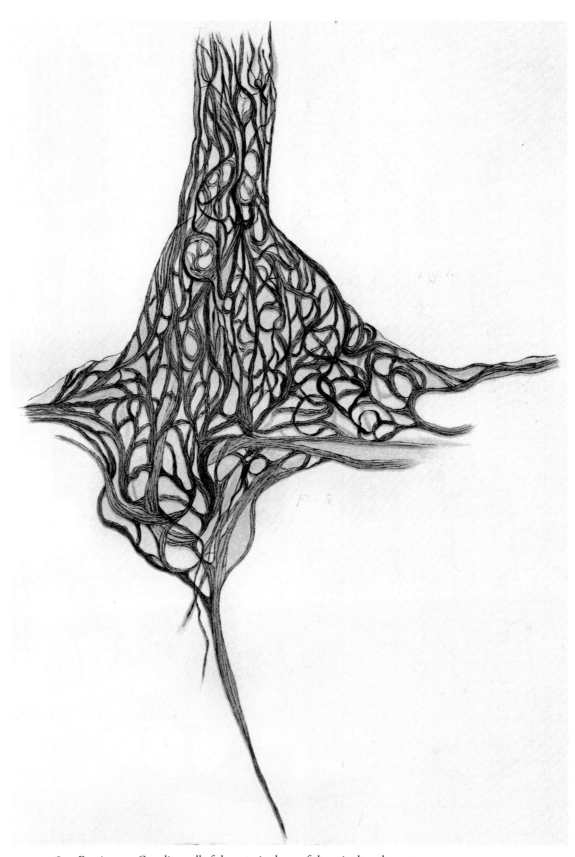

**FIGURE 181.** Rossi, 1909. Ganglion cell of the anterior horn of the spinal cord.

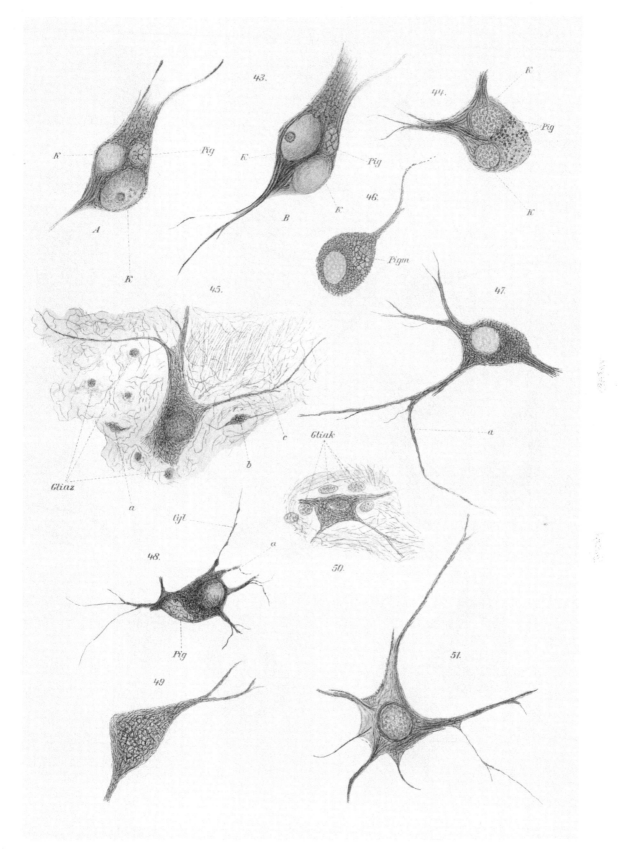

FIGURE 182. Da Fano, 1909. The optic thalamus in psychoses, I.

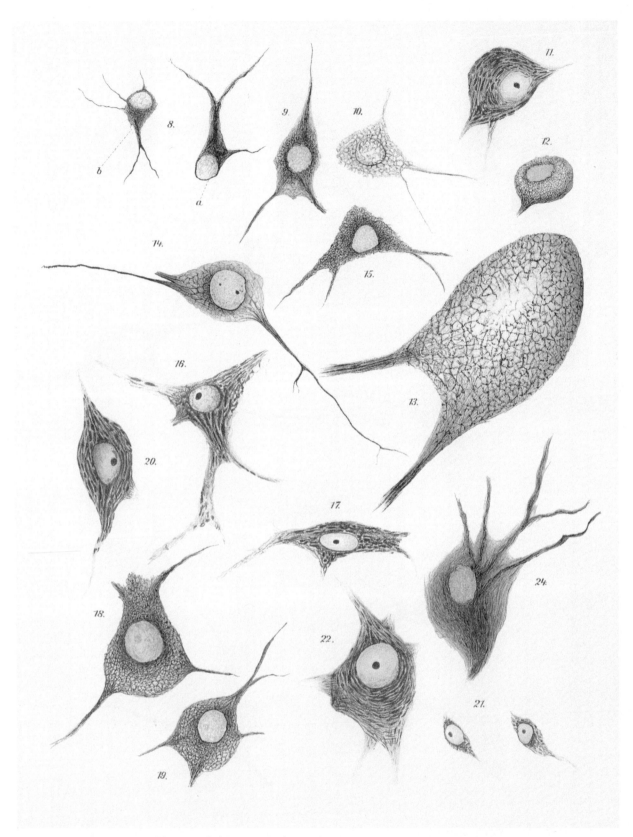

**FIGURE 183.** Da Fano, 1909. The optic thalamus in psychoses, II.

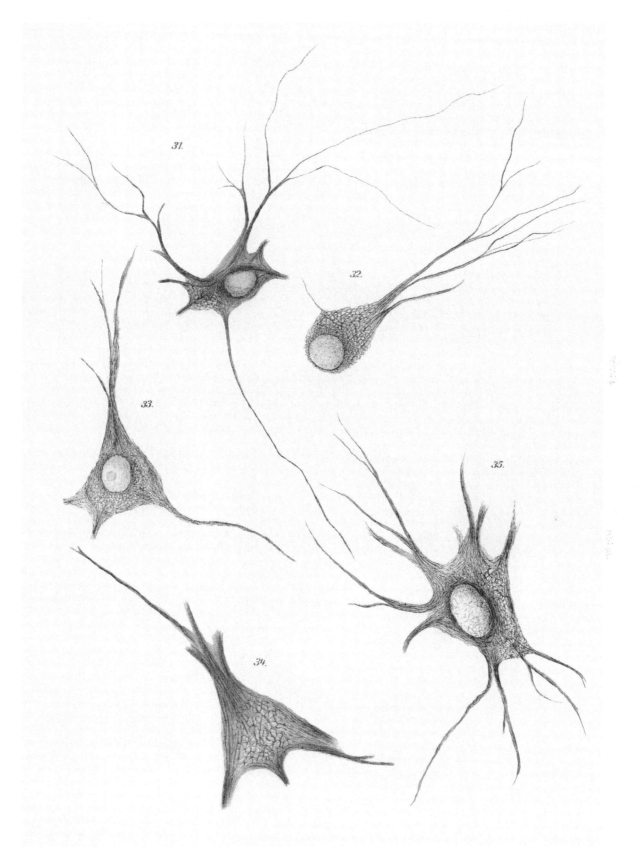

FIGURE 184. Da Fano, 1909. The optic thalamus in psychoses, III.

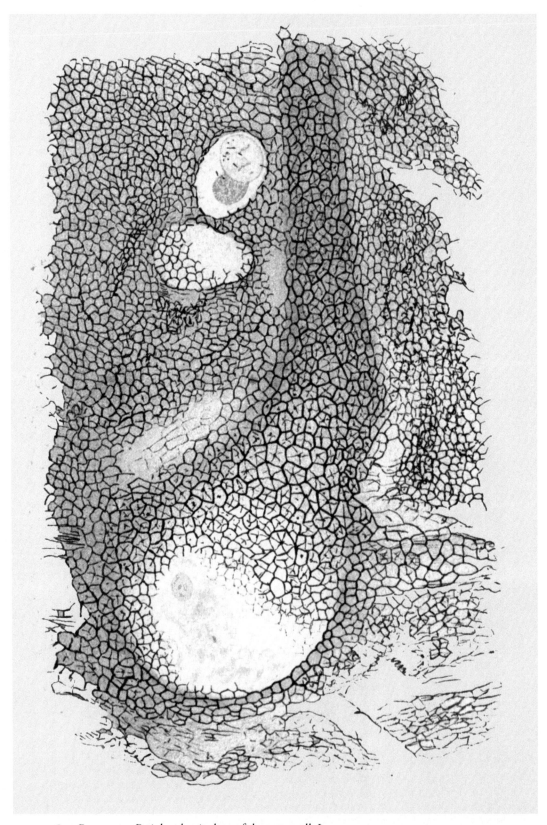

FIGURE 185. Besta, 1910. Peripheral reticulum of the nerve cell, I.

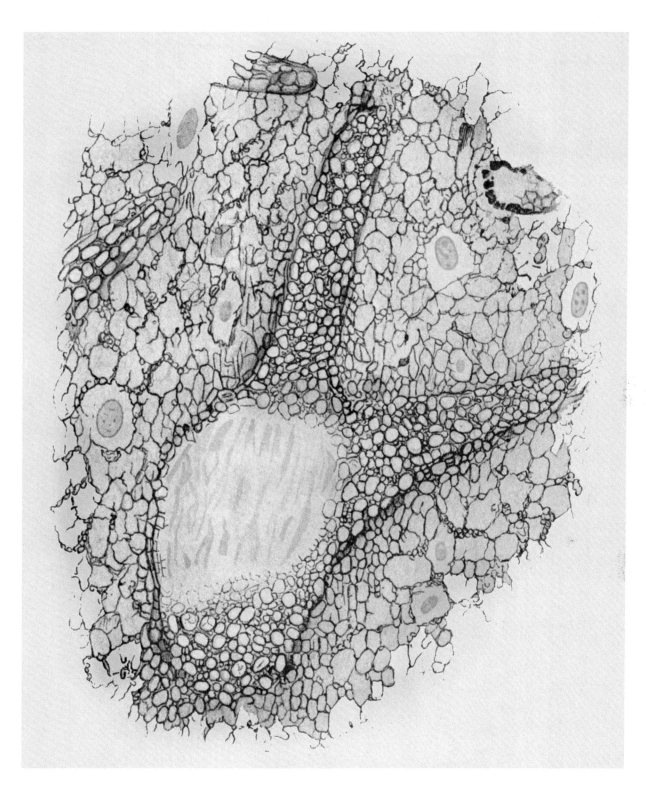

**FIGURE 186.** Besta, 1910. Peripheral reticulum of the nerve cell, II.

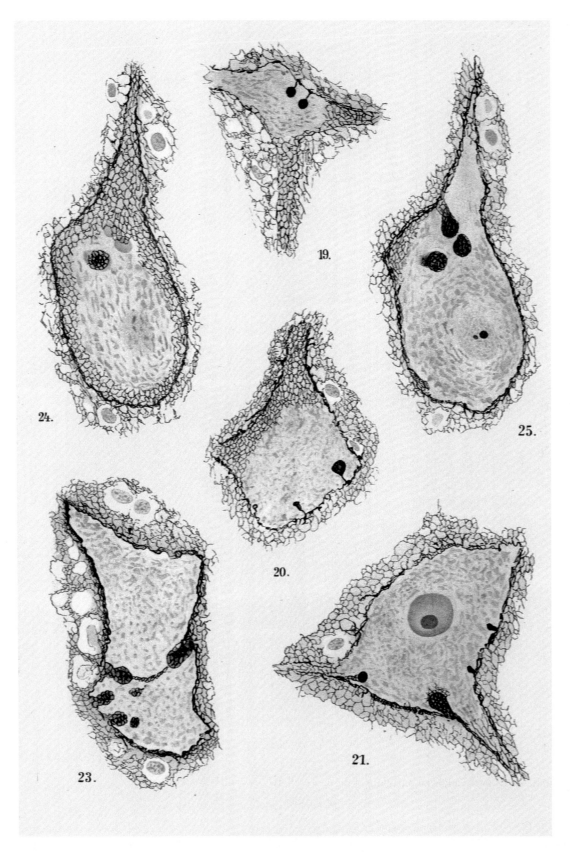

**FIGURE 187.** Besta, 1910. Peripheral reticulum of the nerve cell, III.

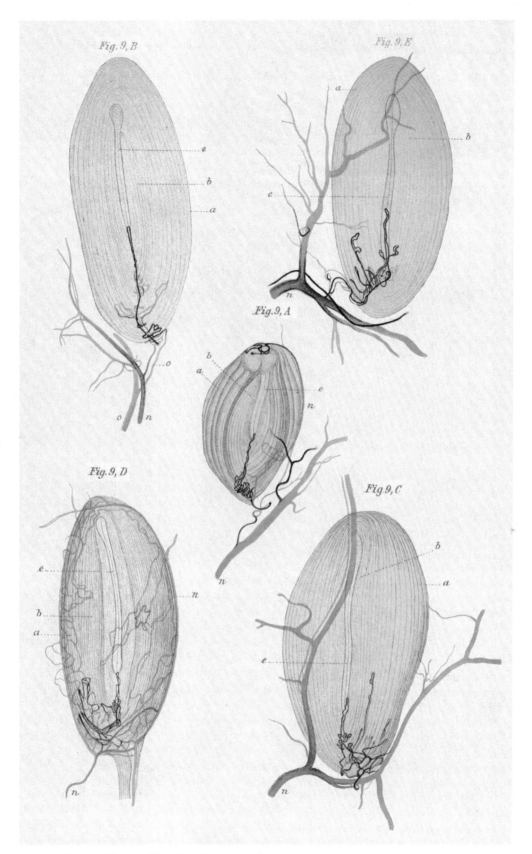

FIGURE 188. Dogiel, 1910. Vater-Pacinian corpuscles.

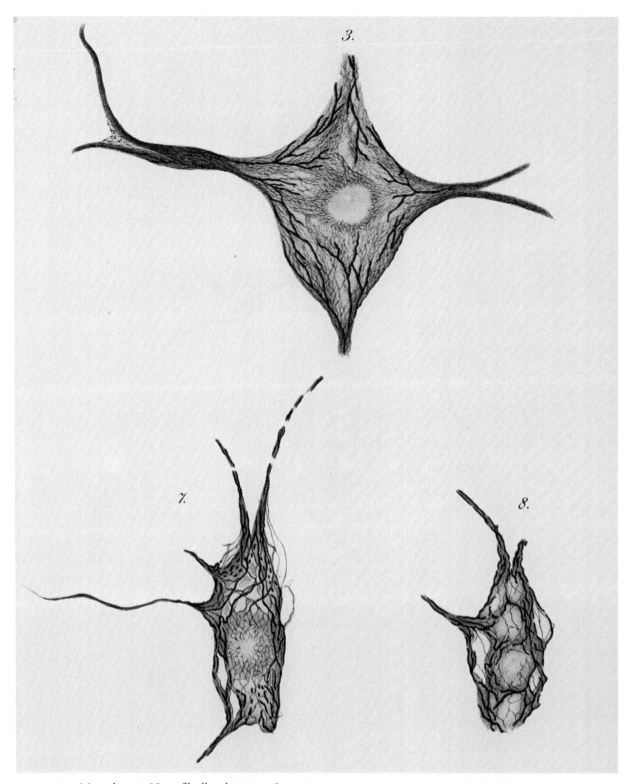

**FIGURE 189.** Mattioli, 1910. Neurofibrillar alterations, I.

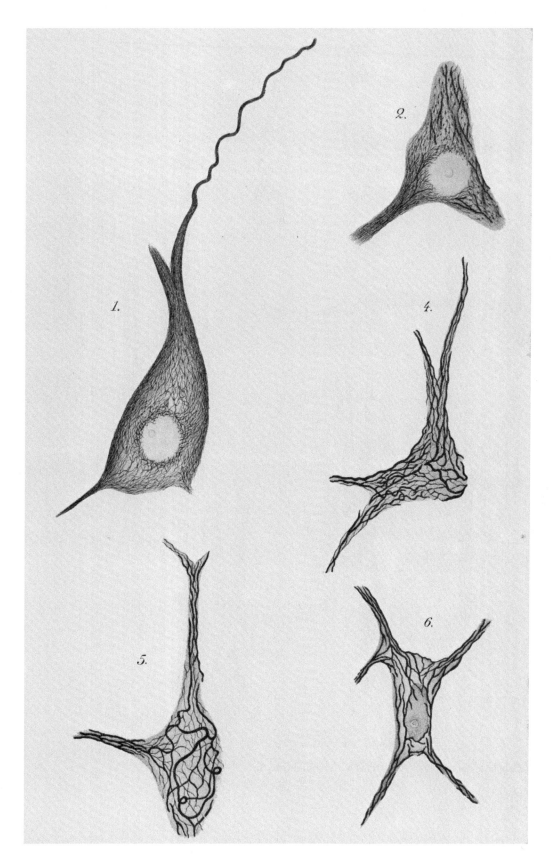

FIGURE 190. Mattioli, 1910. Neurofibrillar alterations, II.

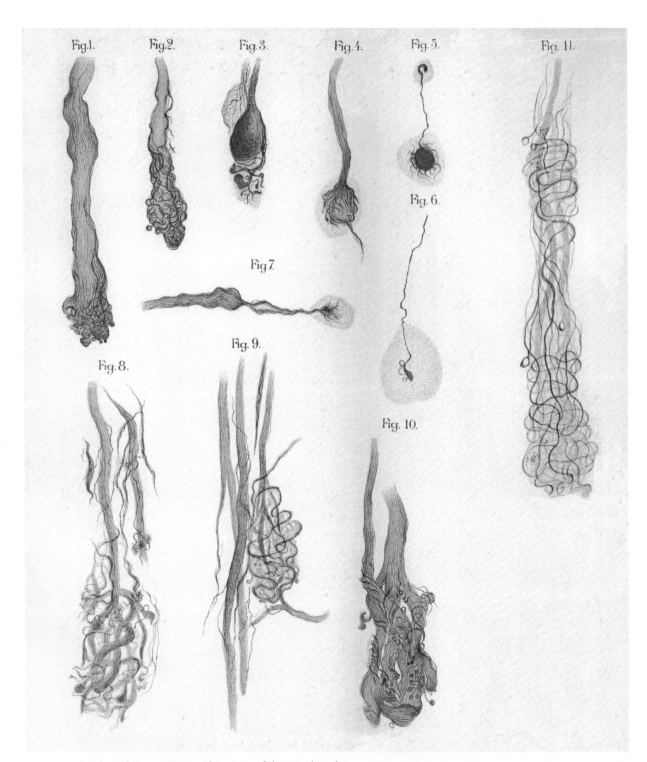

Fig.1.  Fig.2.  Fig.3.  Fig.4.  Fig.5.  Fig. 11.

Fig 7.

Fig. 6.

Fig. 8.  Fig. 9.

Fig. 10.

**FIGURE 191.** Sala and Cortese, 1910. Alterations of the spinal cord, I.

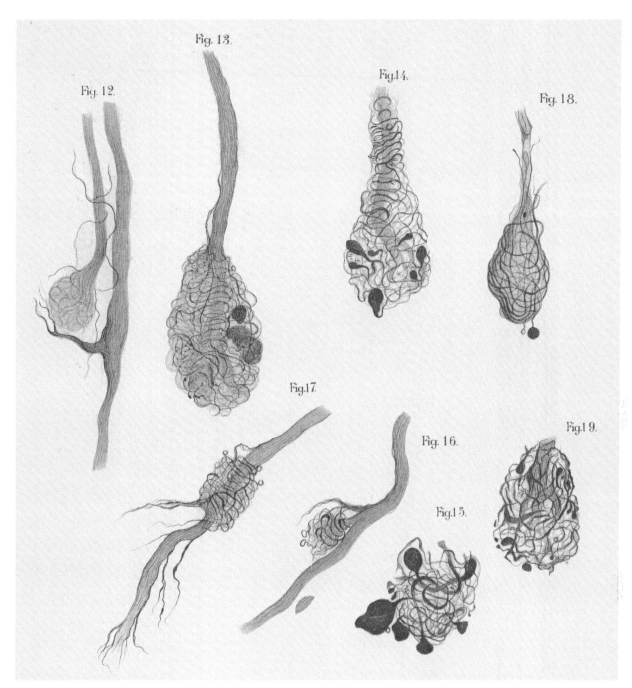

FIGURE 192. Sala and Cortese, 1910. Alterations of the spinal cord, II.

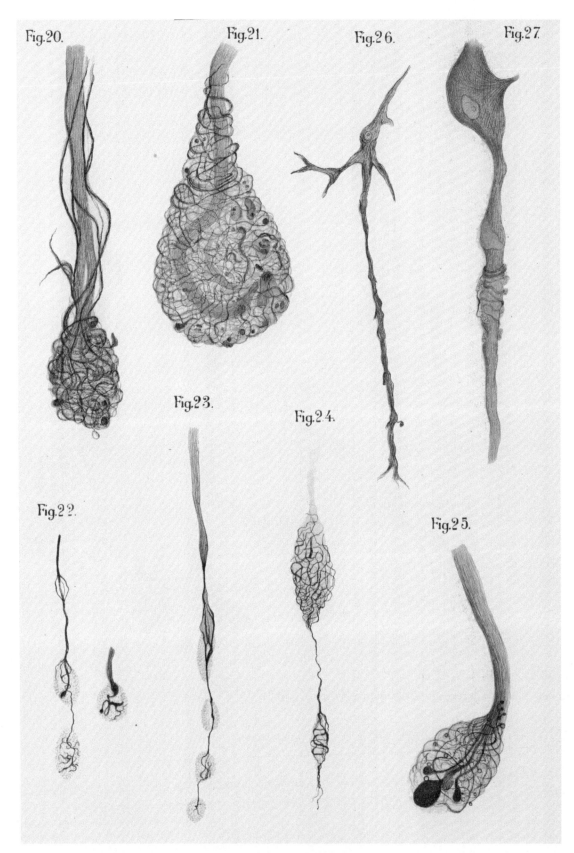

FIGURE 193. Sala and Cortese, 1910. Alterations of the spinal cord, III.

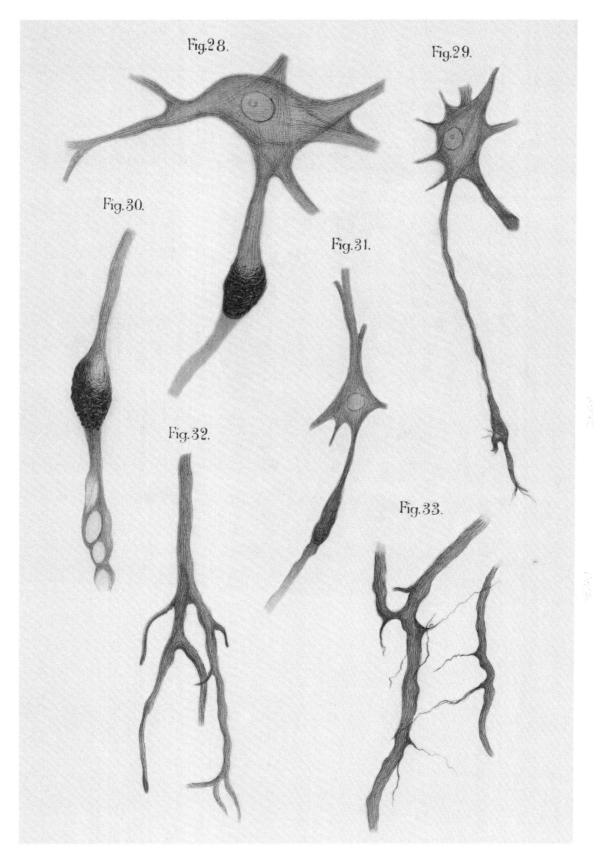

Fig. 28.

Fig. 29.

Fig. 30.

Fig. 31.

Fig. 32.

Fig. 33.

**FIGURE 194.** Sala and Cortese, 1910. Alterations of the spinal cord, IV.

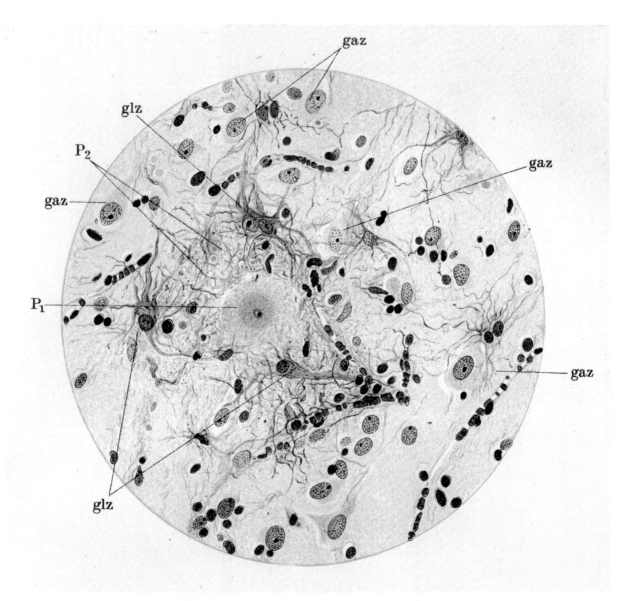

**FIGURE 195.** Alzheimer, 1911. Neuritic plaque.

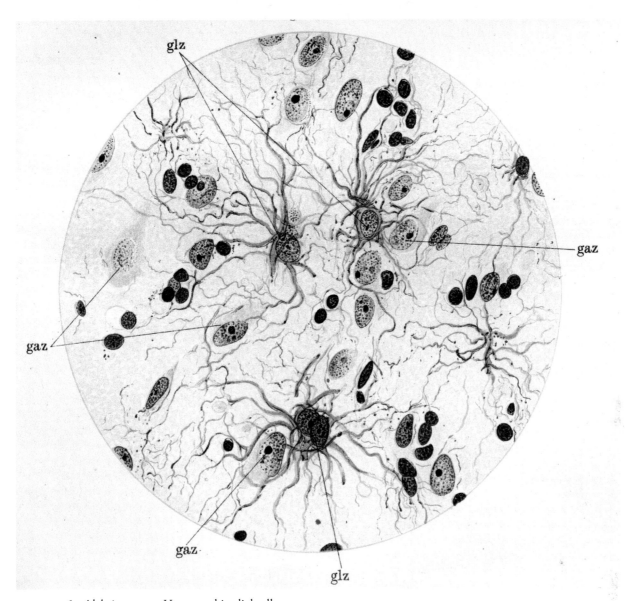

FIGURE 196. Alzheimer, 1911. Hypertrophic glial cells.

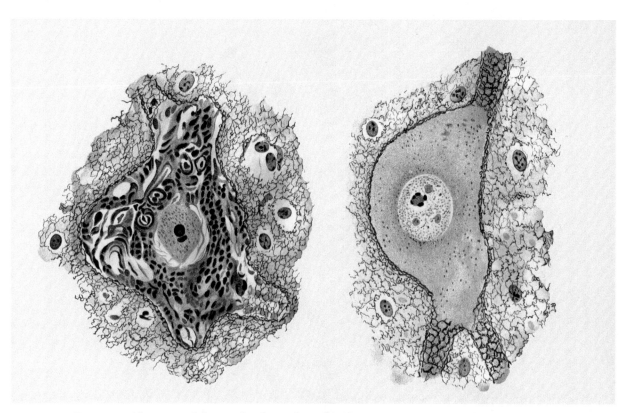

**FIGURE 197.** Besta, 1911. Alterations of the peripheral reticulum of neurons.

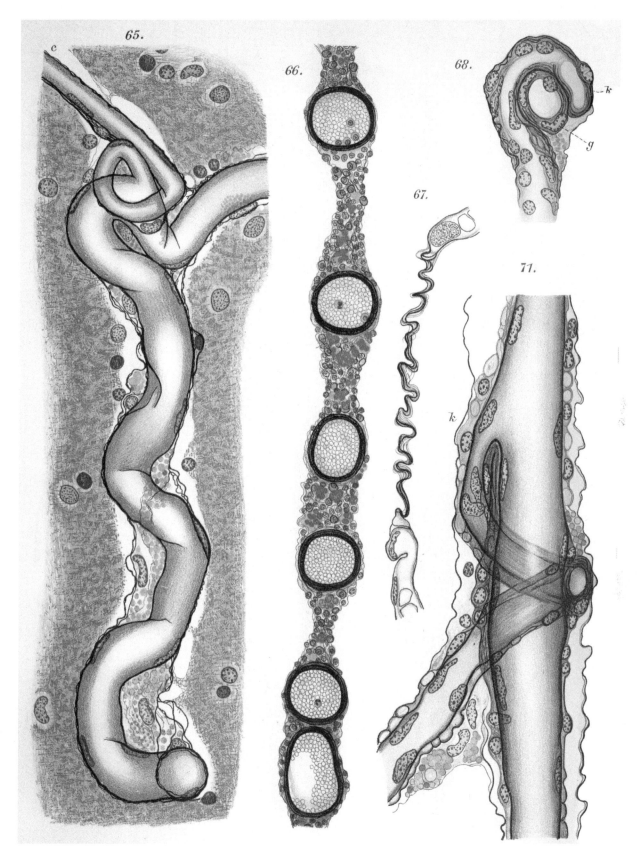

**FIGURE 198.** Cerletti, 1911. Cerebral vessels, I.

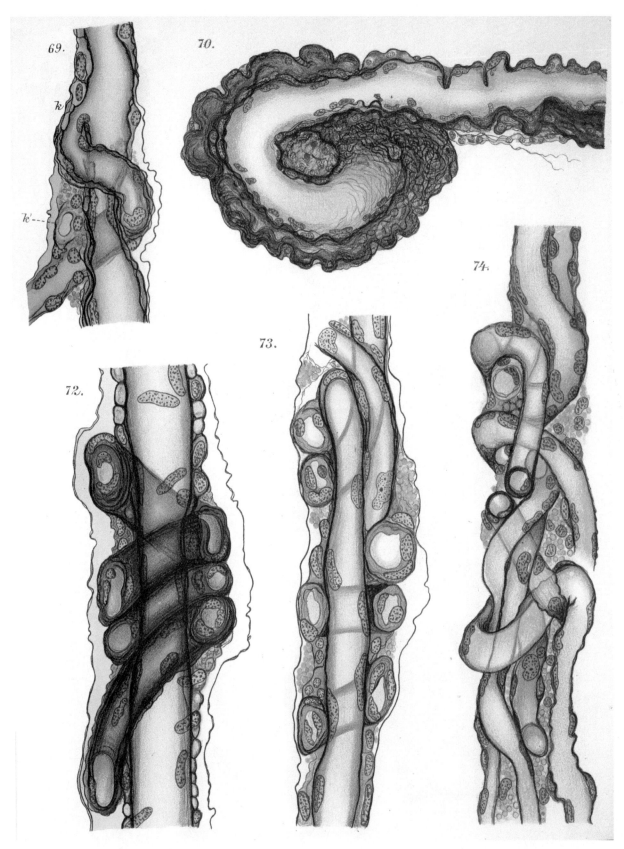

**FIGURE 199.** Cerletti, 1911. Cerebral vessels, II.

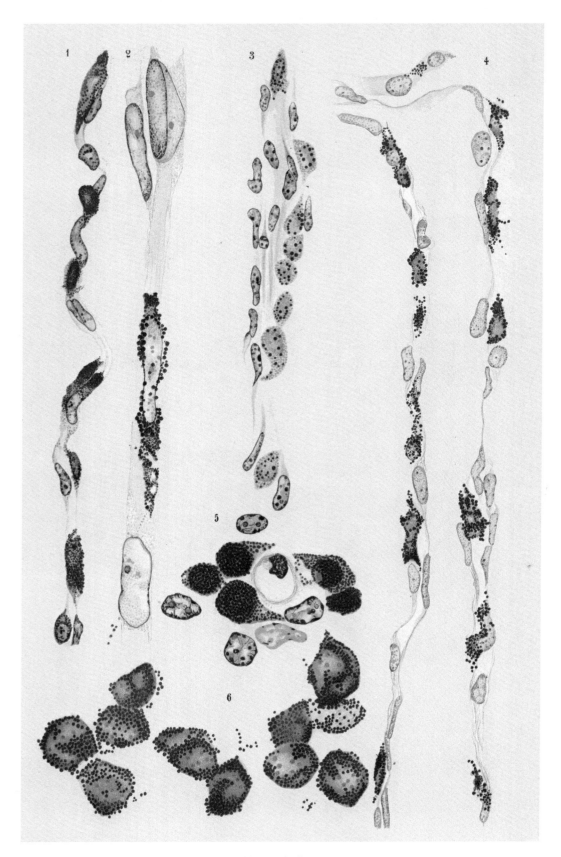

**FIGURE 200.** Cerletti, 1911. Mast cells in the olfactory bulb.

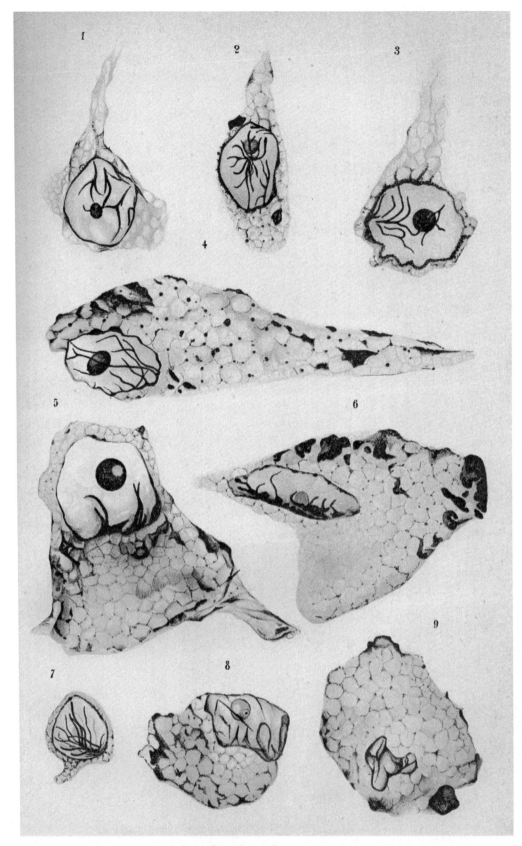

**FIGURE 201.** Cerletti, 1911. Pathology of ganglion cells.

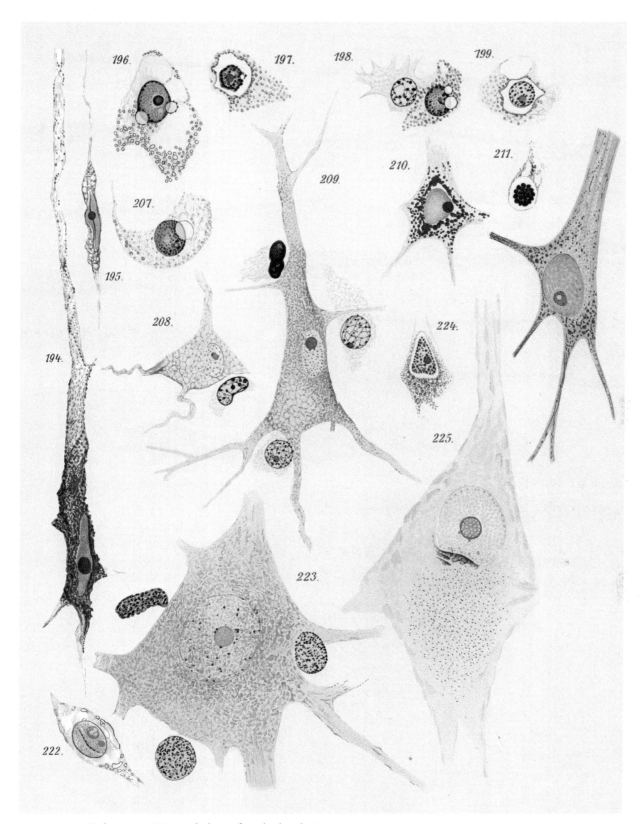

**FIGURE 202.** Cerletti, 1911. Histopathology of cerebral malaria.

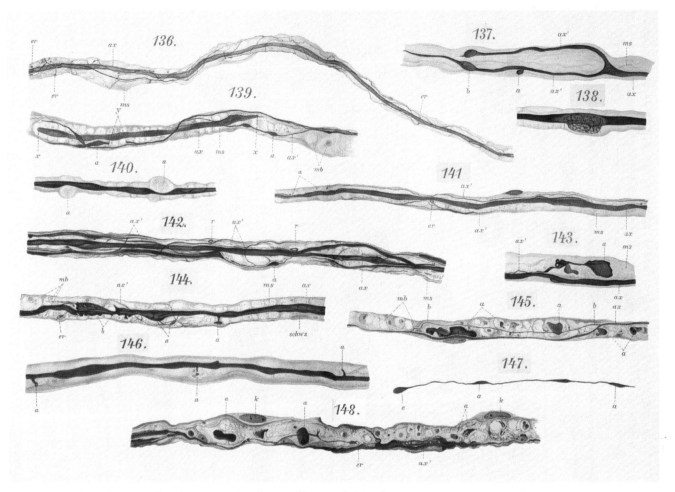

**FIGURE 203.** Doinikow, 1911. Peripheral nerve histology and histopathology, I.

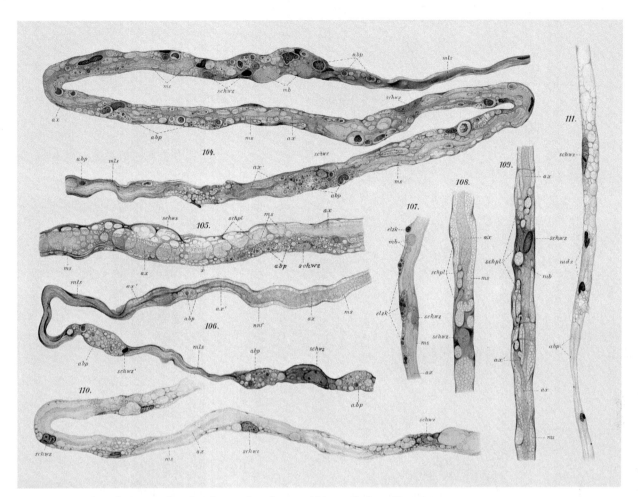

**FIGURE 204.** Doinikow, 1911. Peripheral nerve histology and histopathology, II.

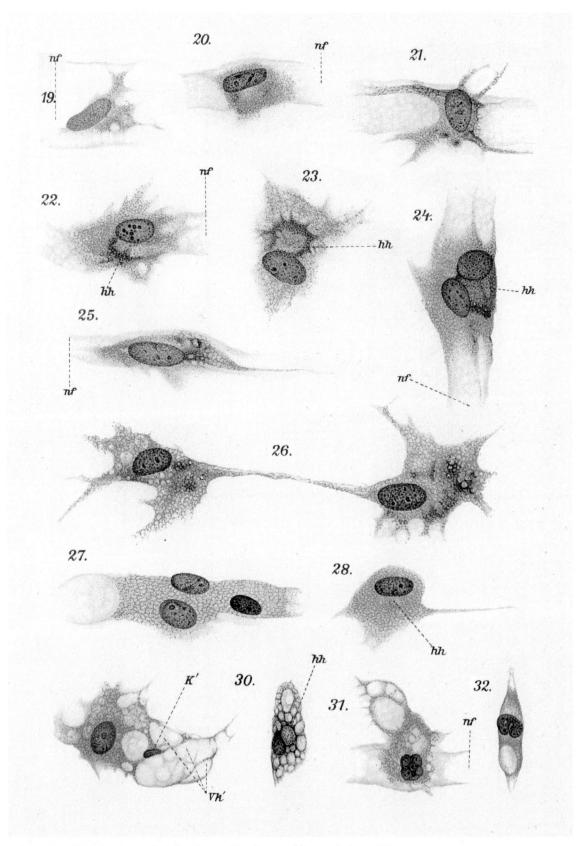

**FIGURE 205.** Doinikow, 1911. Peripheral nerve histology and histopathology, III.

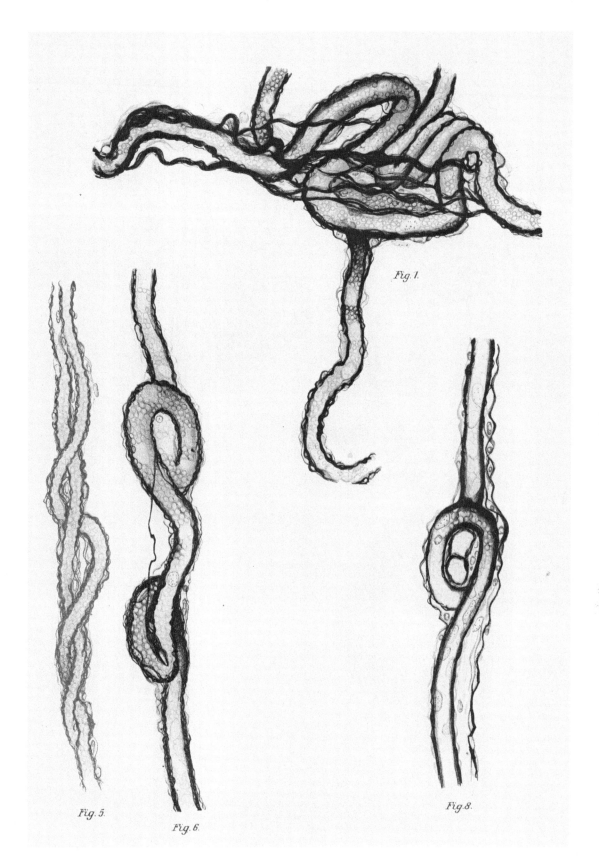

**FIGURE 206.** Lafora, 1911. Histopathology of the spinal cord, I.

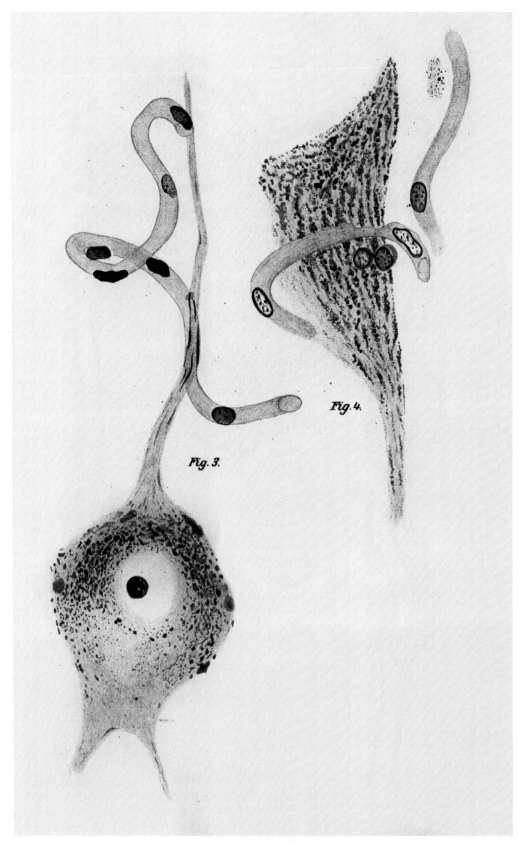

Fig. 3.

Fig. 4.

FIGURE 207. Lafora, 1911. Histopathology of the spinal cord, II.

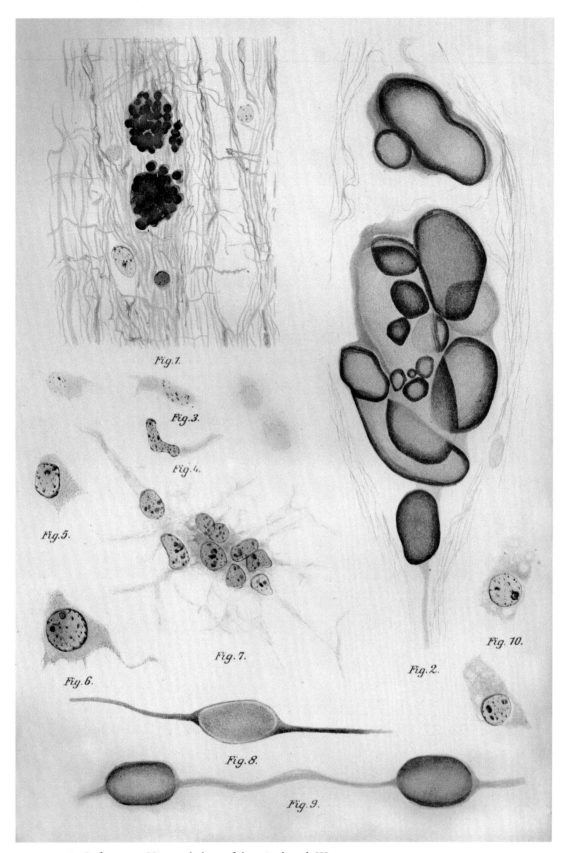

**FIGURE 208.** Lafora, 1911. Histopathology of the spinal cord, III.

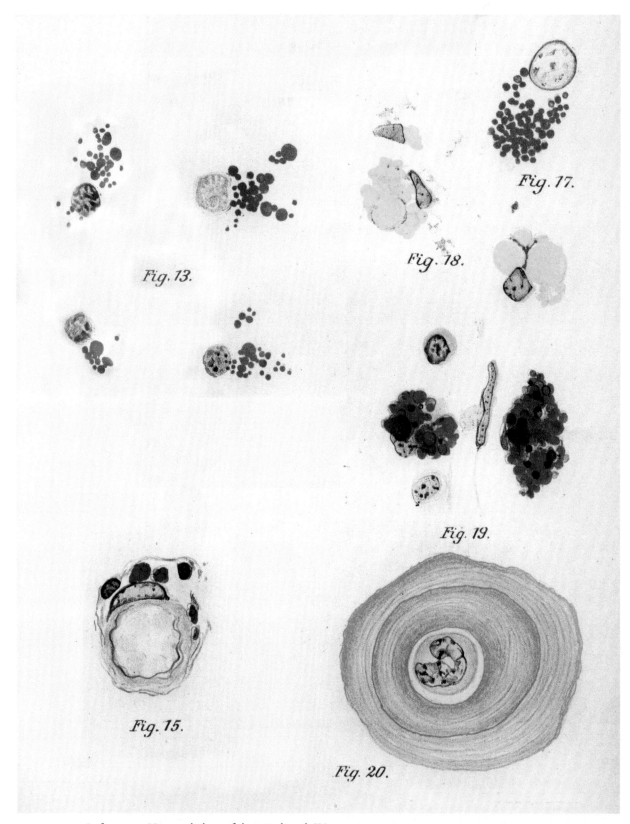

Fig. 13.

Fig. 17.

Fig. 18.

Fig. 19.

Fig. 15.

Fig. 20.

**FIGURE 209.** Lafora, 1911. Histopathology of the spinal cord, IV.

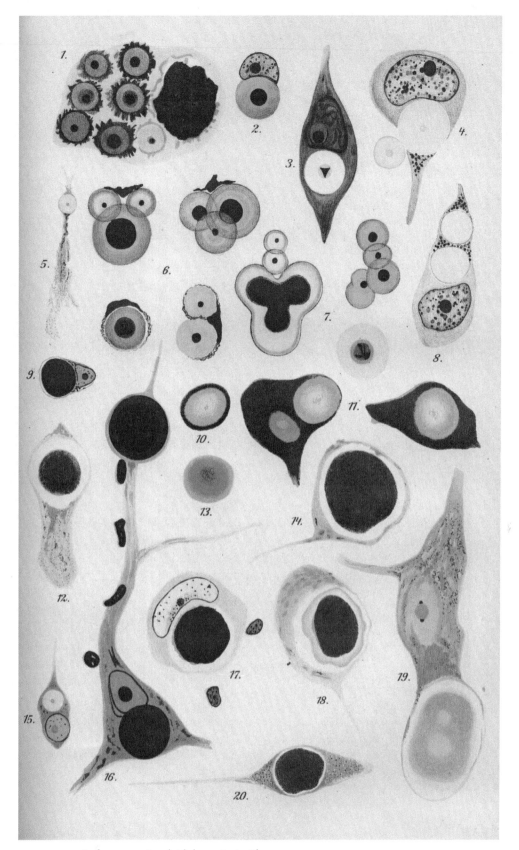

**FIGURE 210.** Lafora, 1911. Amyloid desposits inside neurons.

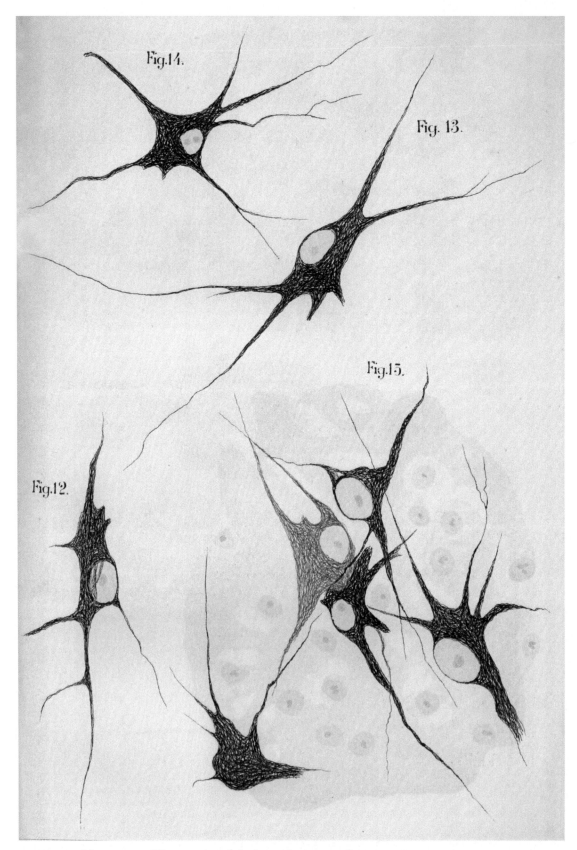

**FIGURE 211.** Marcora, 1911. Histogenesis and the internal structure of neurons.

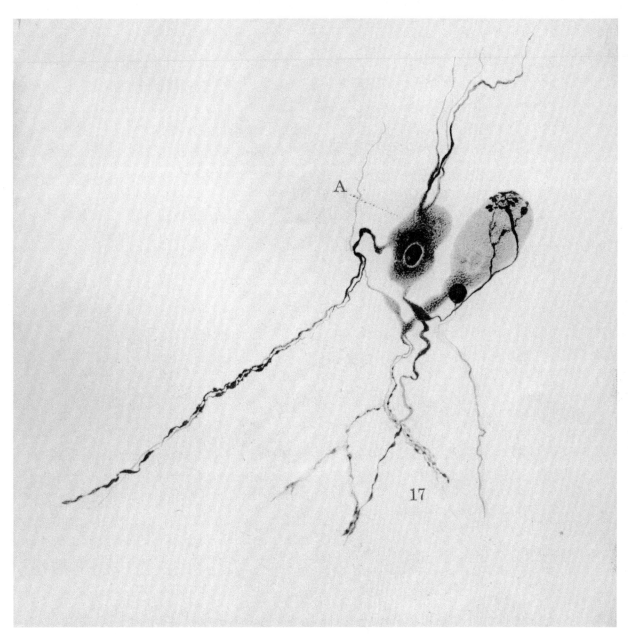

**FIGURE 212.** Michailow, 1911. The regeneration of the neuron, I.

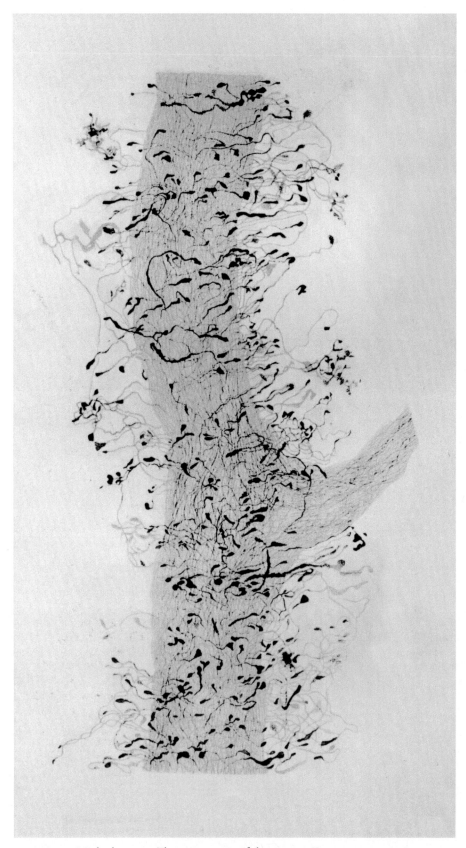

FIGURE 213. Michailow, 1911. The regeneration of the neuron, II.

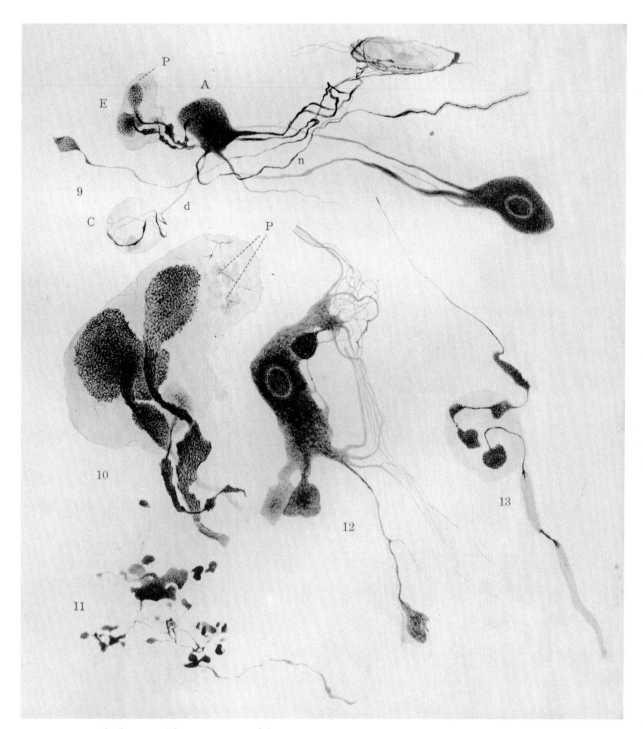

**FIGURE 214.** Michailow, 1911. The regeneration of the neuron, III.

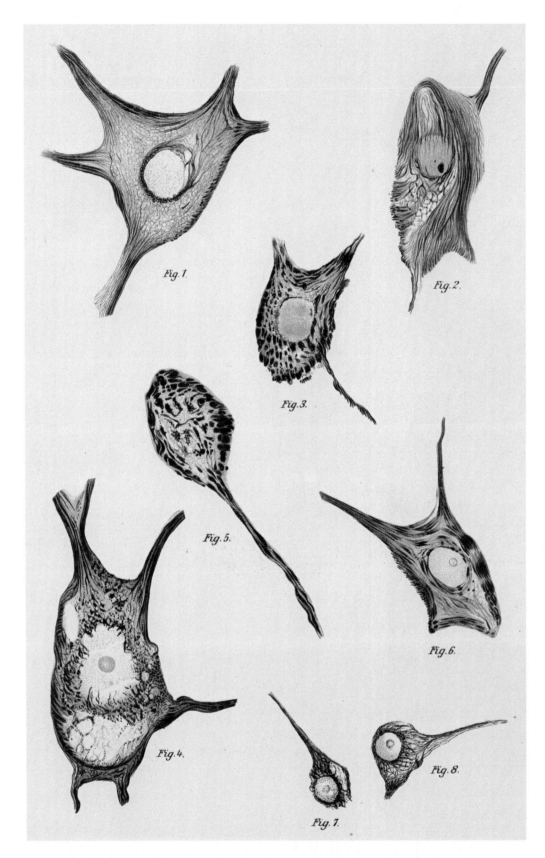

FIGURE 215. Modena and Cavara, 1911. Cytological alterations in polyneuritis and poliomyelitis.

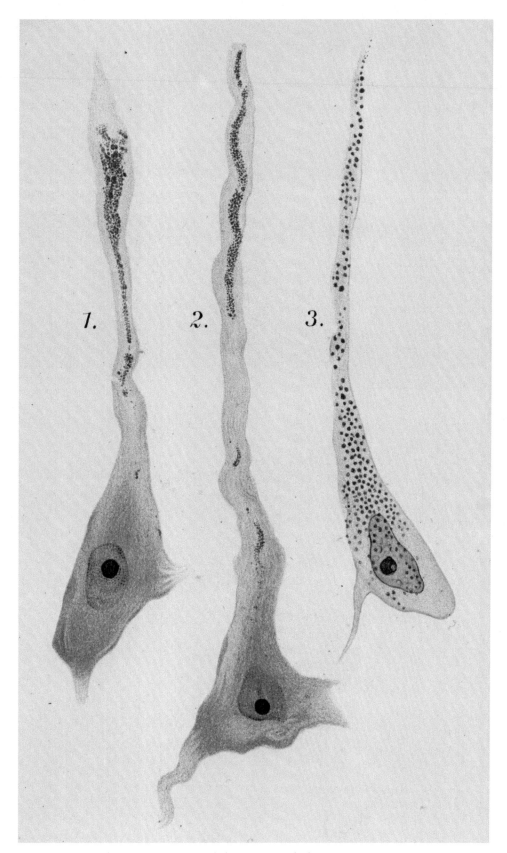

**FIGURE 216.** Simchowicz, 1911. Neuronal changes in senile dementia, I.

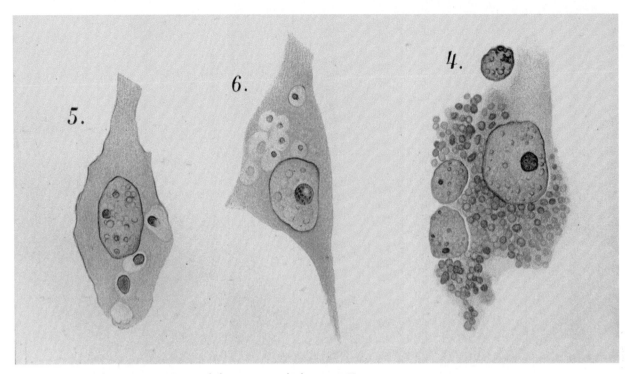

**FIGURE 217.** Simchowicz, 1911. Neuronal changes in senile dementia, II.

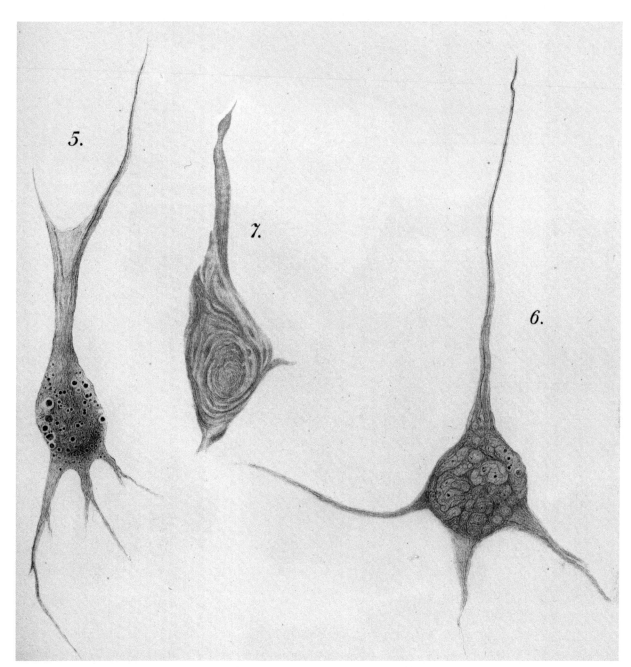

FIGURE 218. Simchowicz, 1911. Neuronal changes in senile dementia, III.

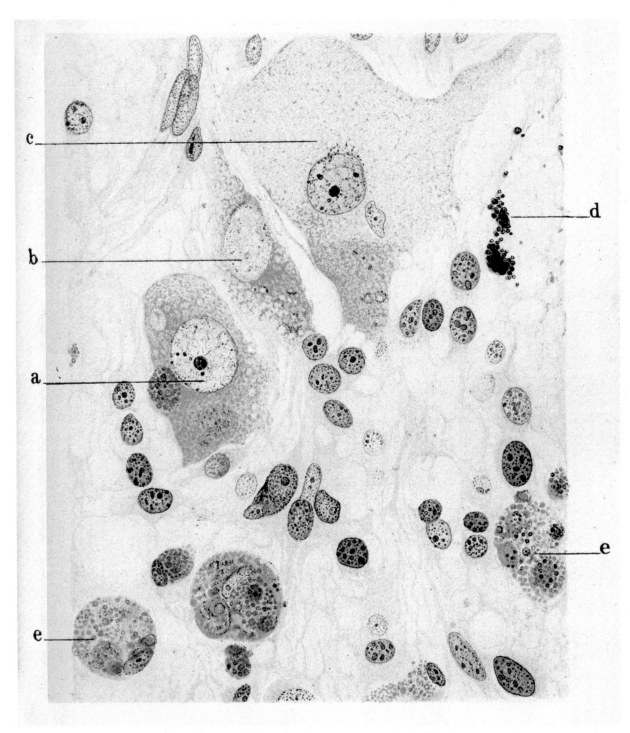

**FIGURE 219.** Von Hoesslin and Alzheimer, 1912. Seudosclerosis of Westphal-Strümpell (dentate nucleus).

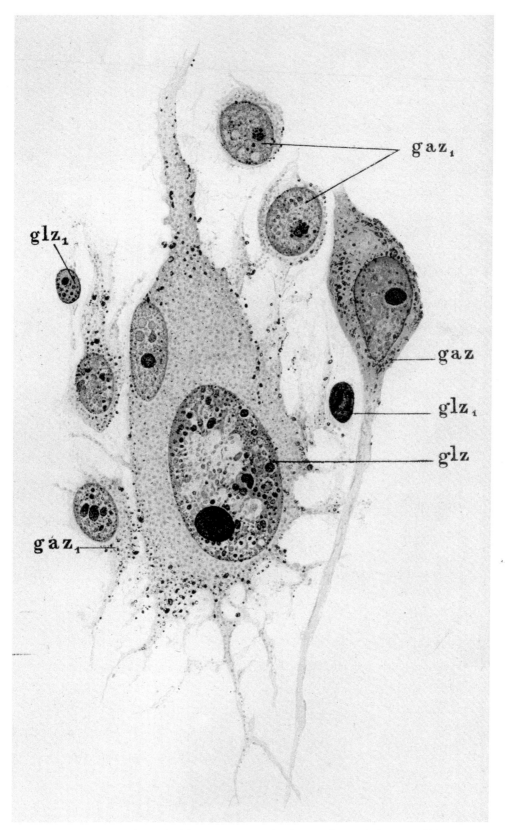

**FIGURE 220.** Von Hoesslin and Alzheimer, 1912. Seudosclerosis of Westphal-Strümpell (corpus striatum).

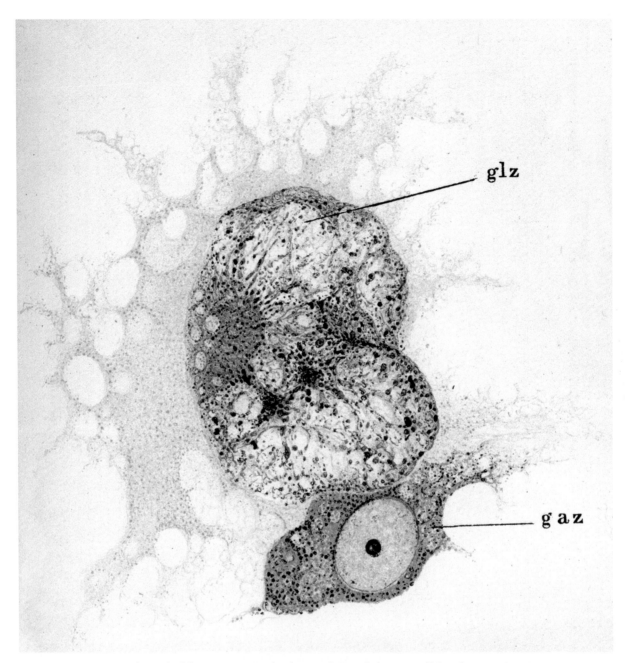

FIGURE 221. Von Hoesslin and Alzheimer, 1912. Seudosclerosis of Westphal-Strümpell (insular cortex).

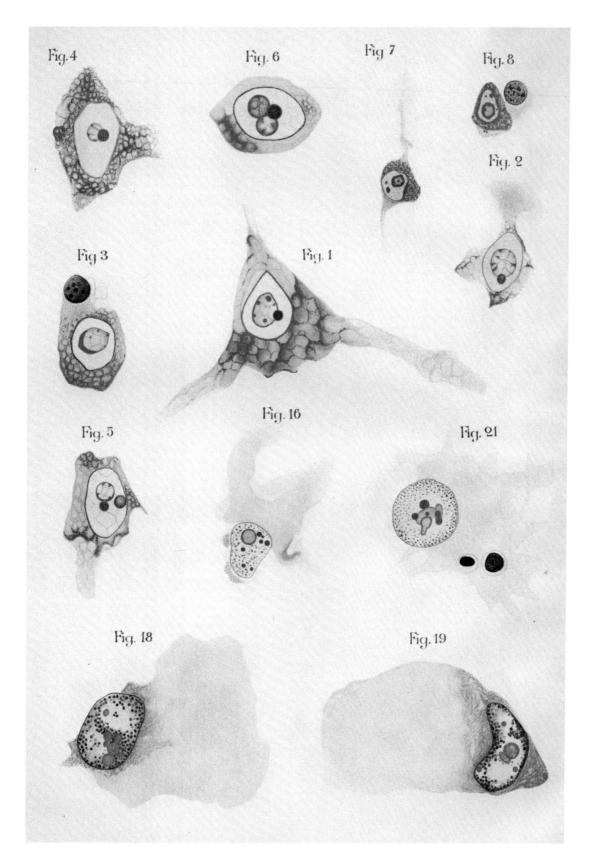

FIGURE 222. Bonfiglio, 1912. Alterations of ganglion cells.

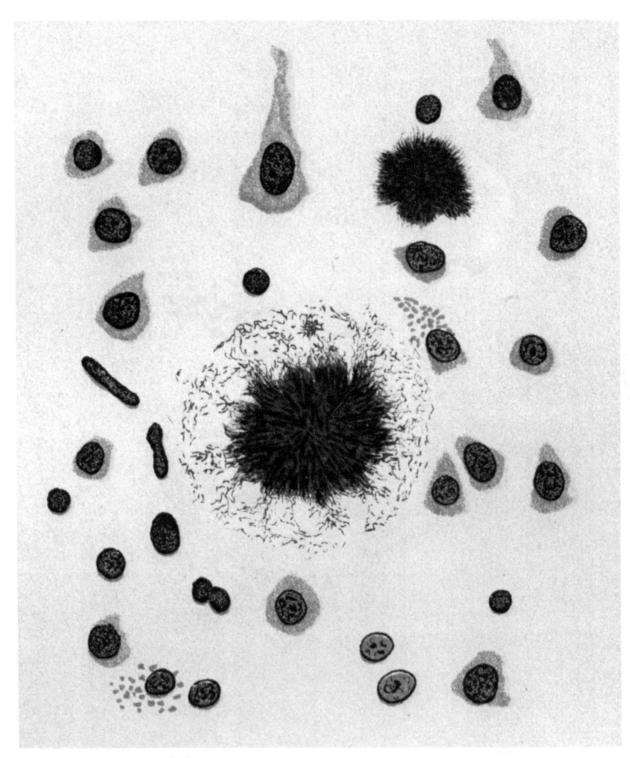

**FIGURE 223.** Fischer, 1912. Senile plaques, I.

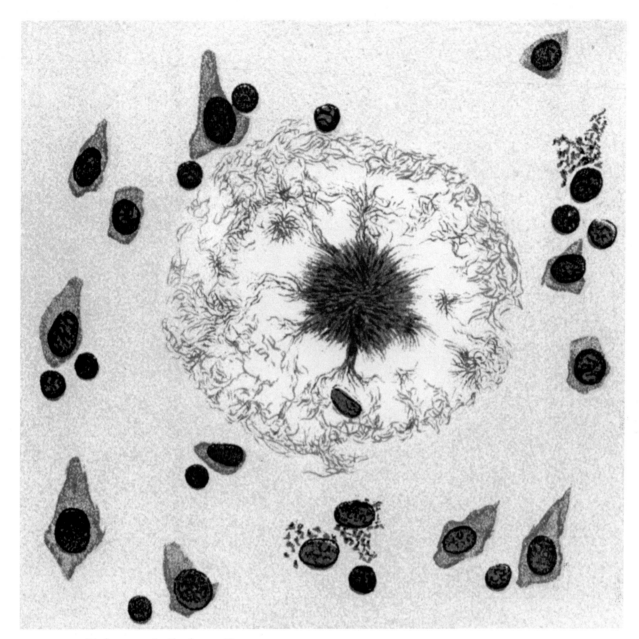

**FIGURE 224.** Fischer, 1912. Senile plaques, II.

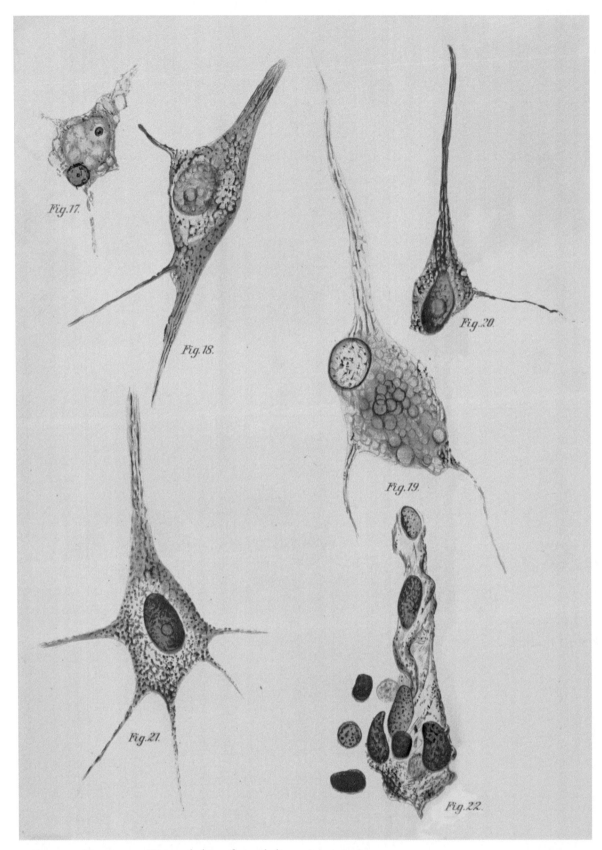

FIGURE 225. Krause, 1912. Histopathology of encephalic cystocercosis, I.

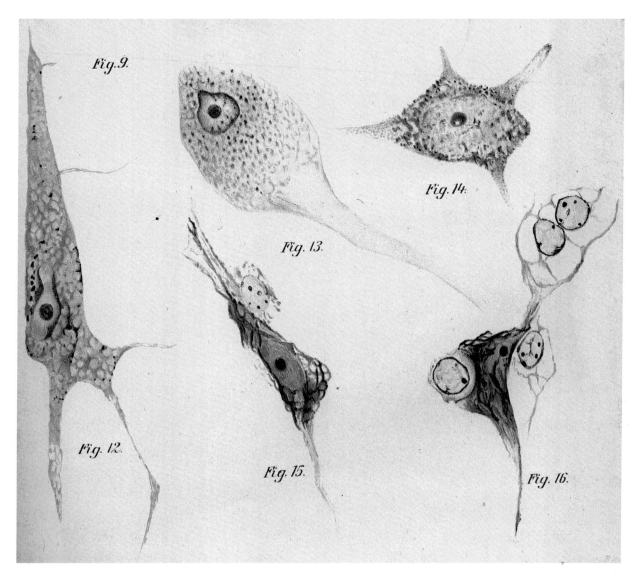

**FIGURE 226.** Krause, 1912. Histopathology of encephalic cystocercosis, II.

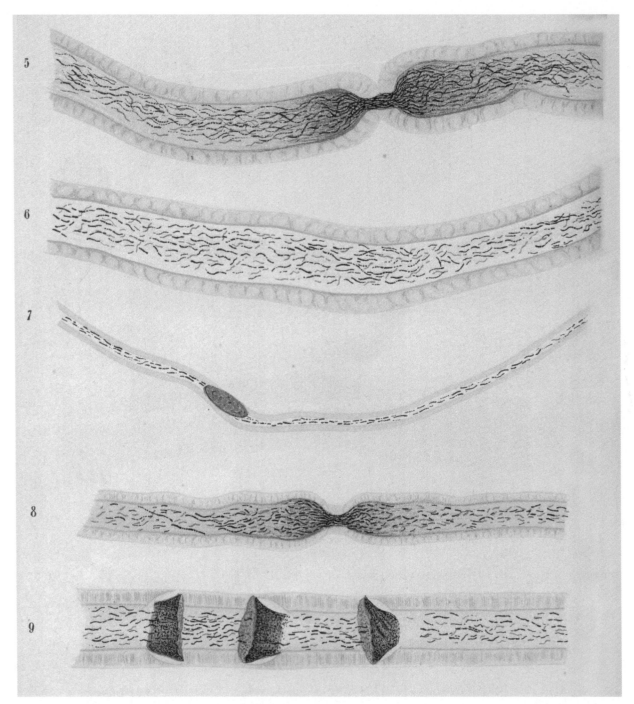

FIGURE 227. Maccabruni, 1912. Fine structure of the nerve fibers, I.

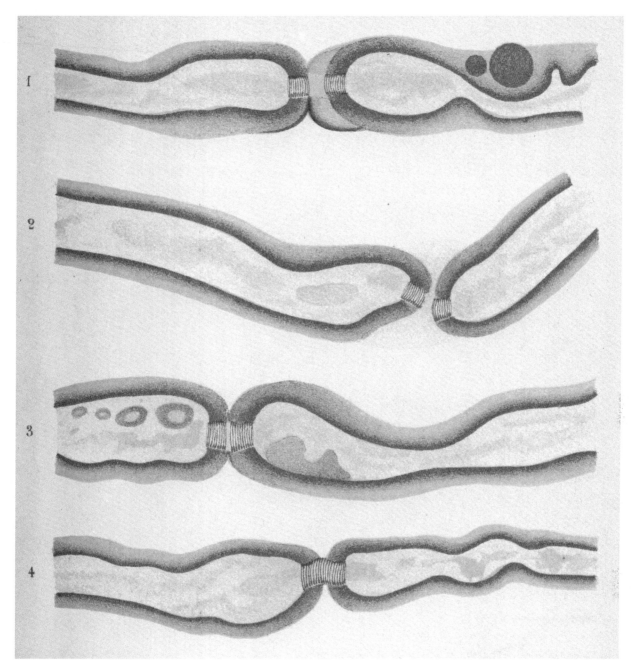

**FIGURE 228.** Maccabruni, 1912. Fine structure of the nerve fibers, II.

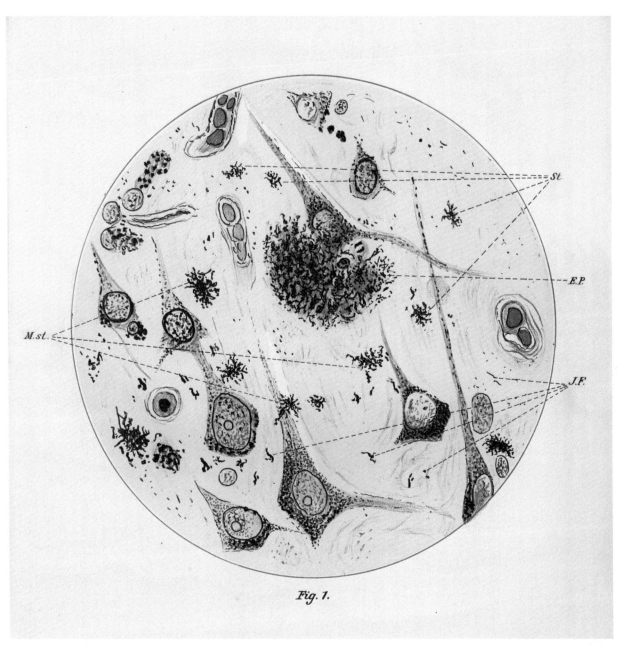

Fig. 1.

**FIGURE 229.** Marinesco and Minea, 1912. Senile plaques, I.

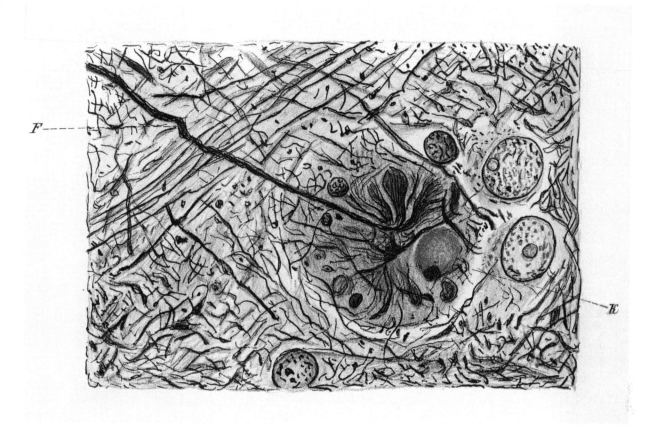

**FIGURE 230.** Marinesco and Minea, 1912. Senile plaques, II.

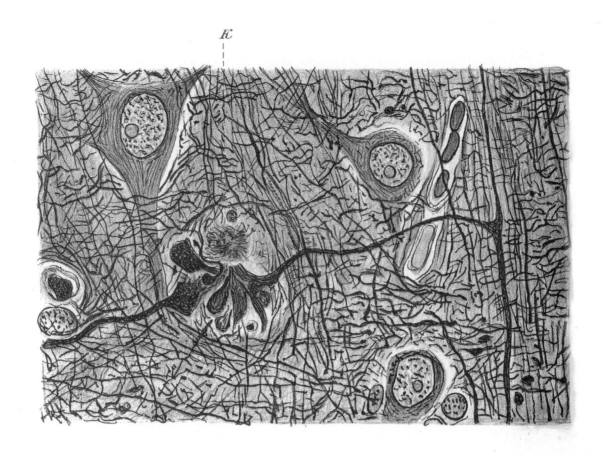

**FIGURE 231.** Marinesco and Minea, 1912. Senile plaques, III.

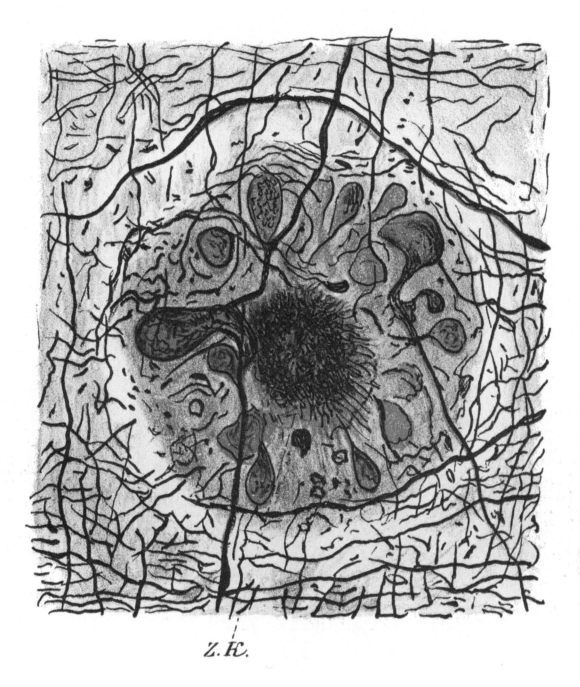

Z. K.

**FIGURE 232.** Marinesco and Minea, 1912. Senile plaques, IV.

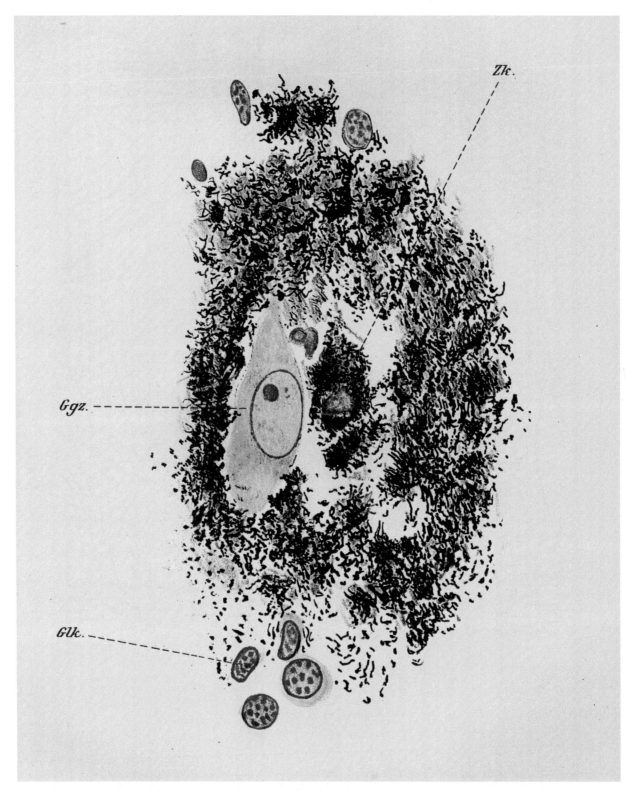

**FIGURE 233.** Marinesco and Minea, 1912. Senile plaques, V.

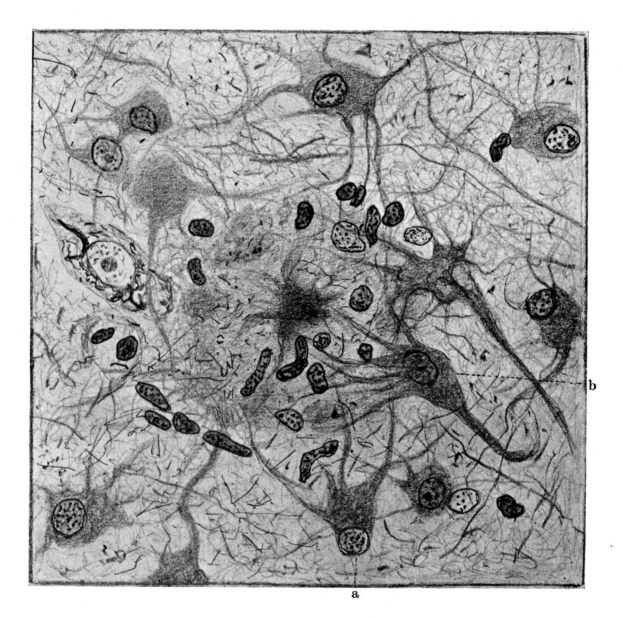

**FIGURE 234.** Marinesco and Minea, 1912. Senile plaques, VI.

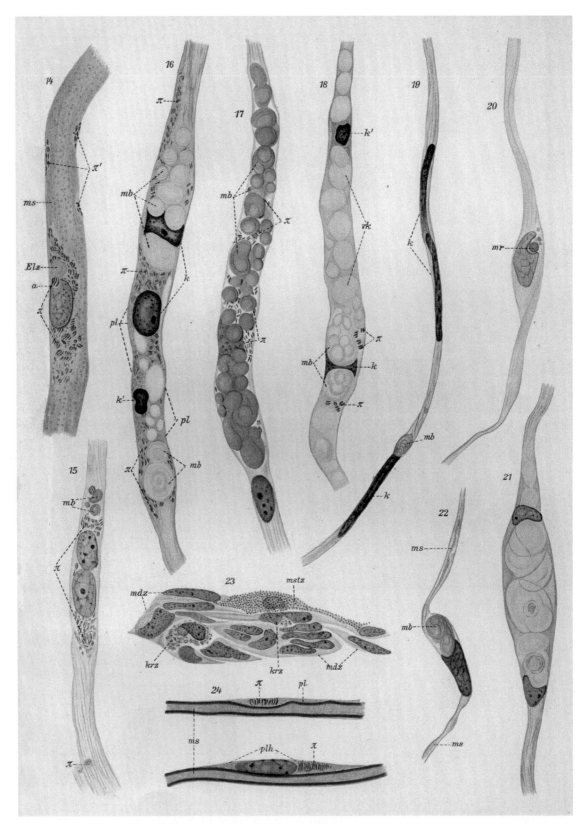

**FIGURE 235.** Rachmanow, 1912. Structure of peripheral nerve fibers, I.

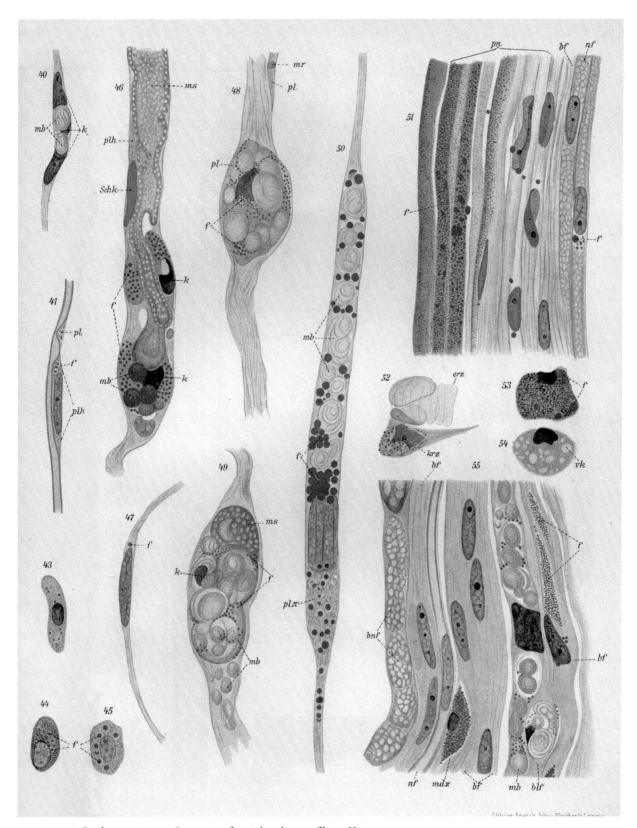

**FIGURE 236.** Rachmanow, 1912. Structure of peripheral nerve fibers, II.

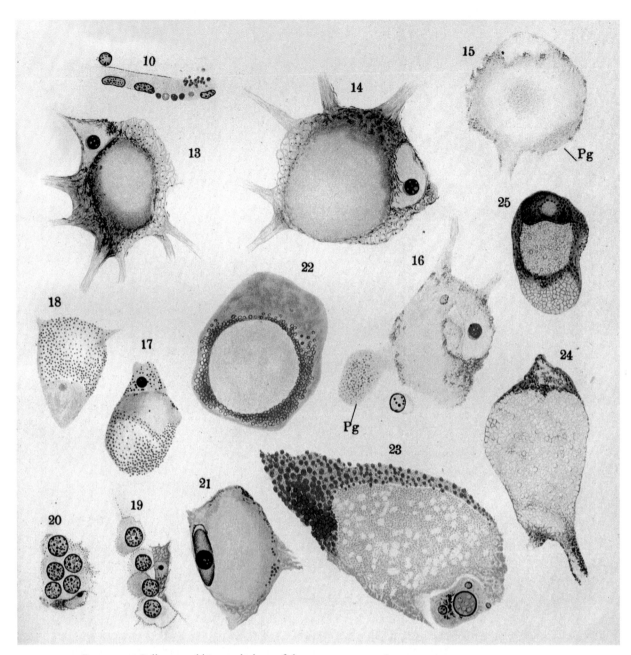

**FIGURE 237.** Rezza, 1912. Pellagra and histopathology of the nervous system, I.

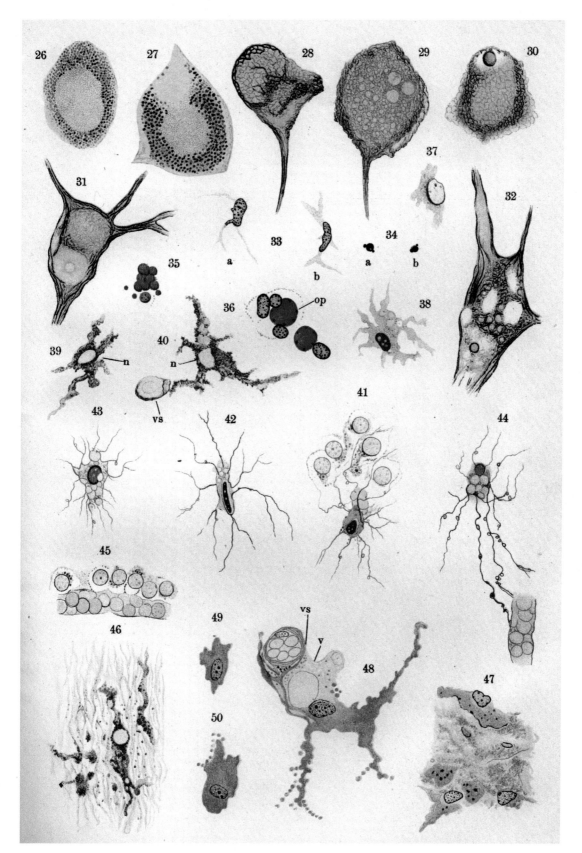

**FIGURE 238.** Rezza, 1912. Pellagra and histopathology of the nervous system, II.

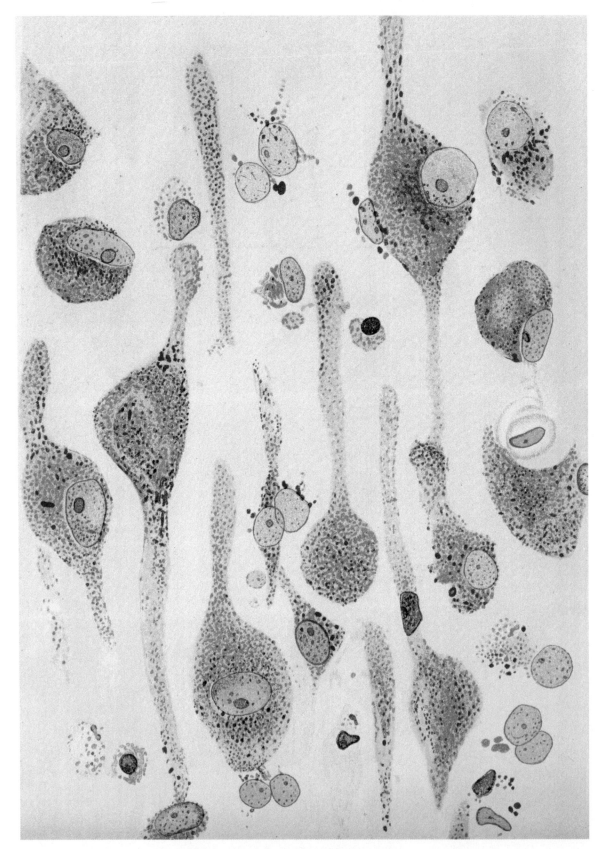

**FIGURE 239.** Schob, 1912. Histopathology of juvenile amaurotic idiocy.

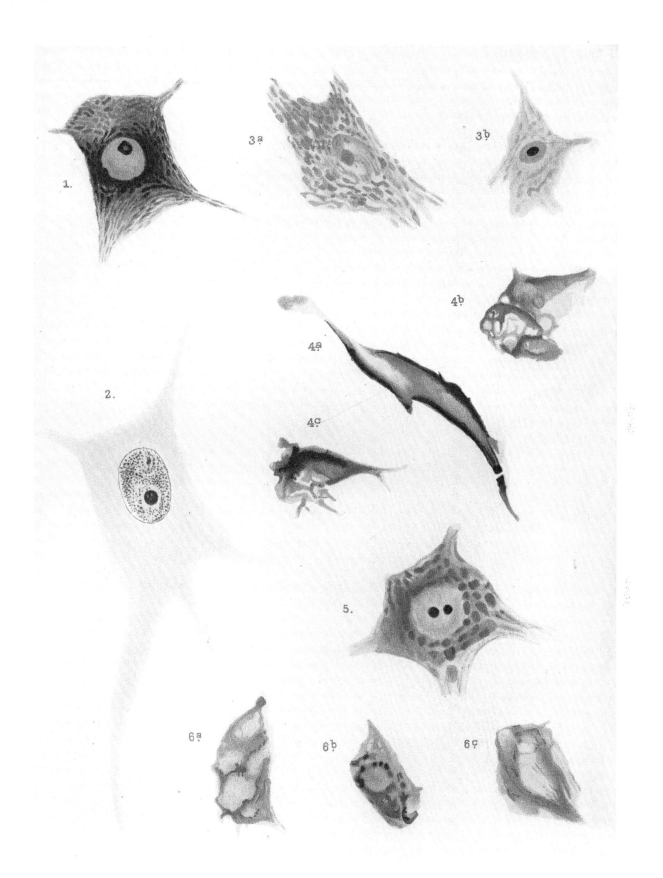

FIGURE 240. Trzebinski, 1912. Spinal cord histopathology, I.

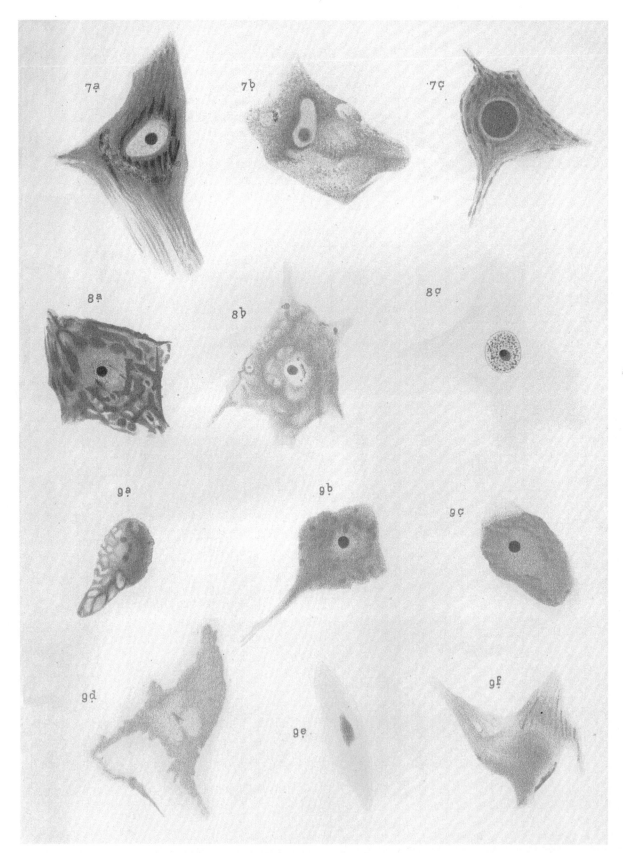

**FIGURE 241.** Trzebinski, 1912. Spinal cord histopathology, II.

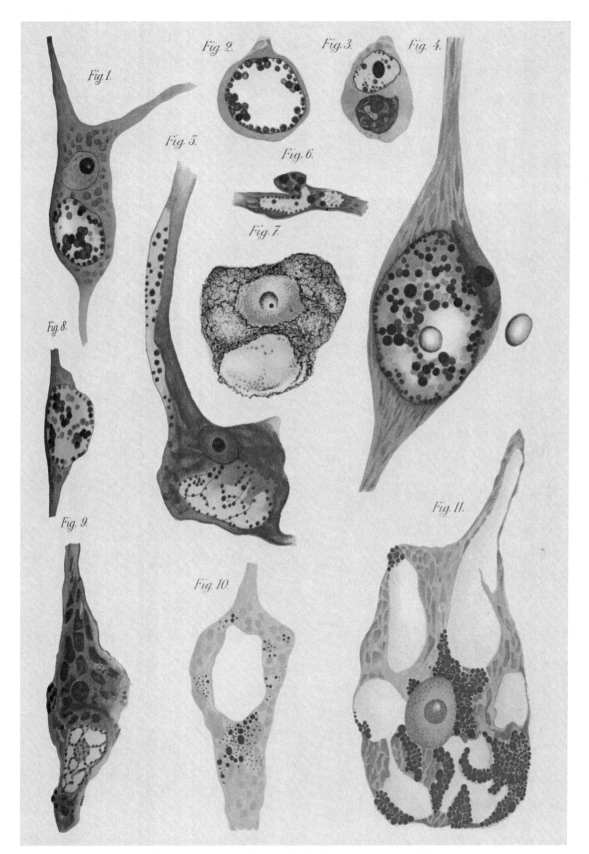

**FIGURE 242.** Rezza, 1913. Changes in neurons of the medulla oblongata in a case of dementia precox.

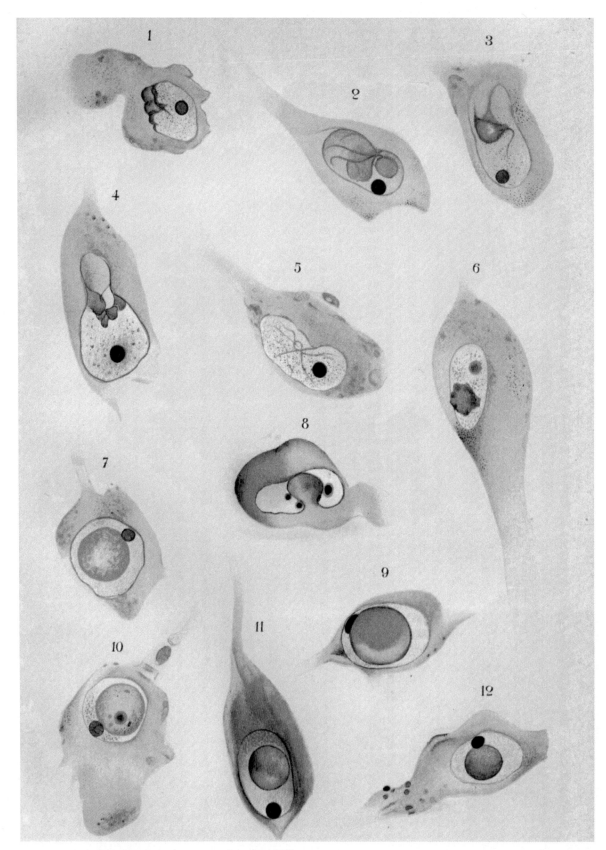

FIGURE 243. Achúcarro, 1913. Alterations of ganglion cells.

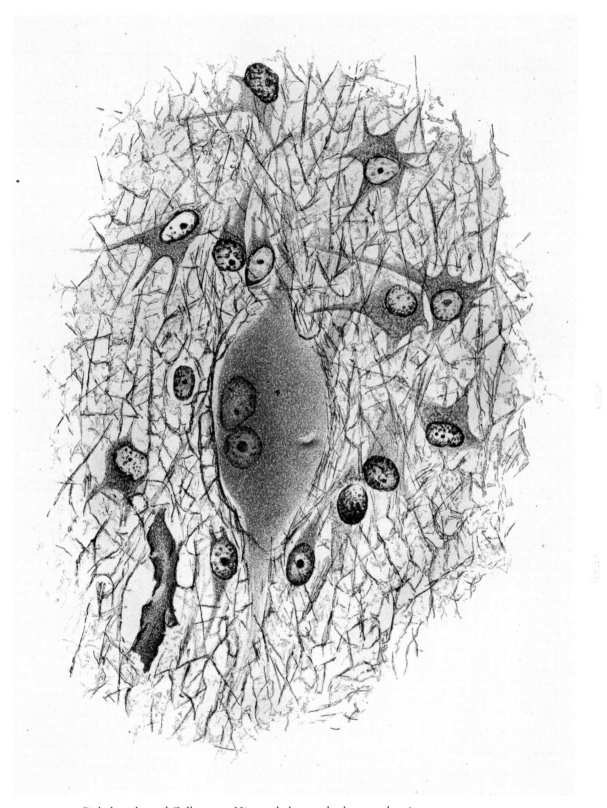

FIGURE 244.  Bielschowsky and Gallus, 1913. Histopathology and tuberous sclerosis.

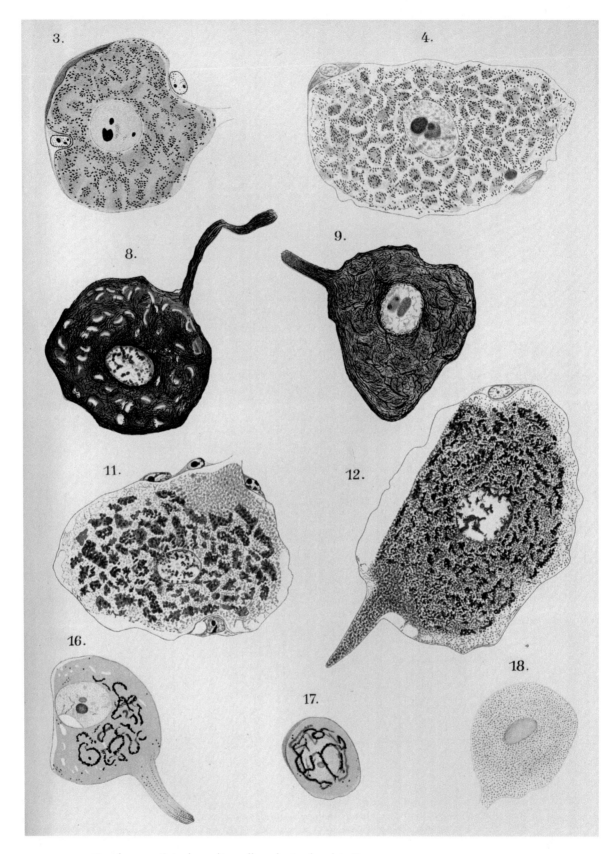

**FIGURE 245.** Cowdry, 1913. Spinal ganglion cells and mitochondria, I.

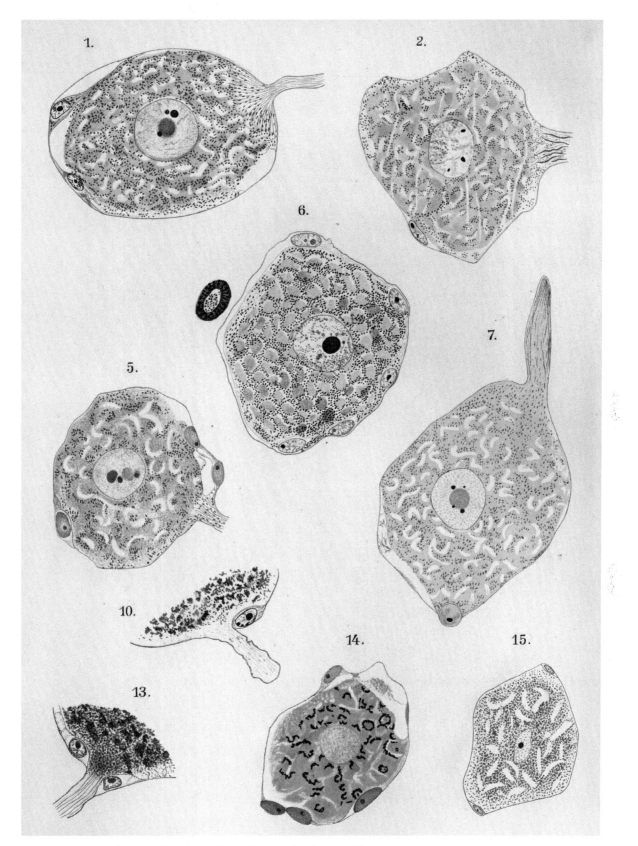

**FIGURE 246.** Cowdry, 1913. Spinal ganglion cells and mitochondria, II.

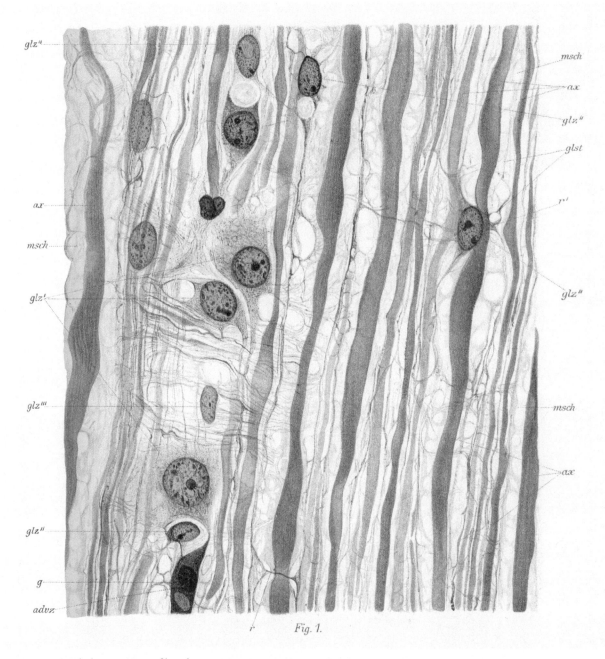

**FIGURE 247.** Jakob, 1913. Nerve fiber degeneration.

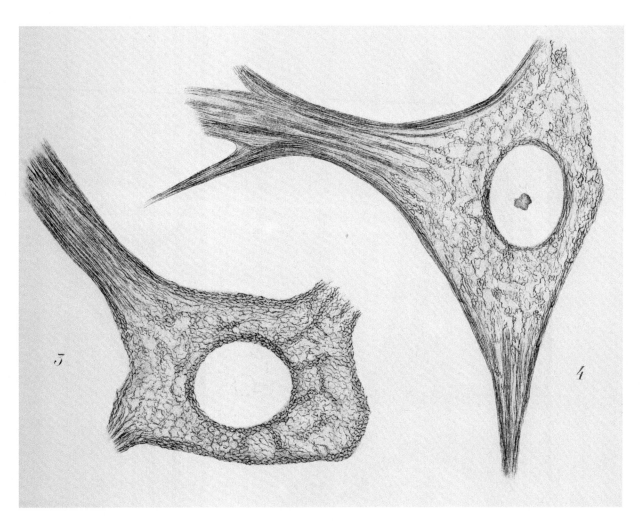

FIGURE 248. Rigotti, 1913. Alteration of the endocellular fibrillary reticulum, I.

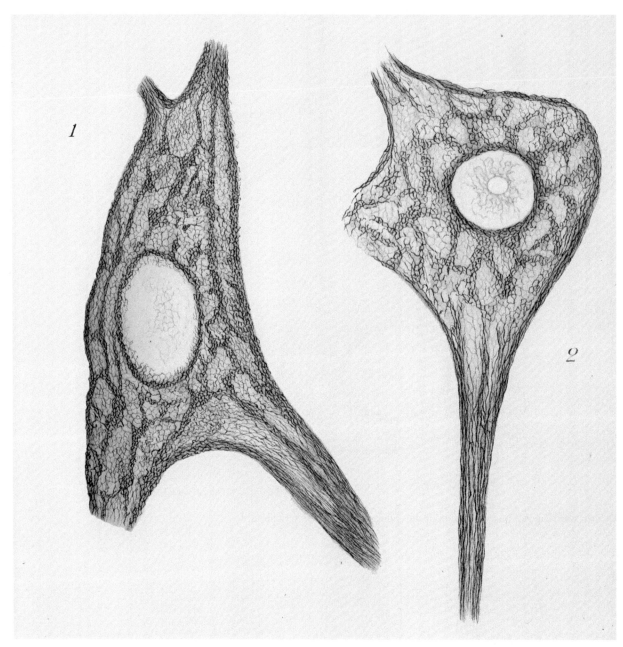

**FIGURE 249.** Rigotti, 1913. Alteration of the endocellular fibrillary reticulum, II.

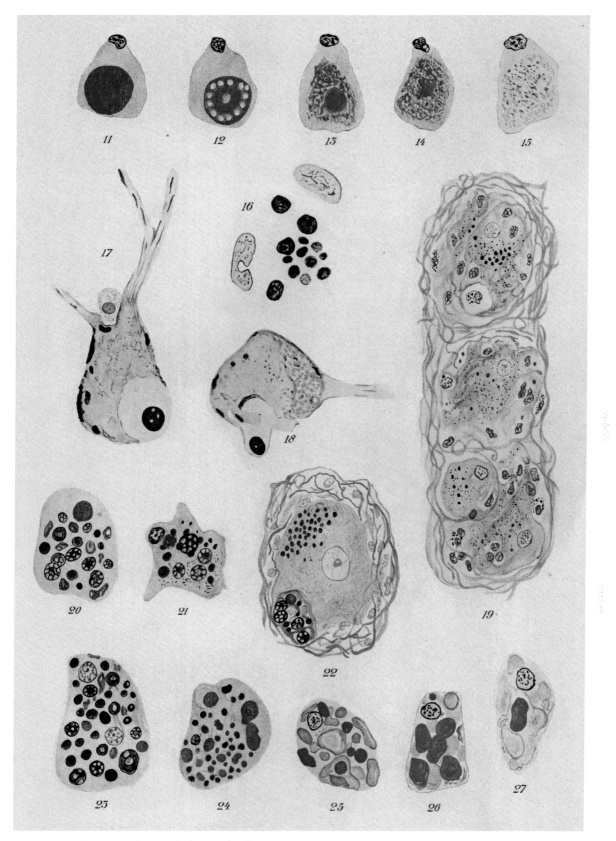

**FIGURE 250.** Rossi, 1913. Histopathology and pellagra.

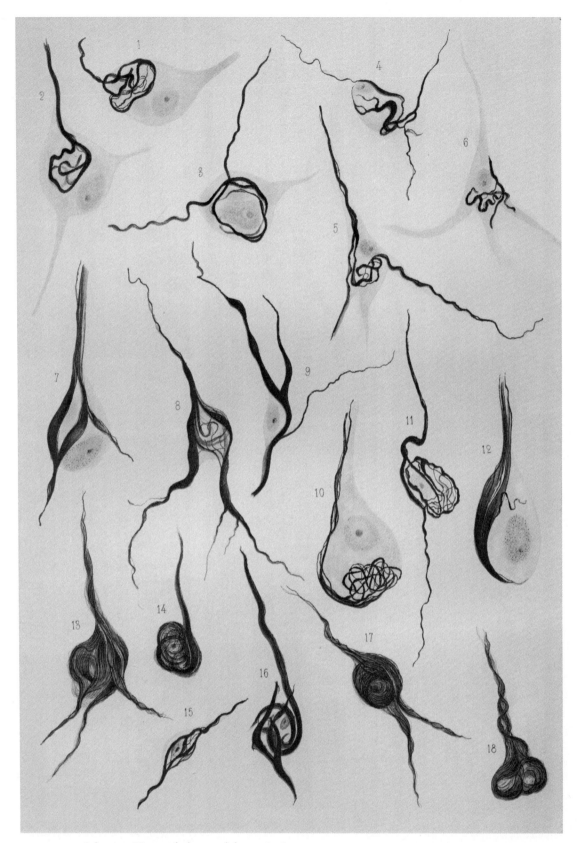

FIGURE 251. Sala, 1913. Histopathology and dementia, I.

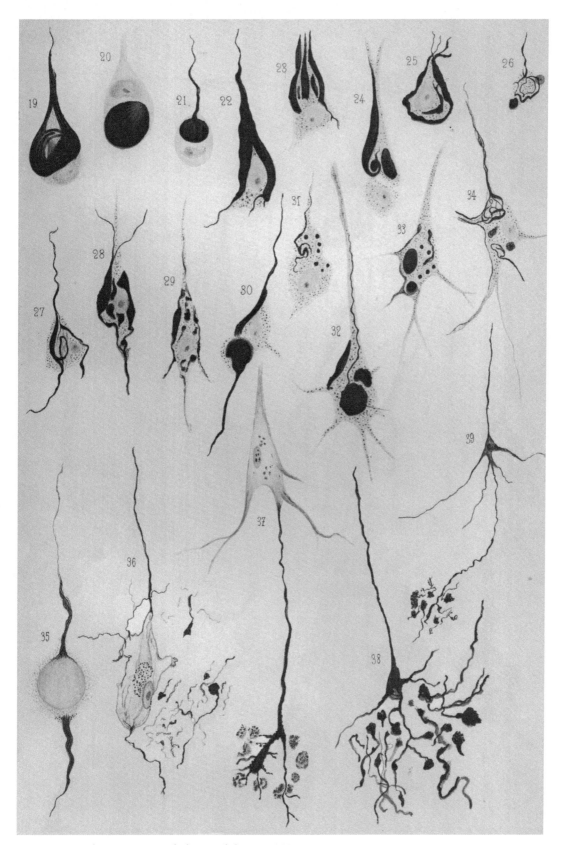

**FIGURE 252.** Sala, 1913. Histopathology and dementia, II.

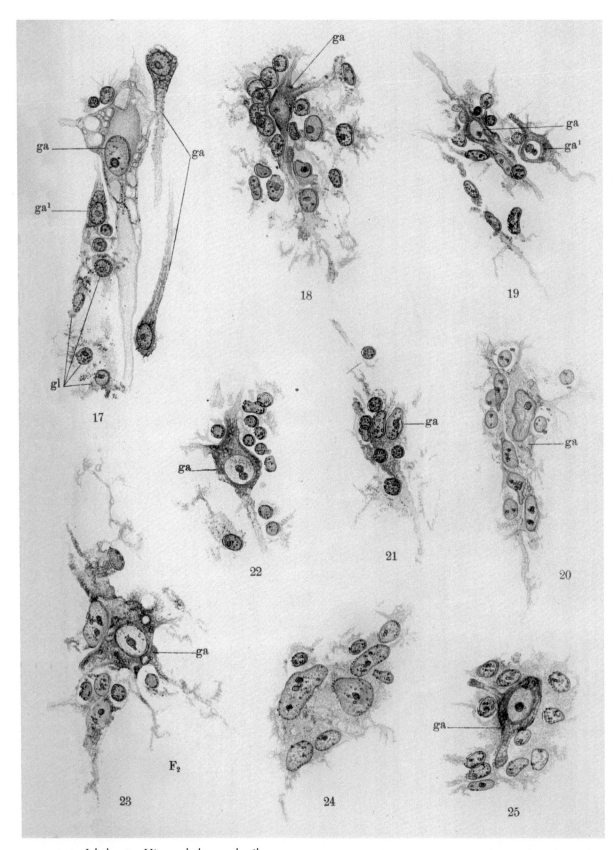

**FIGURE 253.** Jakob, 1914. Histopathology and epilepsy.

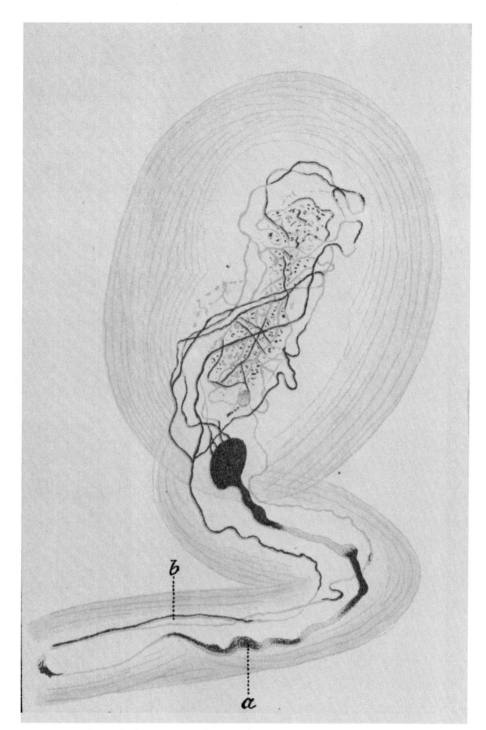

FIGURE 254. Martynoff, 1914. Encapsulated endings, I.

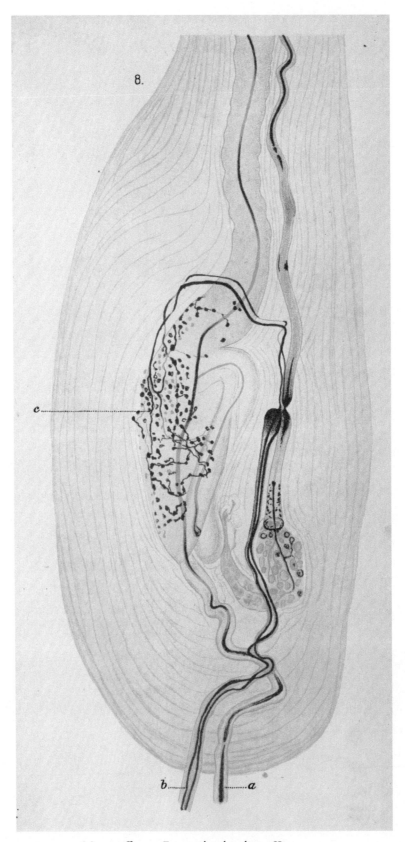

FIGURE 255. Martynoff, 1914. Encapsulated endings, II.

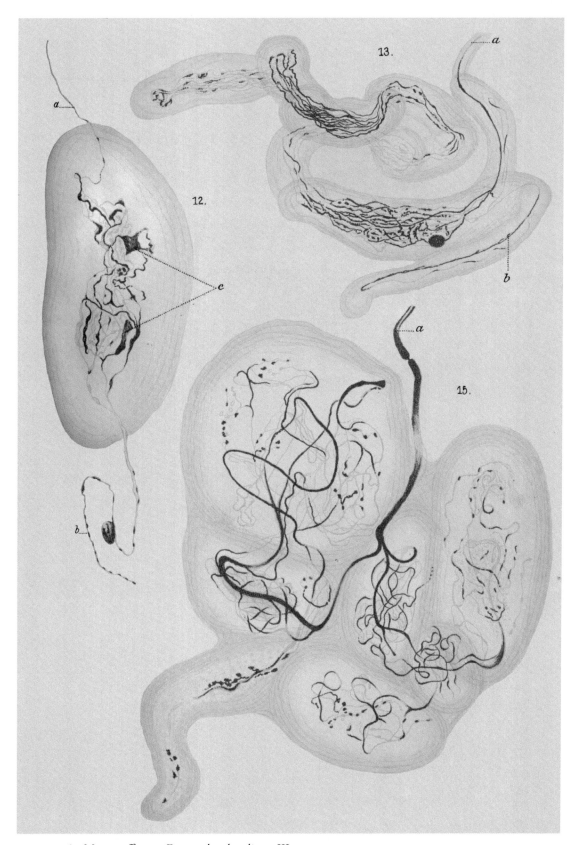

FIGURE 256. Martynoff, 1914. Encapsulated endings, III.

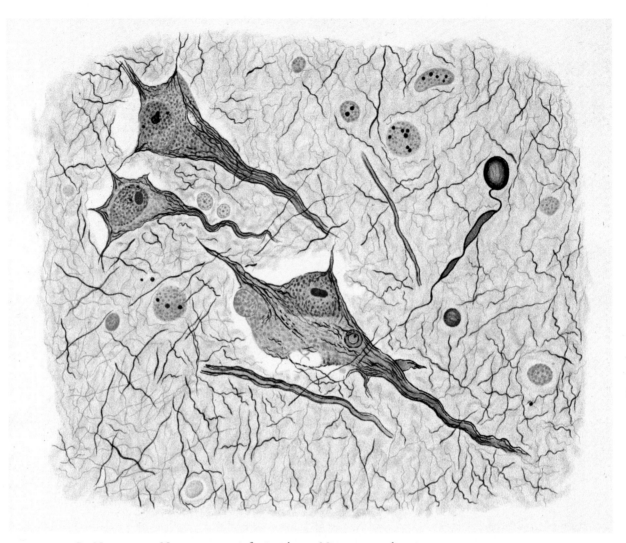

**FIGURE 257.** De Nunno, 1914. Nervous system infection due to *Micrococcus melitensis*.

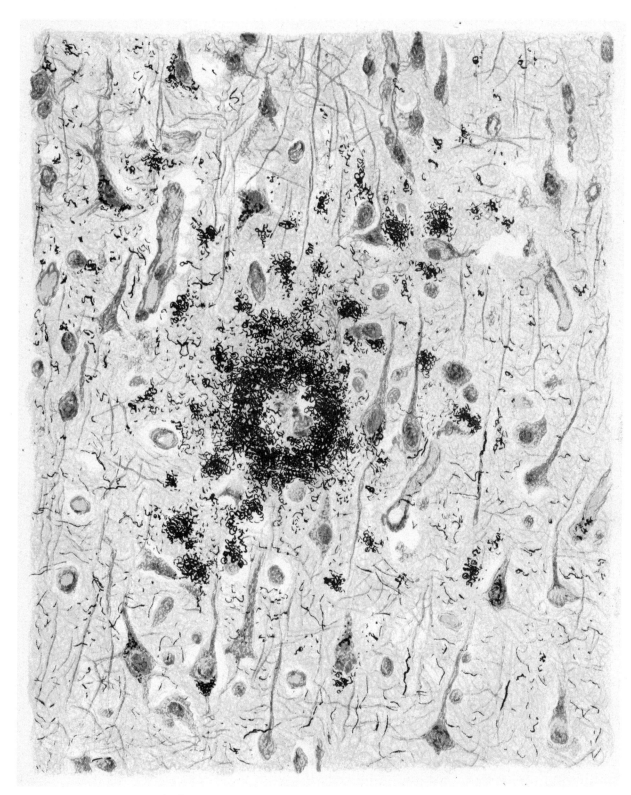

**FIGURE 258.** Cowe, 1915. Senile plaque, I.

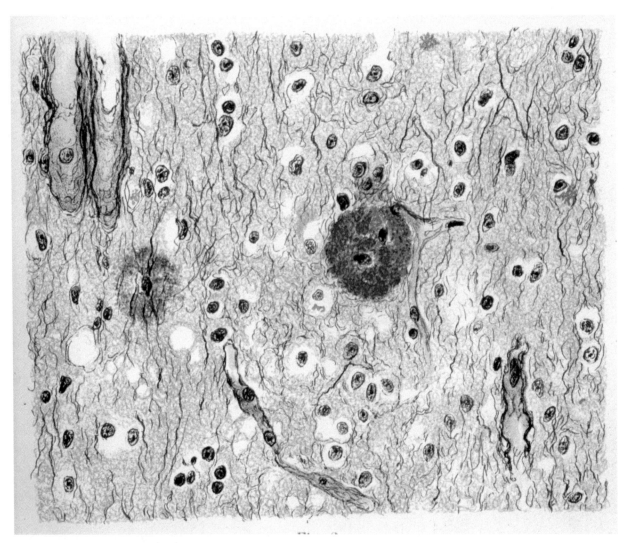

**FIGURE 259.** Cowe, 1915. Senile plaque, II.

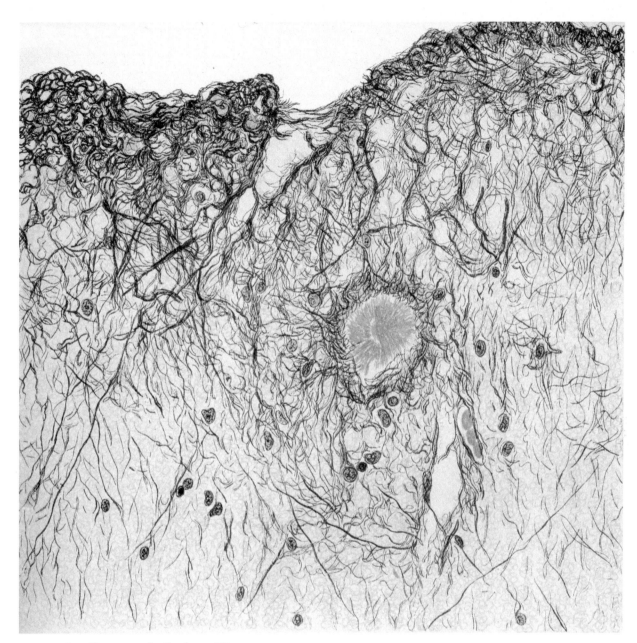

FIGURE 260. Cowe, 1915. Senile plaque, III.

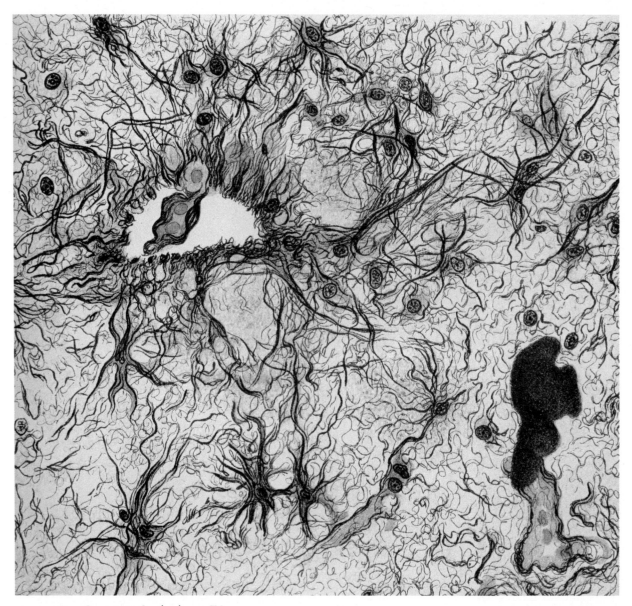

**FIGURE 261.** Cowe, 1915. Senile plaque, IV.

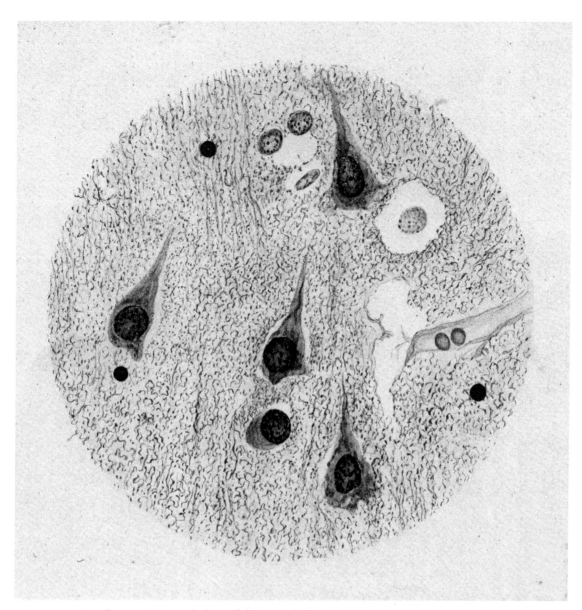

FIGURE 262. Papadia, 1916. Histopathology of the cerebral cortex.

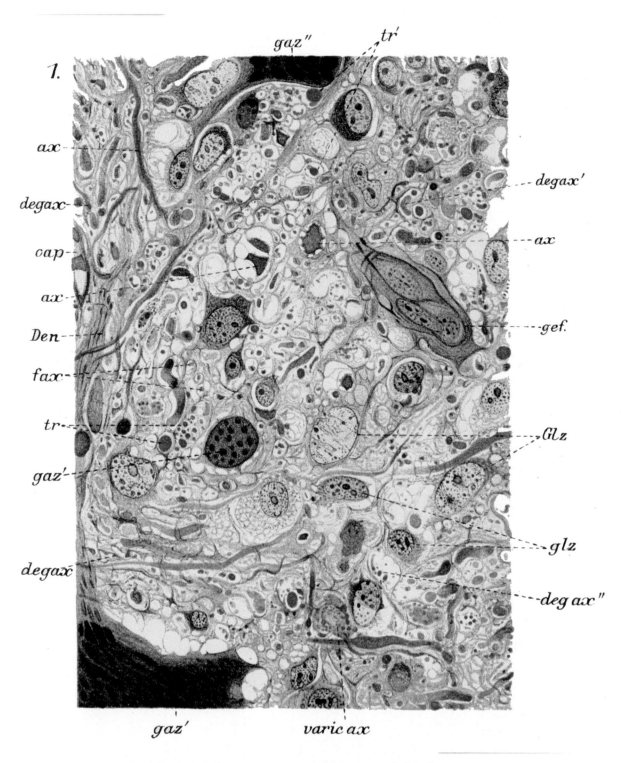

**FIGURE 263.** Lotmar, 1918. Histological alterations in acute myelitis and encephalitis, I.

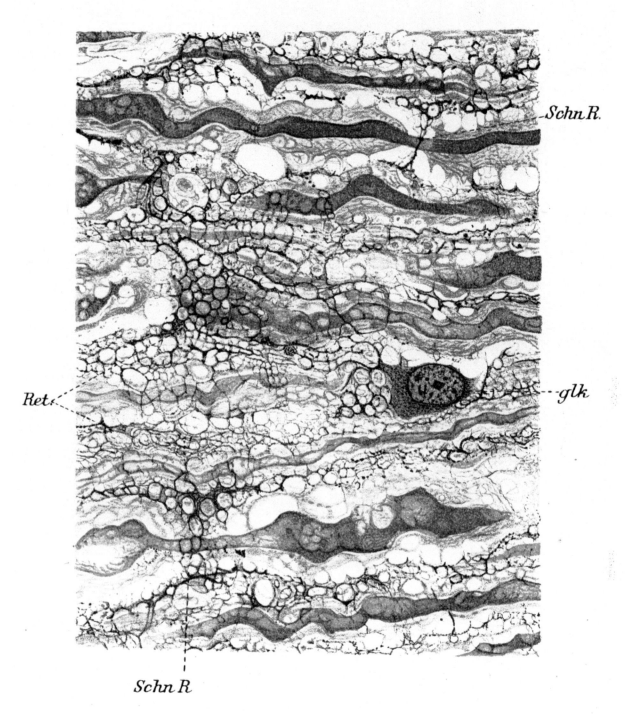

**FIGURE 264.** Lotmar, 1918. Histological alterations in acute myelitis and encephalitis, II.

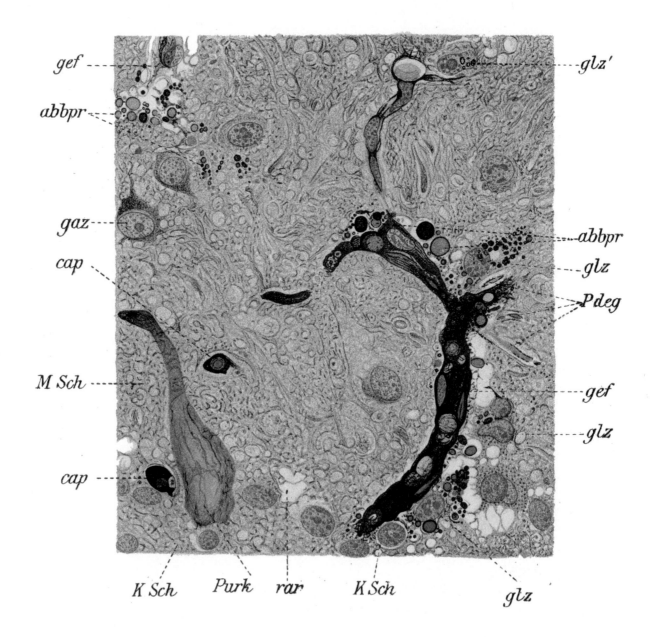

FIGURE 265. Lotmar, 1918. Histological alterations in acute myelitis and encephalitis, III.

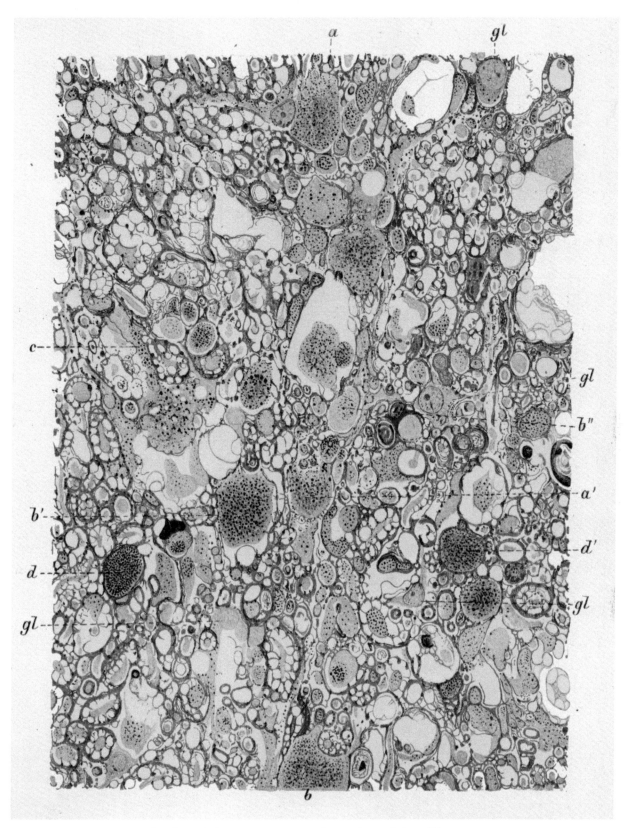

FIGURE 266.  Lotmar, 1918. Histological alterations in acute myelitis and encephalitis, IV.

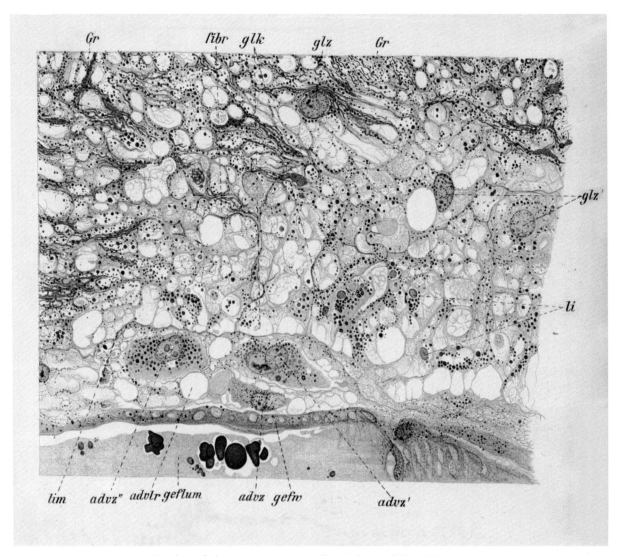

FIGURE 267.   Lotmar, 1918. Histological alterations in acute myelitis and encephalitis, V.

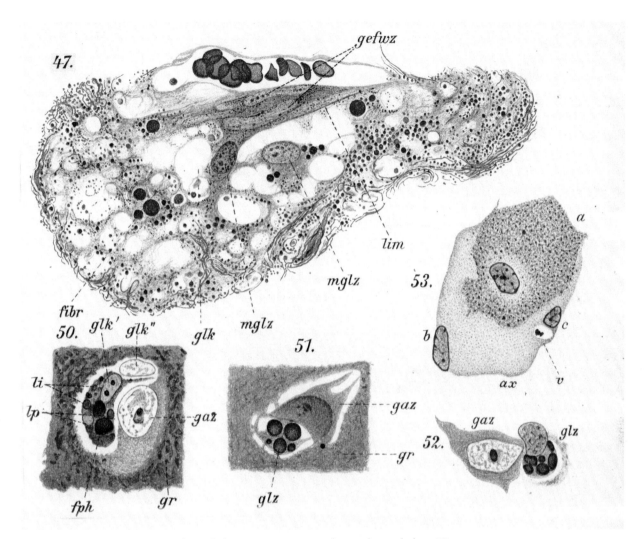

FIGURE 268. Lotmar, 1918. Histological alterations in acute myelitis and encephalitis, VI.

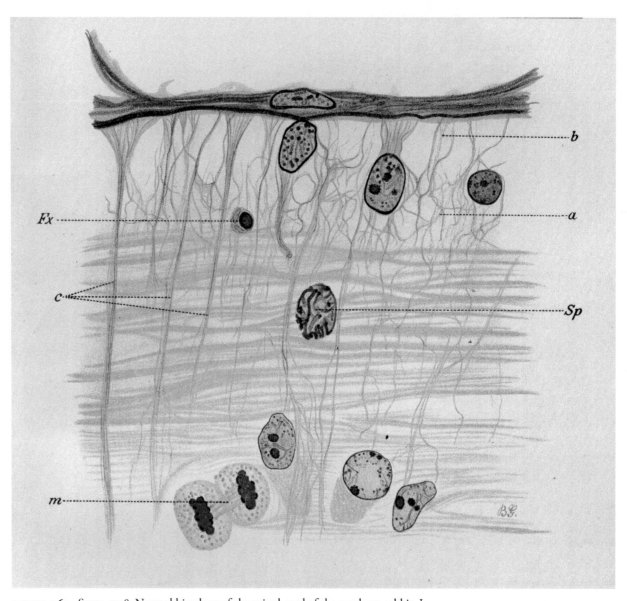

**FIGURE 269.** Spatz, 1918. Normal histology of the spinal cord of the newborn rabbit, I.

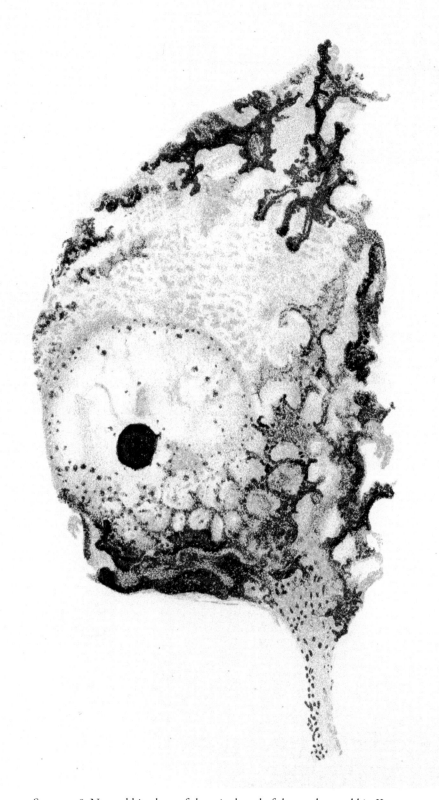

FIGURE 270. Spatz, 1918. Normal histology of the spinal cord of the newborn rabbit, II.

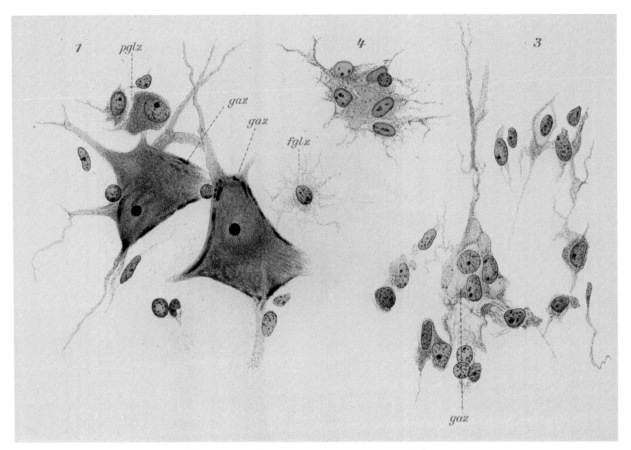

**FIGURE 271.** Creutzfeldt, 1921. Pathological changes in the brain, I.

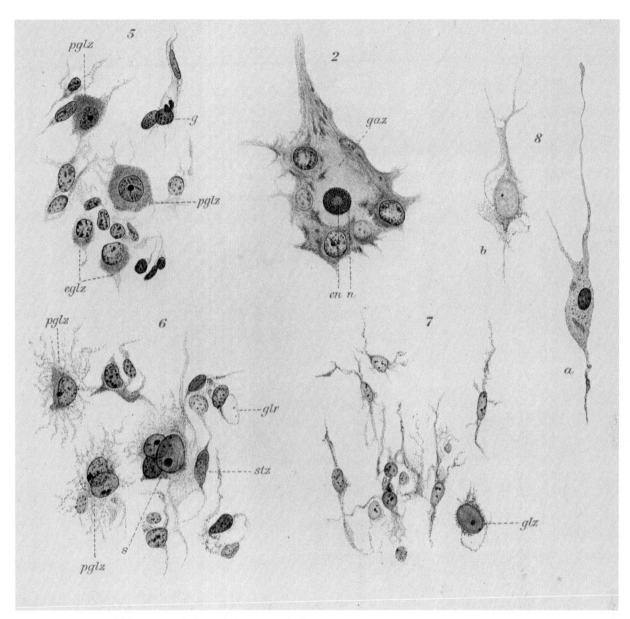

FIGURE 272. Creutzfeldt, 1921. Pathological changes in the brain, II.

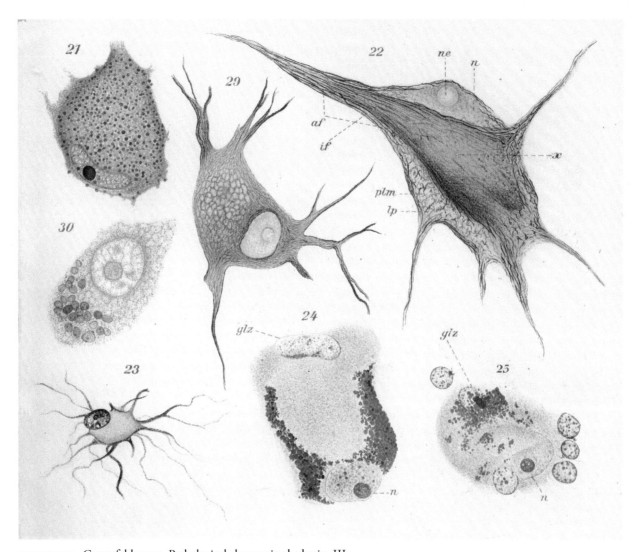

FIGURE 273. Creutzfeldt, 1921. Pathological changes in the brain, III.

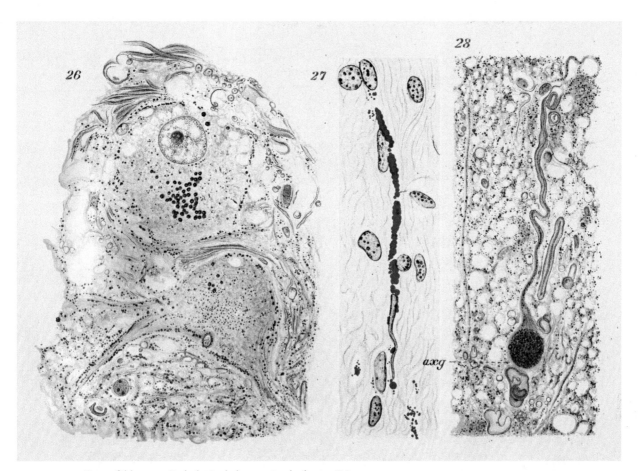

**FIGURE 274.** Creutzfeldt, 1921. Pathological changes in the brain, IV.

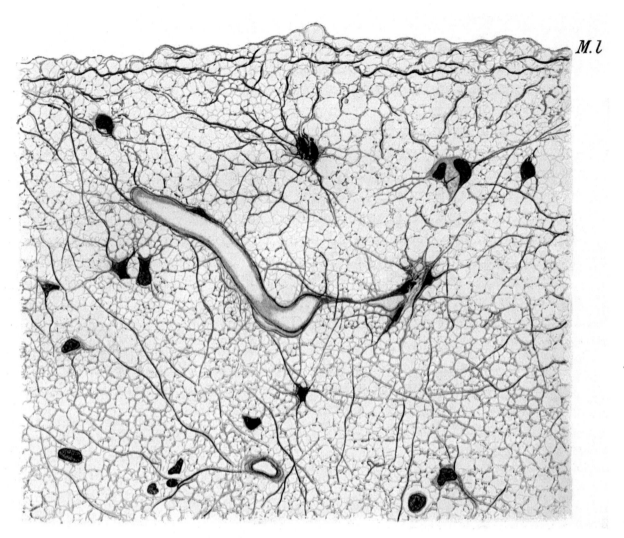

FIGURE 275. Spielmeyer, 1922. Histopathology of the nervous system, I.

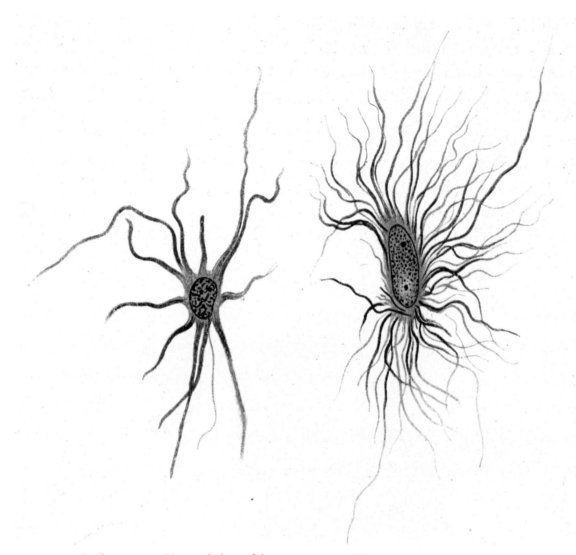

FIGURE 276. Spielmeyer, 1922. Histopathology of the nervous system, II.

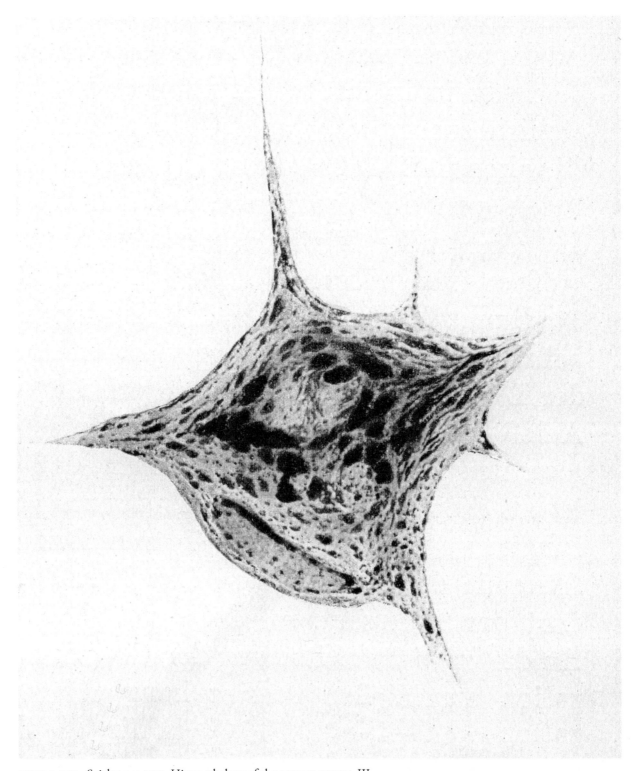

FIGURE 277. Spielmeyer, 1922. Histopathology of the nervous system, III.

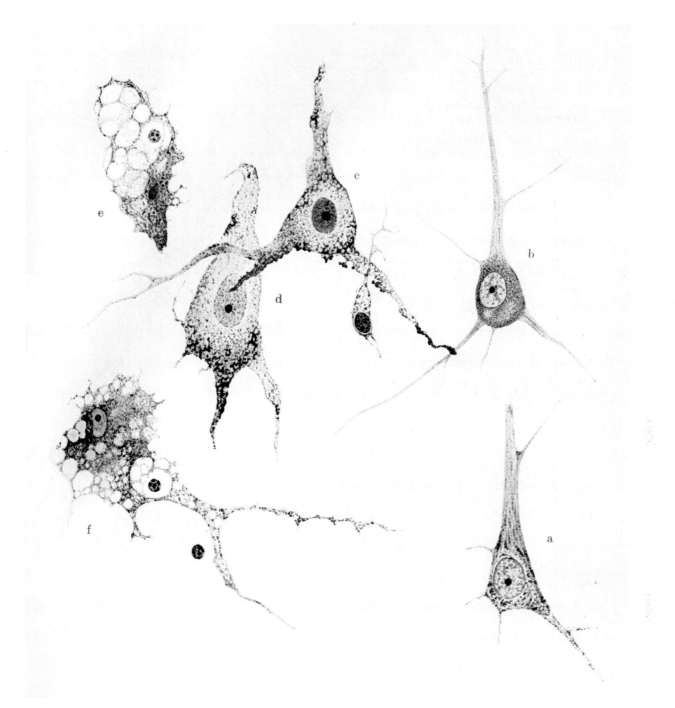

FIGURE 278. Spielmeyer, 1922. Histopathology of the nervous system, IV.

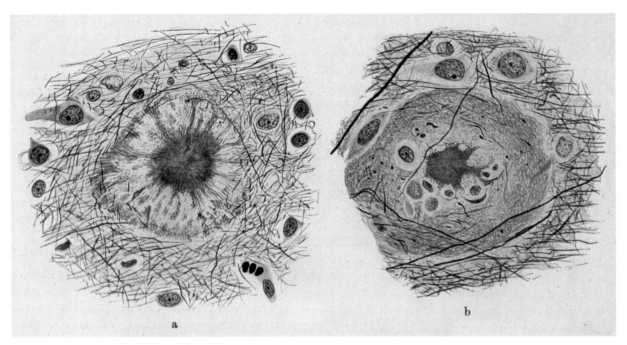

FIGURE 279.   Spielmeyer, 1922. Histopathology of the nervous system, V.

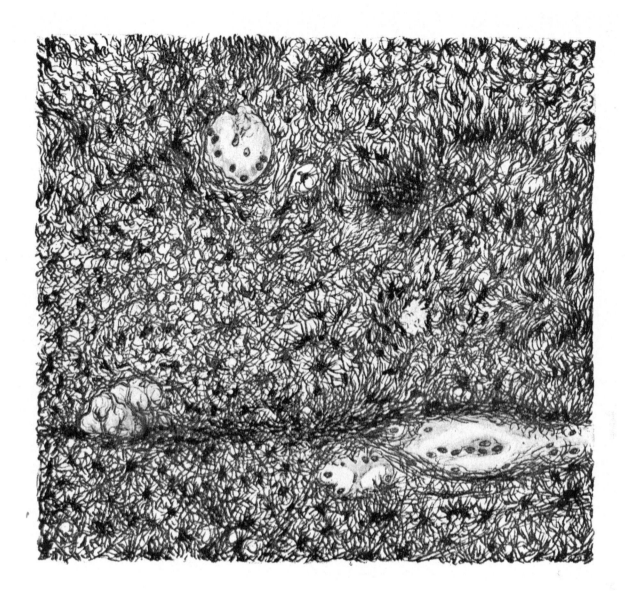

FIGURE 280. Spielmeyer, 1922. Histopathology of the nervous system, VI.

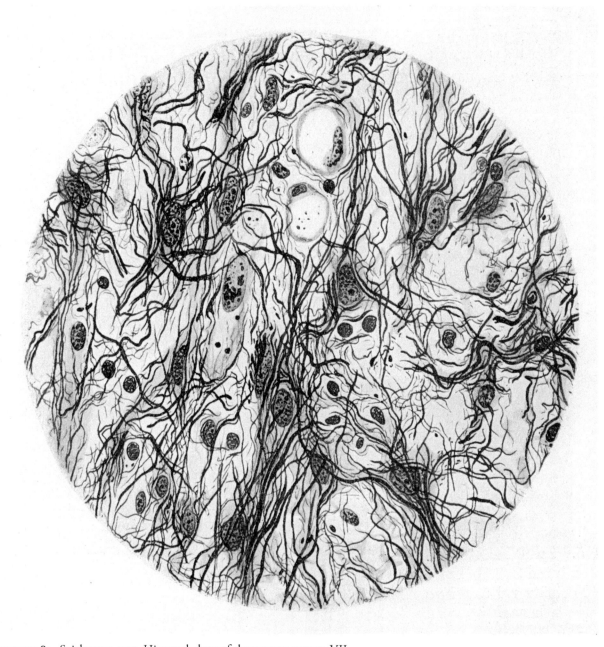

**FIGURE 281.** Spielmeyer, 1922. Histopathology of the nervous system, VII.

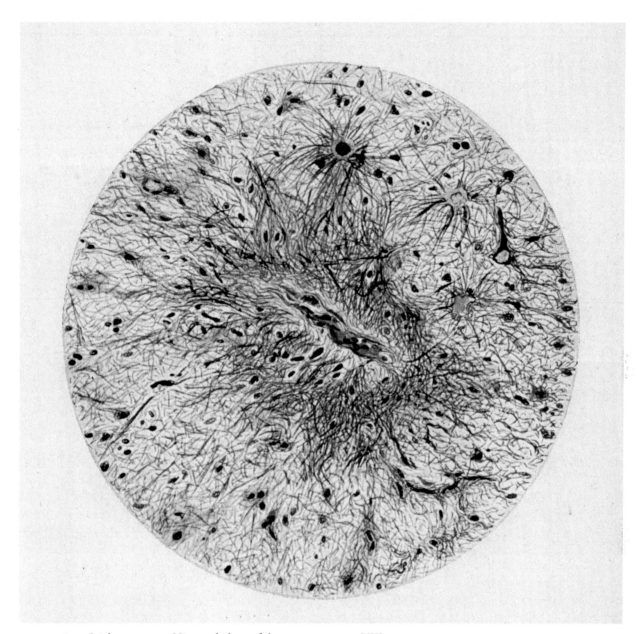

FIGURE 282. Spielmeyer, 1922. Histopathology of the nervous system, VIII.

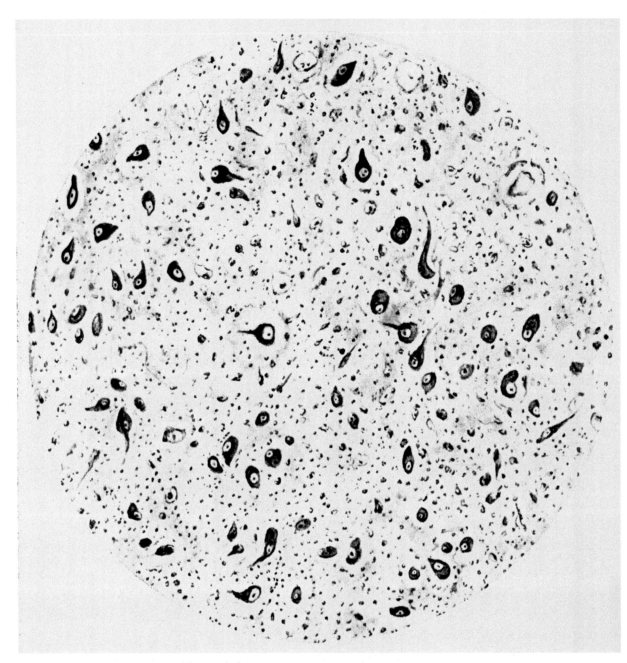

**FIGURE 283.** Bozzi, 1929. Cortical histopathology.

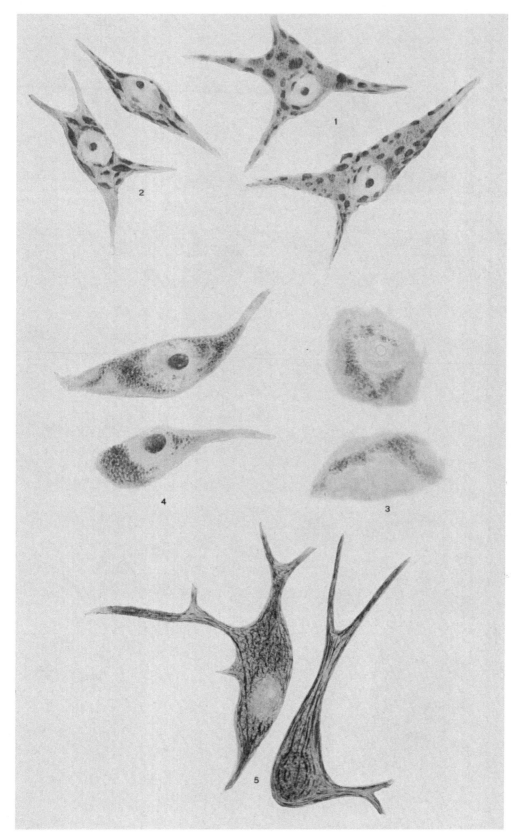

**FIGURE 284.** Emma, 1929. Neurons of the substantia nigra.

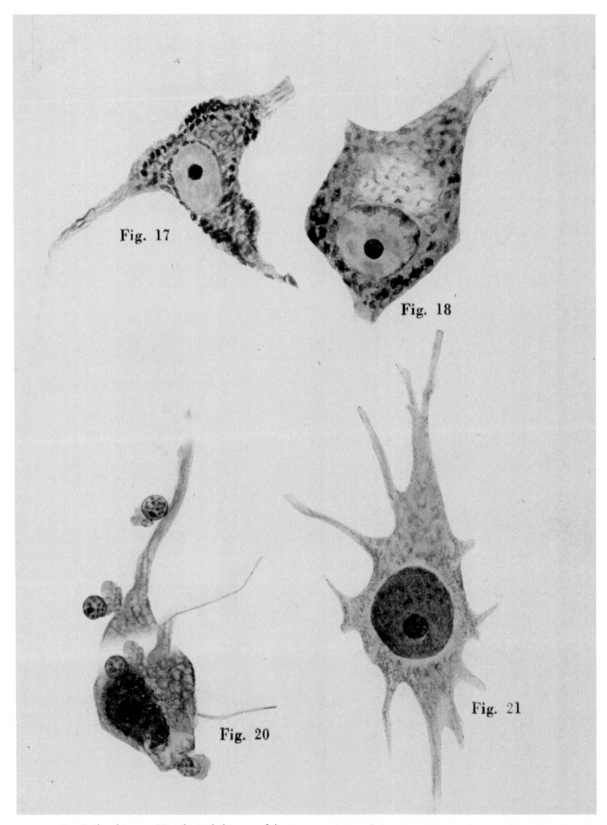

**FIGURE 285.** Berlucchi, 1931. Histological changes of the corpus striatum, I.

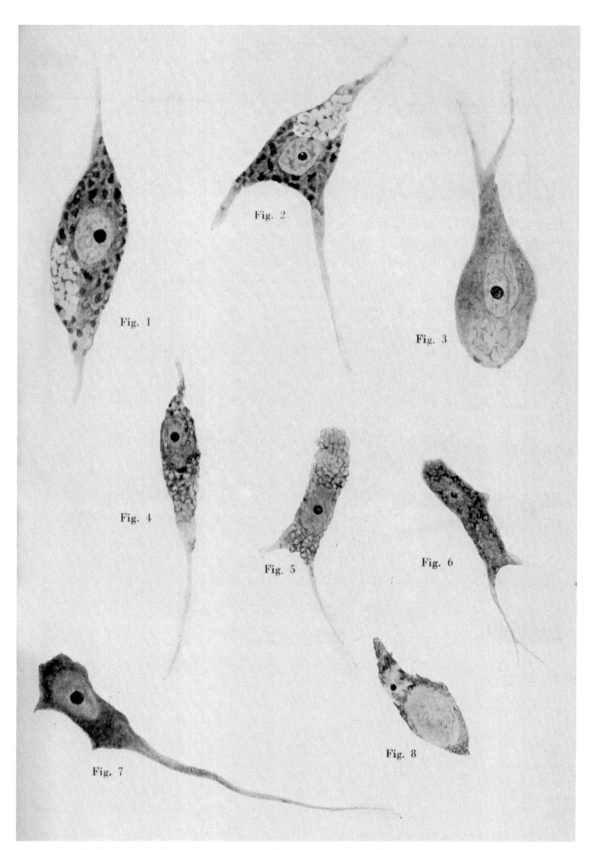

FIGURE 286. Berlucchi, 1931. Histological changes of the corpus striatum, II.

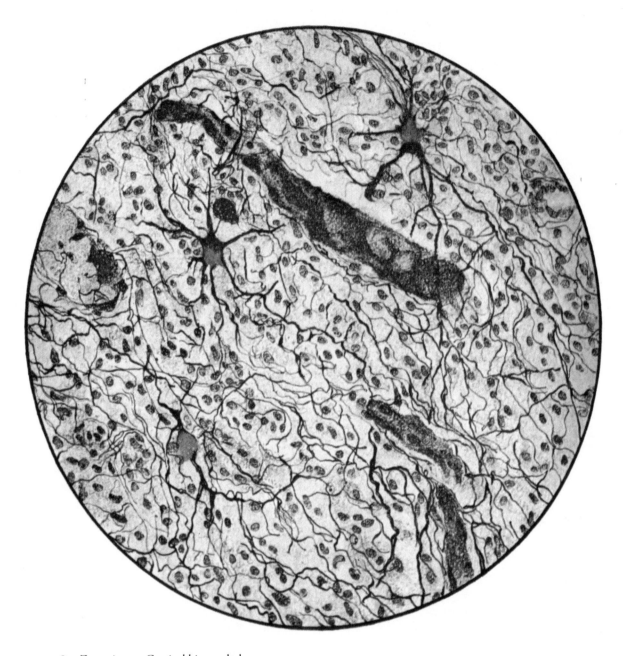

**FIGURE 287.** Zanetti, 1931. Cortical histopathology.

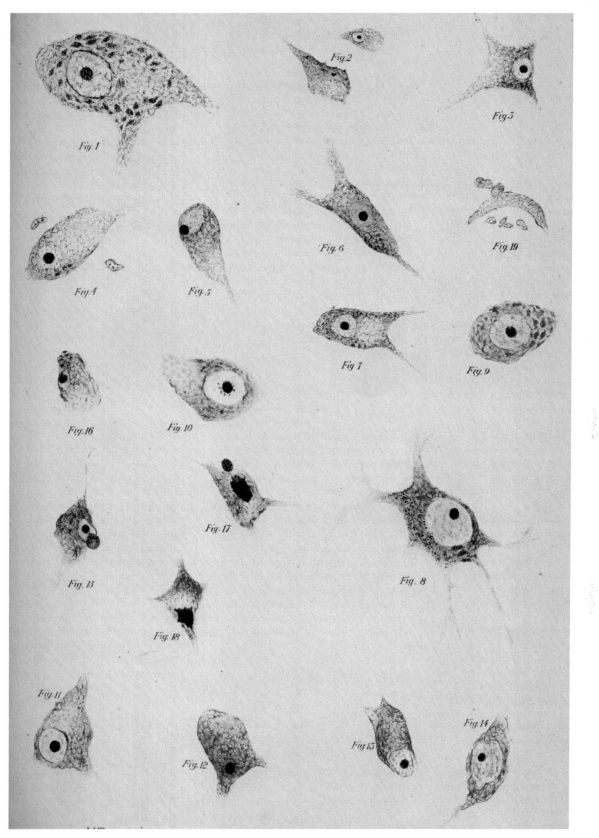

**FIGURE 288.** Tronconi, 1932. Histology and histopathology of the dentate nucleus.

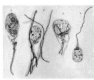

## FIGURE 137.

Smirnow, 1890. Structure of sympathetic nerve cells.

FIG. 1.

Nervenzelle aus dem Grenzstrange des Froschsympathicus. Die Zellkapsel ist vollkommen farblos und enthält Kerne. Die Zelle enthält einen Kern mit Kernkörperchen. Aus dem Zellkörper entspringt ein gerader fibrillärer Fortsatz. Aus den stark gewundenen pericellulären Fäden setzt sich die Spiralfaser zusammen. Letztere ist viel feiner, als die gerade Faser. Spiralfaser und pericelluläre Fäden erscheinen blau. Die Färbung mit Methylenblau ist fixirt mittelst Pikrocarmin. Reichert 8a. Oc. 3. FIG. 2. Nervenzelle aus dem Plexus in der Gaumenschleimhaut des Frosches. Man sieht den hellen bläschenförmigen Kern mit Kernkörperchen. Das gefärbte Oberflächennetz besteht aus sehr feinen varicösen Fäden. Die Varicositäten sind verschieden gross und verschieden geformt und enthalten Tröpfchen, die durch Methylenblau stark gefärbt sind. Aus diesem Netze entwickeln sich 3 gefärbte dünne Fasern, die anfangs mit der geraden, ungefärbten Faser in einer Richtung verlaufen. Eine von ihnen verläuft an ihrer Ursprungsstelle spiralig. Eine andere sehr feine Faser biegt von der geraden Faser ab, um in einem benachbarten Nervenstämmchen in entgegengesetzter Richtung zu verlaufen. In den umgebenden Nervenstämmchen sind nur einige Fasern gefärbt, die meisten sind ungefärbt. Fixirt mit pikrinsaurem Ammoniak. Reichert 8 a. Oc. 3. FIG. 3. Nervenzelle aus dem Grenzstrange des Sympathicus vom Frosch. In der ungefärbten .Zellkapsel sieht man Kerne. In dem hellen runden Kerne sieht man ein stark lichtbrechendes Kernkörperchen. Das feine Oberflächennetz bildet ziemlich regelmässige eckige Maschen. Die Spiralfaser scheint myelinhaltig zu sein und theilt sich in 2 Fasern, die sich an die gerade Faser legen. Methylenblau fixirt mit Jod. Zeiss. Oelimmersion 1/12. Oc. 3. FIG. 4. Nervenzelle aus der Harnblase der Kröte (Bufo vulgaris). In der ungefärbten Zelle liegt der helle runde Kern. Das gefärbte Oberflächennetz geht in die gefärbte Spiralfaser über. Der gerade Fortsatz ist nicht gezeichnet; weil er sehr verschwommen erschien. Die Färbung fixirt mit pikrinsaurem Ammoniak. Reichert 8 a. Ocu. 3. Smirnow, A. (1890) Die Struktur der Nervenzellen im Sympathicus der Amphibien. *Arch. Mikrosk. Anat. 5*, 407–423 [Plate 14].

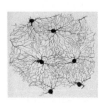

## FIGURE 138.

Dogiel, 1891. Human retinal ganglion cells.

Die Abbildungen sind sämmtlich mit Hülfe der Camera lucida nach Präparaten der Retina gezeichnet, welche durch Methylenblau gefärbt und mit pikrinsaurem Ammoniak oder Ammonium-Pikrat-Osmiumsäure-Mischung fixirt worden waren. Fig. 10. Nervenzellen des zweiten Typus aus dem Gangl. n. opt. *a* Protoplasmafortsätze, welche ein Netz bilden; *b* Axencylinderfortsätze; *c* Zelle des dritten Typus mit Axencylinderfortsatz. Mittlerer Theil der Retina. Flächenpräparat. Reichert, Obj. 6. Dogiel, A. S. (1891) Ueber die nervösen Elemente in der Retina des Menschen. *Arch. Mikrosk. Anat* 38, 317–344 [Figure 10].

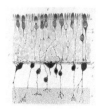

## FIGURE 139.

Dogiel, 1891. Diagram of the structure of the retina.

Die Abbildungen sind sämmtlich mit Hülfe der Camera lucida nach Präparaten der Retina gezeichnet, welche durch Methylenblau gefärbt und mit pikrinsaurem Ammoniak oder Ammonium-Pikrat-Osmiumsäure-Mischung fixirt worden waren. Fig. 1. Querschnitt durch die Retina. 1) Neuroepithelschicht ; 2) äussere reticuläre Schicht ; 3) Körnerschicht; 4) innere reticuläre Schicht; a) Membr.lim. externa; b) Stäbchen; c) Zapfen; d) grosse sternförmige Zellen mit äusseren und inneren Fortsätzen; e) bipolare Zellen mit den äusseren (horizontalen), dem intraepithelialen (f) und dem inneren Fortsatze; letzterer zerfällt in der inneren reticulären Schicht in ein Fibrillenbüschel. Reichert, Obj, 8a. Dogiel, A. S. (1891) Ueber die nervösen Elemente in der Retina des Menschen. *Arch. Mikrosk. Anat.* 38, 317–344 [Plate 19, Figure 1].

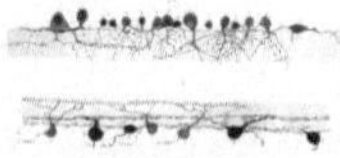

## FIGURE 140.

Dogiel, 1891. Nerve cells of the human retina.

Die Abbildungen sind sämmtlich mit Hülfe der Camera lucida nach Präparaten der Retina gezeichnet, welche durch Methylenblau gefärbt und mit pikrinsaurem Ammoniak oder Ammonium-Pikrat-Osmiumsäure-Mischung fixirt worden waren. Fig. 7. Querschnitt der Retina. 1) Innere reticuläre Schicht; 2) Ganglion nervi optici ; 3) Nervenfaserschicht ; a) Nervenzellen des I. Typus ; b) Nervenzellen des II. Typus; c) Nervenzellen des III. Typus. Protoplasmafortsätze, welche in der inneren reticulären Schicht Nervennetze bilden. Reichert, Obj. 6. Fig. 13. Durchschnitt der Netzhaut: 1) Mittlere gangliöse Schicht (Schicht der W. Müller'schen Spongioblasten); 2) innere reticuläre Schicht; a) grosse Nervenzellen; b) kleine Nervenzellen; c, c',c") Nervenzellen der II. Untergruppe: c) Zellen des 1. Typus; c') Zelle des II. Typus; c") Zellen des III. Typus. Reichert, Obj. 8a. Dogiel, A. S. (1891) Ueber die nervösen Elemente in der Retina des Menschen. *Arch. Mikrosk. Anat.* 38, 317–344 [Plates 20, 22; Figures 7, 13].

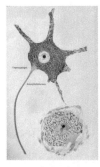

## FIGURE 141.

Held, 1895. Neurons in the spinal cord.

Die Figuren sind alle mit Zeiss homogener Immersion. Apochrom. 2·0, Ap. l·30 gezeichnet worden unter Anwendung von Querlicht und Abbé'schem Zeichenapparat. Die Vergrösserungen sind bei Taf. XII Fig. 1 und Taf. XIII Figg. 1, 8, 9, 10 durch Comp. ocul. 4, bei Taf. XII Fig. 2 und Taf. XIII Figg. 2, 3, 7 durch Ocul. 6, bei Taf. XIII Figg. 4, 5, 6, 11, 12, 13 durch Ocul. 8 erzielt worden. So weit möglich sind auch die feineren Structuren mit dem Abbé'schen Zeichenapparat entworfen worden. Die Angaben über Fixirung, Färbung und Herkunft des Materials sind zur besseren Uebersicht unter die Figuren gedruckt worden. Fig. 1 [up] Multipolare Vorderhornzelle. Rind. Lumbalmark. Paraffinschnitt 10 μ.Alkoh. 96%. Erythtosin-Methylenblau. Fig. 2 [down]. Spinalzelle.Kaninchen. Alkohol 96%. Paraffinschnitt 1-2 μ Erythrosin-Methylenblau. Held, H. (1895) Beiträge zur Structur der Nervenzellen und ihrer Fortsätze. *Arch. Anat. Phys. Anat. Abt.* 396–416 [Figures 1, 2].

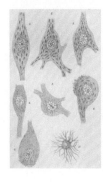

## FIGURE 142.

Arnold, 1898. Cells from the spinal cord of the cow.

1. Isolirte Ganglienzelle aus dem Vorderhorn des Rückenmarks vom Rind; 0,7% Kochsalzlösung; 2. Dasselbe,

Jod-Jodkalilösung 1) 1. c. u. über die feinere Structur der hämoglobinlosen und hämoglobinhaltigen Knochen-Markzellen. Virchow's Archiv Bd. 144. 1896. Es ist in dieser Beziehung ferner zu berücksichtigen, dass die angewandten Conservirungsmethoden auf das morphologische und tinctorielle Verhalten der "Granula" von grossem Einfluss sind; 3. Dasselbe, Jod-Jodkalilösung; 4. Dasselbe, Jod-Jodkalilösung; 5. Dasselbe, Jod-Jodkalilösung; 6. Dasselbe, Jodkalilösung und nachträglicher Zusatz von Jod-Jodkalilösung; 7. Dasselbe, die gleichen Zusatzflüssigkeiten; 8. Protoplasmafortsatz, dieselben Zusatzflüssigkeiten; 9. Centrale Nervenfaser, Zusatzflüssigkeiten wie bei 8; 10. Isolirte Gliazelle, 10% Jod-Jodkalilösung. Arnold, J. (1898) Ueber Structur und Architectur des Zellen. *Arch. Mikrosk. Anat.* 52, 535–552 [Plate 26; Figures 1–7, 10].

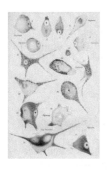

**FIGURE 143.**

Juliusburger and Meyer, 1898. Ganglion cells of the spinal cord.

1–3. Veränderte grosse Ganglienzellen der Centralwindungen (Fall 1). Härtung: Müller-Formol, Färbung: Thionin. Vergr.: Immersion (Zeiss und Winkel); 4. Veränderte grosse Ganglienzelle aus den Centralwindungen (Fall 1). Central restituirte Granula? (Härtung etc. wie oben.); 5. Veränderte Vorderhornzelle aus dem Lendenmark (Fall 1). (Härtung etc. wie oben.); 6. Unveränderte Vorderhornzelle aus dem unteren Lendernmark der rechten Seite. (Härtung etc. wie oben.); 7. Veränderte Vorderhornzelle aus dem unteren Lendenmark der linken Seite. (Härtung etc. wie oben.); 8. Unveränderte grosse Ganglienzelle aus den Centralwindungen der linken Seite. (Härtung etc. wie oben.); 9. Veränderte grosse Ganglienzelle aus den Centralwindungen der rechten Seite. (Härtung etc. wie oben.); 10–12. Veränderte Vorderhornzellen aus dem Lendenmark. (Härtung: Alkohol, Färbung: Məthylenblau [nach Nissl], Imm.: Zeiss.); 13–16. Veränderte Vorderhornzellen aus dem Lendenmark (Härtung etc. wie vorige). Juliusburger, O. and Meyer, E. (1898) Beitrag zur Pathologie der Ganglenzelle. *Monatsschr. Psychiatr. Neurol.* 3, 316–343 [Figures 1–16].

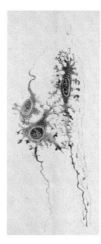

**FIGURE 144.**

Dogiel, 1899. Cells of the Auerbach plexus.

Kleines Ganglion des Auerbach'schen Geflechts aus dem Dünndarm des Meerschweinchens. *a* Ganglienzellen des ersten Typus; die Endverästelungen der Dendriten der Zellen bilden ein Netz. 8a. Dogiel, A. S. (1899) Ueber den Bau der Ganglien in den Geflechten des Darmes und der Gallenblase des Menschen und der Säugethiere. *Arch. Anat. Physiol. Anat. Abt. (Leipzig)* 130–158 [Plate 5, Figure 2].

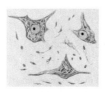

**FIGURE 145.**

Nelis, 1899. Structure of the nerve cell protoplasm, I.

Toutes les figures ont été dessinées a la chambre claire d'Abbé, avec la table spéciale construite par Zeiss, l'objectif à immersion homogène de 2 millimètres et l'oculaire apochromatique n° 4 du même constructeur. Le tube du microscope a été étiré. FIG. 8. Cellules de la corne antérieure de la moelle de Cobaye inoculé de toxines tétaniques. Méthode de Nissl. Nelis, C. (1899) Un nouveau detail de structure du Protoplasme des Cellules nerveuses (état espérimateux du protoplasme). *Bull. Acad. R. Belgique* 37, 102–124 [Figure 8].

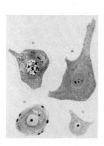

**FIGURE 146.**

Nelis, 1899. Structure of the nerve cell protoplasm, II.

Toutes les figures ont été dessinées a la chambre claire d'Abbé, avec la table spéciale construite par Zeiss, l'objectif à immersion homogène de 2 millimètres et l'oculaire apochromatique n° 4 du même constructeur. Le tube du microscope a été étiré. FIG. 4. Cellule pyramidale de l'écorce cérébrale d'un Chien normal. Méthode de Nissl. FIG. 9. Cellule de la corne antérieure de la moelle d'un Chien enragé. Méthode de Heidenhain. FIG. 10. Cellule pyramidale de l'écorce cérébrale du même Chien enragé. Méthode de Heidenhain. FIG. 11.Cellule d'un ganglion spinal de Lapin inoculé de rage. Méthode de Heidenhain. Nelis, C. (1899) Un nouveau detail de structure du Protoplasme des Cellules nerveuses (état espérimateux du protoplasme). *Bull. Acad. R. Belgique* 37, 102–124 [Figures 4, 9, 10, 11].

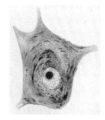

**FIGURE 147.**

Righetti, 1899. Nerve cell of the spinal cord, I.

Cellula radicolare anteriore (midollo lombare). Cromatolisi periferica iniziale. Disposizione eccezionale del pigmento e degli elementi cromatofili a strati alternati concentrici. Righetti, R. (1899) Polinevrite radiculare in un caso di psicosi pellagrosa. *Riv. Patol. Nerv. Ment.* 4, 433–456 [Figure 3].

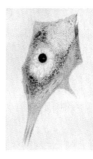

**FIGURE 148.**

Righetti, 1899. Nerve cell of the spinal cord, II.

Cellula radicolare anteriore (midollo lombare). Cromatolisi periferica. Grande zolla di pigmento inclusa fra gli elementi cromatofili superstiti. Righetti, R. (1899) Polinevrite radiculare in un caso di psicosi pellagrosa. *Riv. Patol. Nerv. Ment.* 4, 433–456 [Figure 5].

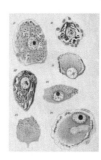

**FIGURE 149.**

Holmgren, 1900. Fine structure of nerve cells, I.

Alle Figuren sind mit dem Abbeschen Zeichenapparat ausgeführt. FIG. 17-19. Spinale Nervenzelle vom Huhn. Rabls Gemisch. Tol.-Erythr. Dieselbe Vergrösserung. FIG. 22. Motorische Nervenzelle desselben Tieres. Übrigens dasselbe. FIG. 23. Spinale Nervenzelle des Frosches. Apàthys Gemisch. Tol.-Erythr. Dieselbe Vergr. FIG 24. Dasselbe. FIG. 26. Sympathische Nervenzelle desselben Tieres. Übrigens dasselbe. Holmgren, E. (1900) Studien in der Feineren Anatomie der Nervezellen. *Anat. Hefte* 15, 1–88 [Figures 17–19, 22–24, 26].

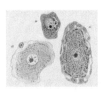

**FIGURE 150.**

Holmgren, 1900. Fine structure of nerve cells, II.

Alle Figuren sind mit dem Abbeschen Zeichenapparat ausgeführt. FIG. 10. Spinale Nervenzelle vom Hund. Rabls Gemisch. Tol.-Erythr. Dieselbe Vergr. FIG. 13. Spinale Nervenzelle von Katze. Rabls Gemisch. Tol.-Erythr. Dieselbe Vergr. FIG. 15. Spinale Nervenzelle vom Pferd. Rabls Gemisch. Tol.-Erythr. Dieselbe Vergr. Holmgren, E. (1900) Studien in der Feineren Anatomie der Nervezellen. *Anat. Hefte* 15, 1–88 [Figures 10, 13, 15].

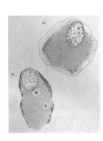

**FIGURE 151.**

Holmgren, 1900. Fine structure of nerve cells, III.

Alle Figuren sind mit dem Abbeschen Zeichenapparat ausgeführt. FIG. 62. Spinale Nervenzelle von Acanthias. Rabls Gemisch. Ammoniummolybdanat-Toluidin. Dieselbe Vergr. FIG. 64. Dasselbe. Tol.-Erythr. Holmgren, E. (1900) Studien in der Feineren Anatomie der Nervezellen. *Anat. Hefte* 15, 1–88 [Figures 62, 64].

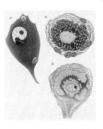

**FIGURE 152.**

Holmgren, 1900. Fine structure of nerve cells, IV.

Alle Figuren sind mit dem Abbeschen Zeichenapparat ausgeführt. FIG. 35. Nervenzelle von Medulla oblongata von Petromyzon. Apàthys Gemisch. Tol.-Erythr. Dieselbe Vergr. FIG. 36. Nervenzelle von Schlundganglion von Astacus fluviatilis. Rabls Gemisch. Tol.-Erythr. Dieselbe Vergr. FIG. 39. Nervenzelle von Schlundganglion von Hirudo medicinalis. Rabls Gemisch. Tol.-Erythr. Dieselbe Vergr. Holmgren, E. (1900) Studien in der Feineren Anatomie der Nervezellen. *Anat. Hefte* 15, 1–88 [Figures 35, 36, 39].

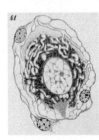

**FIGURE 153.**

Holmgren, 1900. Fine structure of nerve cells, V.

Alle Figuren sind mit dem Abbeschen Zeichenapparat ausgeführt. FIG. 41.

Elektrisierte spinale Nervenzelle vom Kaninchen. Rabls Gemisch. Tol.- Erythr. Dieselbe Vergr. Holmgren, E. (1900) Studien in der Feineren Anatomie der Nervezellen. *Anat. Hefte* 15, 1–88 [Figure 41].

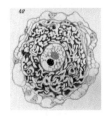

**FIGURE 154.**

Holmgren, 1900. Fine structure of nerve cells, VI.

Alle Figuren sind mit dem Abbeschen Zeichenapparat ausgeführt. FIG. 42. Elektrisierte spinale Nervenzelle vom Huhn. Rabls Gemisch Tol.-Erythr. Dieselbe Vergr. Holmgren, E. (1900) Studien in der Feineren Anatomie der Nervezellen. *Anat. Hefte* 15, 1–88 [Figure 42].

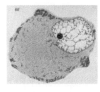

**FIGURE 155.**

Holmgren, 1900. Fine structure of nerve cells, VII.

Alle Figuren sind mit dem Abbeschen Zeichenapparat ausgeführt. FIG. 66. Spinale Nervenzelle von Acanthias. Rabls Gemisch. Ammoniummolybdanat-Toluidin. Dieselbe Vergr. Holmgren, E. (1900) Studien in der Feineren Anatomie der Nervezellen. *Anat. Hefte* 15, 1–88 [Figure 66].

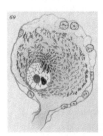

**FIGURE 156.**

Holmgren, 1900. Fine structure of nerve cells, VIII.

Alle Figuren sind mit dem Abbeschen Zeichenapparat ausgeführt. FIG. 60. Spinale Nervenzelle vom Huhn. Rabls Gemisch. Tol.-Erythr. Dieselbe Vergr. Holmgren, E. (1900) Studien in der Feineren Anatomie der Nervezellen. *Anat. Hefte* 15, 1–88 [Figure 60].

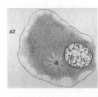

**FIGURE 157.**

Holmgren, 1900. Fine structure of nerve cells, IX.

Alle Figuren sind mit dem Abbeschen Zeichenapparat ausgeführt. FIG. 63. Spinale Nervenzelle von Acanthias. Rabls Gemisch. Ammoniummolybdanat-Toluidin. Dieselbe Vergr. Holmgren, E. (1900) Studien in der Feineren Anatomie der Nervezellen. *Anat. Hefte* 15, 1–88 [Figure 63].

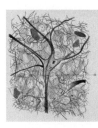

**FIGURE 158.**

Dimitrova, 1901. Structure of the pineal gland.

Toutes les figures de cette planche out été dessinées d'après des préparations colorées par la méthode de WEIGERT sauf la FIG. 2 qui est reproduite d'après une coupe traitée par l'hématoxyline ferrique. Pour ne pas compliquer le tirage en couleurs nous lui avons donné les mèmes teintes qu'aux autres. Tous les dessins ont été faits avec l'objectif. à immersion 1/12 Leitz et l'oculaire 6. FIG. 7. Dessinée d'après une préparation très différenciée. a, cellule névroglique. Noyaux clairs à fines granulations; noyaux clairs à grosses granulations et noyaux foncée à granulations. (Homme). Dimitrova, Z. (1901) Recherches sur la structure de la glande pinéale chez quelques mammifères. *Névraxe* 2, 257–321 [Figure 7].

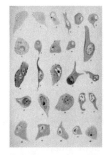

**FIGURE 159.**

Kolster, 1901. Structure of anterior horn cells of the spinal cord, I.

Figs. 1–10. Vorderhornzellen von Cottus scorpius und quadricornus. Vergrösserung Zeiss Apochromat. 2,0. Kompensationsokular 8. Figs. 11–21. Vorderhornzellen von Rana temporaria. Vergrösserung Zeiss Apochr 2,0. Kompensationsokular 12. Figs. 22–26. Vorderhornzellen von Tropidonatus natrix. Vergrösserung Zeiss Apochr. 2,0. Kompensationsokular 8. Kolster, R. (1901) Über centralgebilde in vorderhornzellen der wirbeltiere. *Anat. Hefte* 16, 151–230 [Figures 1–26].

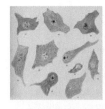

**FIGURE 160.**

Kolster, 1901. Structure of anterior horn cells of the spinal cord, II.

Figs. 68–77. Vorderhornzellen von Bos taurus. Vergrösserung Zeiss Apochr. 2,0. Kompensationsokular 8. Kolster, R. (1901) Über centralgebilde in vorderhornzellen der wirbeltiere. *Anat. Hefte* 16, 151–230 [Figures 68–77].

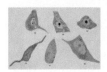

**FIGURE 161.**

Kolster, 1901. Structure of anterior horn cells of the spinal cord, III.

Figs. 79-81. Vorderhornzellen von Homo, 6 Monate alt. Vergrösserung Zeiss Apochr. 2,0. Kompensationsokular 8. Figs. 82–84. Vorderhornzellen von Homo, ca. 40 Jahr alt. Vergrösserung Zeiss Apochr. 2,0. Kompensationsokular 8. Kolster, R. (1901). Über centralgebilde in vorderhornzellen der wirbeltiere. *Anat. Hefte* 16, 151–230 [Figures 79–84].

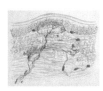

FIGURE 162.

Leontowitsch, 1901. Innervation of human skin, I.

Rücken der I. Fingerphalanx. Papille mit Nerven von der Seite. Schräger Schnitt mit dem Doppelmesser. Die Gewölbe *a* und *b*, die aus Verästelungen der feinen markhaltigen Nerven der Cutis *c* entstehen, liegen in benachbarten Papillen derart, dass *a* dem Auge näher als *b* ist, welch letzteres durch eine Bindegewebeschicht durchschimmert. Bearbeitung wie Figur 1. S.-Apochr. 2,5. Comp. Oc. 2. Leontowitsch, A. (1901) Die Innervation der menschlichen Haut. Internationale Monatsschrift für anatomie und Physiologie. *Int. Monatsschr. Anat. Physiol.* 18, 142–310 [Figure 22].

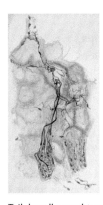

FIGURE 163.

Leontowitsch, 1901. Innervation of human skin, II.

II. Stadium der Haarentwickelung. Haarschaft bereits sichtbar. Talgdrüsen bei keiner Verdunkelung des Gesichtsfeldes sichtbar. Der markhaltige Nerv *e* zerfällt in Zweige; ein Teil derselben geht zur Haut (zu *b*) und besitzt an einigen Zweigen ovale Kerne, der andere Teil geht zum Haare. Hier wurde auch ein Teil der Epithelzellen der Anlage gefärbt. Links von *e* kleiner Haarschaft, rechts ein abgeschnittenes Stück eines anderen Haares. Die Leisten sind um so deutlicher, je näher zu den Haaren. Leontowitsch, A. (1901) Die Innervation der menschlichen Haut. Internationale Monatsschrift für anatomie und Physiologie. *Int. Monatsschr. Anat. Physiol.* 18, 142–310 [Figure 44].

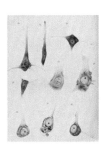

FIGURE 164.

Van Durme, 1901. Different functional states of pyramidal cells.

IV Zone des grandes cellules pyramidales.

FIG. 24. 25, 26, et 27. Cellules obscures ou à l'état de repos. FIG. 28, 29, et 30. Cellule claires ou en pleine activité. FIG. 31. Cellule claire avec quelques gros blocs de chromatine. Van Durme, P. (1901) Etude des différents états fonctionnels de la cellule nerveuse corticale au moyen de la méthode de Nissl. *Névraxe* 2, 113–172 [Figures 24–31].

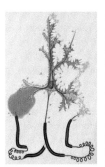

FIGURE 165.

Nissl, 1903. Schematic drawing of the elemental structure of the nervous system.

Schematische Abbildungen, welche theils illustriren, was wir vom elementaren Aufbau des Nervensystems der Wirbelthiere thatsächlich wissen (Fig. 5 A linke Hälfte), und anderntheils zeigen sollen, wie man sich den elementaren Aufbau des Nervensystems vorstellen kann. Vergl. Text Kap. XX. Die Zelle 5 A ist die Ursprungszelle eines markhaltigen Nerven *h-i*, welcher aus dem Nervenfortsatz *cc-f* hervorgeht und nach einem grauen Centrum *aa* zieht, wo die markhaltige Faser *hi* und *hi'* ihre Markscheide bei *i* und *i'* verliert. Die graue Substanz *aa* ist nur an einer Stelle in grauer Farbe angedeutet (auf der rechten Seite α in Form eines Gitters). Der Einfachheit halber endigt die Markfaser *hi* und *hi'* im Schema 5 A in demselben Grau, wo ihre Ursprungszelle liegt. Die Zelle 5 A ist also sowohl als Ursprungszelle der Markfaser *hi* wie auch als eine Nervenzelle des Graues gedacht, in dem die Markfaser *hi* endigt. Die Zelle 5 A entspricht z. B. der Zelle A 3 in Fig. 6, das Grau der Ursprungszelle 5 *A* dem Grau von *A* in Fig. 6, die Markfaser *hi* der Markfaser *b*$_4$ in Fig.6, das Endgrau von *hi* dem Grau in *B*, Fig. 6. Zelle 5 A ist auch eine Nervenzelle des Endgraues, entspricht also in Fig. 6 der Zelle B$_1$ oder B$_2$. Ein und dieselbe Zelle 5 A stellt also sowohl die Zelle A$_3$, Fig. 6, auch Zelle B$_1$oder B$_2$ Fig. 6 dar. Linke Hälfte von 5 A stellt, wie die Fig. 6, in bildlicher Weise den wirklichen Umfang unseres derzeitigen Wissens dar. Siehe kap. XX. Die schwarzen Linien in 5 A sind die Nervenzellenneurofibrillen. Bei *d* endigt eine Neurofibrille an der Oberfläche des Hauptdendriten und verschwindet an dieser Stelle; die röthliche zackige Umrahmung bedeutet die pericellulären GOLGI' schen Netze, welche die Zelle völlig umgeben; bei *c* hört das GOLGI' schen Netz auf und bildet zwischen *c-c* ein Loch, um dem Nervenfortsatz den Durchtritt zu ermöglichen. *b* entspricht der glatten inneren, der

Zelloberfläche anliegenden Fläche der GOLGI' schen Netze, *b'* sind Balken des GOLGI' schen Netzes, die nach aussen nicht mehr vollständig Maschenräume umschliessen und sich in der grauen Substanz verlieren; bei *f* endigt die Zellleibssubstanz des Nervenfortsatzes; *f-g* ist der Draht der dicht aneinander gepressten Nervenfortsatzneurofibrillen; bei *g* beginnt die perifibrilläre Substanz des Axencylinders (oder das Axoplasma oder Axostroma), in welche die Axencylinderneurofibrillen eingebettet sind; bei *h* beginnt die Markscheide, bei *i* verliert der Axencylinder seine Markscheide; *a* stellt das nervöse Grau des grauen Centrums dar, in welchem die Markfaser *hi* die Markscheide verliert. *ik* deutet an, dass die Neurofibrillen des markhaltigen Axencylinders mit dem nervösen Grau in Beziehung treten. Nissl, F. (1903) *Die Neuronenlehre und ihre Anhänger.* Jena: Verlag von Gustav Fischer [Figure 5A].

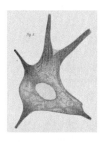

FIGURE 166.

Donaggio, 1904. Endocellular fibrillary reticulum.

Le sezioni, dello spessore di 3, 4, 5, μ, sono state esaminate con l'obiettivo a immersione Leitz $^1/_{16}$. *a, b, d,* = prolungamenti protoplasmatici; *c* = cilindrasse. *Fig.* 1, 2, 3, 4, *Tav. VIII.* Cellule delle corna anteriori nel midollo spinale di coniglio adulto. Nella *fig.* 3, addensamento che dal cercine perinucleare si estende all' origine del cilindrasse. Oc. 4. Met. III. (piridina pura). Donaggio, A. (1904) Il reticolo fibrillare endocellulare e il cilindrasse della cellula nervosa dei vertebrati e metodi vari di colorazione elettiva del reticolo endocellulare e del reticolo periferico basati sull'azione della piridina sul tessuto nervoso. *Riv. Sper. Freniat. Med. Leg.* 30, 397–443 [Figure 3].

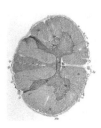

FIGURE 167.

Sobotta, 1906. Human spinal cord, I.

Sección transversal de la médula espinal humana en la región del inflamiento cervical. Aumento, 8: 1. La preparación proviene de un adulto, y fué conservada dos horas y media después de la muerte. Técnica: Líquido de Müller. Carmin sódico. La figura da una vista topográfica de la médula espinal, de la repartición de la sustancia gris y de la blanca, de la división en cordones, de la pía madre.

Explicación de las indicaciones: *bg = Vasos sanguíneos; ca = Columna anterior (cuerno anterior); cma = Comisura anterior; x = Sitio del conducto central obliterado; cp = Columna posterior (cuerno posterior); fa = Cordón anterior (funniculus anterior); fam = Fisura mediana anterior; fc = Cordón de Burdach (funniculus cuneatus); fg = Cordón de Goll (funniculus gracilis); fl = Cordón lateral (funniculus lateralis); fr = Formación reticular; pm = Pía mater; ra = Raiz anterior (fibras radiculares anteriores, ventrales ó motoras); rp = Raiz posterior (fibras radiculares posteriores, dorsales ó sensitivas); sg = Sustancia gelatinosa de Rolando; sp = Septum mediano posterior.* Sobotta, J. (1906) *Atlas y elementos de histología y anatomía microscópica,* trans. J. Póu Orfila. Madrid: Librería Académica [Plate 13].

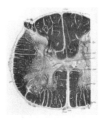

**FIGURE 168.**

Sobotta, 1906. Human spinal cord, II.

Sección transversal de la médula humana á la altura del inflamiento lumbar (representados los dos tercios). Aumento, 15 : 1. La preparación proviene de un cadáver fresco (conservado dos horas y media después de la muerte). La figura muestra la mayor parte de la sección transversal de la médula, con la pía madre que la rodea. Las fibras nerviosas meduladas están coloreadas. en azul oscuro, los núcleos en rojo. Se ve la distribución de las fibras nerviosas meduladas en la sustancia gris y en la sustancia blanca. Técnica: Líquido de Müller. Coloración de las vainas de mielina por el método de Weigert-Pal. Carmín aluminoso. Explicación de las indicaciones*: caa = Comisura blanca anterior; Cc = Resto del conducto central (obliterado); fma= Fisura mediana anterior; gl = Envoltura neuróglica externa; Gz = Células nerviosas del cuerno anterior; nd = Núcleo dorsal; pm = Pía madre; Ra = Raiz anterior; Rp = Raiz posterior; sg = Sustancia gelatinosa de Rolándo; smp= Septum mediano posterior.* Sobotta, J. (1906) *Atlas y elementos de histología y anatomía microscópica,* trans. J. Póu Orfila. Madrid: Librería Académica [Plate 14].

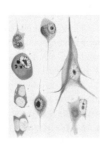

**FIGURE 169.**

Fragnito, 1907. Ganglion cells of the spinal cord, I.

Tutte le figure, eccetto la 5.ª e la 6.ª , provengono da preparati allestiti col metodo

V del Donaggio, e sono state ritratte, tutte, con l'obbiettivo apocromatico 1,5 mm. ap. 1,30 Zeiss e l'oculare compensatore 12. Fig. 1. Cellula binucleata di ganglio intervertebrale di un embrione di pollo di 9 giorni. I nuclei sono ambidue floridi. Fig. 2. Cellula di ganglio intervertebrale di un embrione di pollo di 11 giorni. Ha un nucleo florido, e accosto ad esso, al suo lato sinistro, una zolla ovoidale di sostanza tinta in violetto (*Zolla fibrillogena),* in mezzo alla quale tre blocchi di sostanza (nucleolare?) di color viola cupo. Nucleo e zolla fibrillogena sono circondati da abbondante citoplasma tinto in bluastro. Fig.3. Cellula di gannglio intervertebrale di embrione di pollo di 11 giorni. Nella massa protoplasmatica tinta in bluastro e di figura ovoidale si osservano due formazioni di grandezza presso che uguale e tinte in viola cupo: l' una è il nucleo, l' altra la zolla fibrillogena. Dal polo inferiore di quest'ultima portano a1cuni filamenti fibrillari che raggiungono il prolungamento, nel quale si continnano. Fig. 4. Cellula di ganglio intervertebrale di embrione di pollo di 11 giorni. Dalla sostanza fibrillogena accollata al lato destro del nucleo partono filamenti che raggiungono i due prolungamenti cellulari. Figs. 5, 6. Rappresentano ciascuna una colonia nevroblastica del corno anteriore del midollo spinale di embrione di pollo al nono giorno di covatura, con un nucleo florido *n* a contorni netti ed un altro che accenna a scomparire. Fissazione in sublimato; colorazione al bleu di metilene. Fig. 7. Cellula del corno anteriore del midollo spinale di embrione di pollo di 11 giorni. Il nucleo è eccentrico, come accollato al margine destro della massa protoplasmatica tinta in bluastro. Nel centro di quest' ultima si nota la *zolla fibrillogena* tinta in viola cupo e con margini sfumati. Fig. 13. Cellula del corno posteriore di embrione di pollo di 14 giorni. Grossi fasci di fibrille lunghe tinti in violetto attraversano il citoplasma tolorito in bleu. Non si osservano formazioni reticolari. Fragnito, O. (1907) Le Fibrille e la sostanza fibrillogena nelle cellule ganglionari dei vertebrati. *Ann. Nevrol.* 25, 209–224 [Figures 1–7, 13].

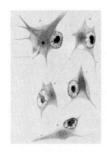

**FIGURE 170.**

Fragnito, 1907. Ganglion cells of the spinal cord, II.

Tutte le figure, eccetto la 5.ª e la 6.ª , provengono da preparati allestiti col metodo V del Donaggio, e sono state ritratte, tutte, con l'obbiettivo apocromatico 1,5 mm. ap. 1,30 Zeiss e l'oculare compensatore 12. FIG.

8. *Idem* - Nel centro della zolla fibrillogena, a destra del nucleo, si osservano dieci massette di sostanza nucleare. Dalla zolla partono filamenti, che si avviano al prolungamento. FIG. 9. *Idem*-La zolla fibrillogena, a destra del nucleo, ha forma triangolare e si continua in tre prolungamenti. Nella zolla e nei prolungamenti si osservano filamenti fibrillari alquanto tozzi. FIG. 10. *Idem* - Dalla zolla fibrillogena posta a sinistra del nucleo, partono filamenti fibrillari che si continuano in due prolungamenti. FIG. 11. *Idem* - Nucleo eccentrico. La zolla fibrillogena, occupante la parte centrale del citoplasma, è conformata a fuso, e si continua per un estremo con un grosso protoplasmatico (*a*) e dall'altro con il cilindrasse *c.* Nel centro e negli estremi della zolla fibrillogena s' inizia la differenziazione della fibrilla. FIG. 12. *Idem* - Nucleo eccentrico. Le fibrille del cilindrasse *c* e di, quasi tutti i protoplasmatici affluiscono verso il centro del citoplasma, dove non è più identificabile chiaramente la zolla fibrillogena. Al posto di questa, si notano un accenno di rete ed un blocco di sostanza granulosa (nucleolare?) intensamente colorata. Fragnito, O. (1907) Le Fibrille e la sostanza fibrillogena nelle cellule ganglionari dei vertebrati. *Ann. Nevrol.* 25, 209–224 [Figures 8–12].

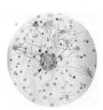

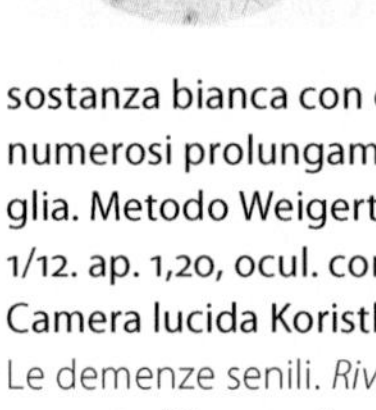

**FIGURE 171.**

Franceschi, 1907. Neuroglial cells and a blood vessel in the white matter.

Caso VIII. Lobo frontale. Vaso della sostanza bianca con cui predono contatto numerosi prolungamenti di celhule di nevroglia. Metodo Weigert, Micr. Zeiss, obiett. imm. 1/12. ap. 1,20, ocul. comp. 4, tubo mm. 150. Camera lucida Koristka. Franceschi, F. (1907) Le demenze senili. *Riv. Patol. Nerv. Ment.* 12, 445–469 [Figure 14].

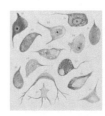

**FIGURE 172.**

Sciuti, 1907. Nerve cell alterations, I.

FIG. 20 Cellula del nucleo di Goll; caso II. Lesione iniziale del reticolo, parziale degenerazione pigmentaria e fibrillolisi, inversione della tingibilità del nucleo ed ingrossamento di esso, nucleolo ingrossato, colorato intensamente, con un vacuolo. - Metodo neurofibrillare Donaggio. - Oc. 4 comp. - Obb. 1, 5 imm. Apert. 1,30, t. all. 16 Zeiss. FIG. 21 Cellula del nucleo di Bourdach; caso VII Stato di degenerazione pigmentaria e di parziale fibrillolisi, parziale conservazione del cercine fibrillare periferico e perinucleare, ingrossamento del nucleo ed inversione della sua tingibilità, nucleolo ingrossato e vacuolizzato. - Colorazione ed ingrandimento come sopra. FIG. 22 Cellula del nudeo di GOLL; caso II. Spezzettamento delle fibrille, degenerazione pigmentaria, difformità del nucleo. - Colorazione ed ingrandimento come sopra. FIG. 23. Cellula del nucleo di GOLL; caso IV Degenerazione pigmentaria e parziale fibrillolisi; relativa conservazione del cercine fibrillare periferico e delle fibrille dei prolungamenti; ingrossamento e difformità del nucleo .- Colorazione ed ingrandimento come sopra. FIG. 24 Cellula del nucleo di GOLL; caso VI. Grave fibrillolisi e degenerazione pigmentaria; raggrinzamento e difformità del nucleo. Colorazione ed ingrandimento come sopra. FIG. 25 Cellula del nucleo di BOURDAH; caso II. Spezzettamento delle fibrille, rarefazione del reticolo, degenerazione pigmentaria. - Colorazione ed ingrandimento come sopra. FIG. 26 Cellula del nucleo di GOLL; caso II. Aggrovigliamento del reticolo, parziale fibrillolisi. Colorazione ed ingrandimento come sopra. FIGS. 27 e 28 Cellule del nucleo di GOLL; caso III. Fibrillolisi parziale, degenerazione pigmentaria, ingrossamento, difformità, inversione della colorazione del nucleo. Colorazione ed ingrandimento come sopra. FIG. 29 Cellula del nucleo di GOLL; caso VI. Parziale fibrillolisi.- Colorazione ed ingrandimento come sopra. FIG. 30 Cellula del nucleo di GOLL; caso II. Parziale fibrillolisi, conservazione delle fibrille che vanno ai prolungamenti. - Colorazione ed ingrandimento come sopra. FIG. 31 Cellula del nucleo di GOLL; caso II. Spezzettamento delle fibrille, degenerazione pigmentaria. - Colorazione ed ingrandimento come sopra. FIGS. 37 e 38 Cellule del talamo ottico; caso IV. Fibrillolisi; residuano quasi integre poche fibrille che passano da un prolungamento ad un altro. - Metodo fotografico CAJAL. - Oc. 4 Obb. 8 KORISTKA. Sciuti, M. (1907) *Le fine alterazioni degli elementi nervosi. Ann. Nevrol. 25, 77–188; 225–241; 393–473 [Figures 20–31, 37–38].*

## FIGURE 173.
### Sciuti, 1907. Nerve cell alterations, II.

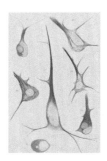

FIG. 47 Cellula media piramidale della terza circonvoluzione frontale; caso IV. Degenerazione pigmentaria, fibrillolisi, inversione della tingibilità del nucleo. Colorazione ed ingrandimento come sopra. FIG. 48 Cellula piramidale media della circonvoluzione parietale ascendente; caso II. Ingrossamento e spezzettamento delle fibrille. Colorazione ed ingrandimento come sopra. FIG. 49-Cellula piramidale media della circonvoluzione frontale ascendente; aso II. Fibrillolisi parziale, degenerazione pigmentaria, conservazione di alcuni fascetti di fibrille che dal prolungamento apicale vanno ad uno della base; ingrossamento e difformità del nucleo. Colorazione ed ingrandimento come sopra. FIG. 50 Cellula piramidale media della prima circonvoluzione temporale; caso II. Fibrillolisi, persistenza di fascetti di fibrille lunghe che passano da un prolungamento all'altro. Colorazione ed ingrandimento come sopra. FIG. 51 Cellula dello strato polimorfo della circonvoluzione frontale ascendente; caso X. Degenerazione granulare, spezzettamento delle fibrille. Colorazione ed ingrandimento come sopra. FIG. 52 Cellula piramidale media della terza circonvoluzione frontale; caso IV. Stato di aggrovigliamento del reticolo, degenerazione pigmentaria con fibrillolisi alla base della cellula. Colorazione ed ingrandimento come sopra. FIG. 53 Cellula gigante della circonvoluzione frontale ascendente; caso II. Parziale fibrillolisi attorno al nucleo ed alla base; degenerazione pigmentaria; persistenza delle fibrille lunghe; atrofia dei prolungamenti della base. Colorazione ed ingrandimento come sopra. Sciuti, M. (1907) *Le fine alterazioni degli elementi nervosi nella paralisi progressiva. Ann. Nevrol. 25, 77–188; 225–241; 393–473 [Figures 47–53].*

## FIGURE 174.
### Gurewitsch, 1908. Internal structure of nerve cells.

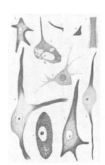

FIG. 1. Zelle aus dem Vorderhorn des Rückenmarkes eines Kaninchens (normal). Färbung nach der Methode III Donaggio. Immersion. Vergrößerung 1000. Es sind sichtbar das fibrilläre Netz, die perinukleare Verdichtung und lange Fibrillen. FIG. 2. Zelle aus dem Vorderhorn des Rückenmarkes eines Kaninchens. Methode III Donaggio. Immersion. Vergrößerung 800. Es ist unter anderem zu sehen der Übergang der langen Fibrillen aus einem Fortsatze in den anderen. FIG. 3. Zelle aus der Großhirnrinde eines Kaninchens. Methode VII Donaggio. Immers.Vergrößerung 1300. Perizelluläres Netz. FIG. 4. Perizelluläres Netz ringsum eines Dendriten einer Vorderhornzelle des Rückenmarkes eines Hundes. Methode VII Donaggio. Immers. Vergrößerung 1300. FIG.

5. Zelle aus dem Rückenmarke eines Hundes (Inanition). Es sind Vakuolen und Körnelug der Fibrillen zu sehen, die stellenweise schon in Körnchen zerfallen sind. Methode III Donaggio. Immersion. Vergrößerung 1000. FIG. 6. Zelle aus dem Rückenmarke eines Meerschweinchens, das durch Blei vergiftet wurde. Es sind ungleichmäßige Verdickungen der Fibrillen sichtbar. Diese Verdickungen sind nicht voneinander isoliert, sondern durch feine Fibrillärfäden vereinigt. Methode III Donaggio. Immersion. Vergrößerung 1300. FIG. 7. Dendrit einer Vorderhornzelle eines Meerschweinchens, welches mit Blei vergiftet wurde. Die Fibrillen sind etwas verdickt und als ob sie zerrissen sind. Meth. III Donaggio. Immersion. Vergrößerung 800. FIG. 8. Vorderhornzelle vom Rückenmarke eines Kaninchens, welches acht Stunden nach der Kompression der Aorta getötet wurde. Partielle Zerstörung des Fibrillärnetzes bei guter Erhaltung der langen Fibrillen. Methode III Donaggio. Immersion. Vergrößerung 1300. FIG. 9. Strangzelle vom Rückenmarke eines Kaninchens, welches 12 Stunden nach der Kompression der Aorta getötet wurde. Das Netz im Zellkörper ist nicht gefärbt; die Fibrillen in den Fortsätzen sind gut erhalten. Meth. III Donaggio. Immersion. Vergrößerung 1000. FIG. 10. Zelle aus dem Rückenmarke eines Kaninchens, welches 16 Stunden nach der Kompression der Aorta getötet wurde; sie ist geschrumpft (ringsum ein perizellulärer Raum), auch der Kern ist geschrumpft. Der größte Teil der Zelle ist körnig; in den Fortsätzen sind Fibrillenreste vorhanden. Methode III Donaggio. Immersion. Vergrößerung 800. Gurewitsch, M. J. (1908) *Zur Morphologie des fibrillären Apparates der Nervezellen im normalen und pathologischen Zustande. Folia Neurobiol. 2, 197–210 [Figures 1–10].*

## FIGURE 175.
### Calligaris, 1908. Cells of the locus coeruleus, I.

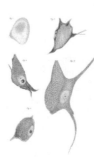

Micr. *Seibert* Oc. III. - Ob 1/12 Imm. om. FIG. 1. Zelle des Locus coeruleus - 60 Jahre. Nigrosinfärbung. FIG. 2. Idem - 37 Jahre. Nisslsche Methode. FIG. 3. Idem - 50 Jahre. Romanowskysche Methode. FIG. 4. Idem - 73 Jahre. Herxheimersche Methode. FIG. 5. Idem - 54 Jahre. Bielschowskysche Methode. Calligaris, G. (1908) *Beitrag zum Studium der Zellen des "Locus coeruleus" und der Substantia nigra. Monatsschr. Psychiatr. Neurol. 24, 339–353 [Figures 1–5].*

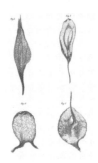

### FIGURE 176.

Calligaris, 1908. Cells of the locus coeruleus, II.

Micr. *Seibert* Oc. III. - Ob 1/12 Imm. om. FIG. 7. Zelle des Locus coeruleus - 69 Jahre. Donaggios Methode. FIG. 8. Idem - 61 Jahre. Donaggios Methode. FIG. 9. Idem - 61 Jahre. Donaggios Methode. Calligaris, G. (1908) Beitrag zum Studium der Zellen des "Locus coeruleus" und der Substantia nigra. *Monatsschr. Psychiatr. Neurol.* 24, 339–353 [Figures 7–9].

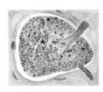

### FIGURE 177.

Luna, 1908. Sympathetic ganglion.

Kleinzellige Ganglien (Cajalsche Methode). Ok. 3 Huyghens, 1/12. Ölimm. om. Koristka. Luna, E. (1908) Über Anordnung und Struktur der sympathischen Ganglien in der menschlichen Prostata. *Folia Neurobiol.* 2, 220–223 [Figure 2].

### FIGURE 178.

Michailow, 1908. Intracardiac nervous system.

Ein kleines Ganglion. Pericapsuläre Geflechte. Pferd Reichert 7 a. Michailow, S. (1908) Zur Frage über den feineren Bau des intracardialen Nervensystems der Säugetiere. *Int. Monatsschr. Anat. Physiol.* 25, 44–89 [Figure 14]

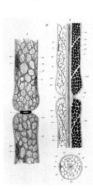

### FIGURE 179.

Nemiloff, 1908. Nerve fibers I.

Fig. 31. Schema des Baues einer markhaltigen Nervenfaser, eines Fisches. A = Nervenfaser in toto; B = Längsschnitt; auf der linken Seite ist die Faser nach der Methylenblaufärbung dargestellt; auf der rechten Seite ist das Mark geschwärzt, wie nach Osmiumsäurefixierung mit den Lantermanschen Einkerbungen angegeben. C = Querschnitt durch eine Nervenfaser in der Höhe einer sog. Zelle der Schwannschen Scheide; sz = sog. Zellen der Schwannschen Scheide; n = deren Kern; ss = Schwannsche Scheide; sp = Fortsätze der sog. Zellen der Schwannschen Scheide oder das Markscheidengerüst; le = gröbere Scheidewände des protoplasmatischen Skelettes der Markscheide, die schräg zum Achsenzylinder angeordnet die sog. Zwischentrichter bilden; leo = helle Streifen auf den mit Osmiumsäure behandelten Fasern; dieselben entsprechen den gröberen, schrägen Scheidewänden (le) des Markmantels und den Lantermanschen Erkerbungen; mo = das durch Osmiumsäure geschwärzte Mark; ax = Achsenzylinder; pa = periaxialer Raum um den Achsenzylinder; gs = Gerinnsel-scheide; pf =- derperipherische in Fibrillen nicht differenzierte Teil des Achsenzylinders; f = Fibrillen des Achsenzylinders; r = ringförmige Verdickung der Schwannschen Scheide an einem Ranvierschen Schnürringe; o = Hohlraum der ringförmigen Verdickung der Schwannschen Scheide; bk = doppelkegelförmige Verdickung des Achsenzylinders, welche durch die an dieser Stelle abgehobene Gerinnselscheide gebildet wird. Nemiloff, A. (1908) Einige Beobachtungen über den Bau des Nervengewebes bei Ganoïden und Knochenfischen. Teil II. Der Bau der Nervenfasern. *Arch. Mikrosk. Anat. Entwicklungsgesch.* 72, 575–606 [Plate 32, Figure 32].

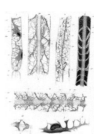

### FIGURE 180.

Nemiloff, 1908. Nerve fibers, II.

FIG. 5. Zwei sog.Zellen der Schwannschen Scheide. n = Kern; sz = Zellprotoplasma; f = Fibrillen des Zellprotoplasma; gr = Körnchen im Zellprotoplasma; pr = Ranvierscher Schnürring (schwach gefärbt); ax=Achsenzylinder (kaum gefärbt). Nervenfaser von Lota vulgaris. Methylenblau. Zeiss' homog. Immers. 1/12; Zeichenokular von Leitz. Fig. 7. Eine sog. Zelle der Schwannschen Scheide mit ihren Verzweigungen. n = Kern; p = Protoplasma; dr = Zellfortsätze. Nervenfaser von Lota vulgaris. Methylenblau. Zeiss' homogene Immers. 1/12; Kamera lucida von Abbé. Fig. 8. Das Neurokeratinnetz einer markhaltigen Nervenfaser. Ss = Schwannsche Scheide; ax = Achsenzylinder; pn = Neurokeratinnetz; n = Kern einer sog. Zelle der Schwannschen Scheide. - Längsdurchschnitt einer in Chromessigsäure fixierten und mit Hämatoxylin nach Heidenhain und Bordeaux - R. gefärbten Nervenfaser von Lota vulgaris. Zeiss' homog. Immers. 1/12; Zeichenokular von Leitz. Fig. 9. Neurokeratinnetz einer markhaltigen Nervenfaser. Szs = Schwannsche Scheide; tr = dickere Scheidewände des Netzes, die, schräg zum Achsenzylinder gerichtet, um denselben einen Tricher bilden; pn = Neurokeratinnetz; ax = Achsenzylinder. Längsschnitt durch eine markhaltige Nervenfaser. Fixiert in Chromessigsäure, gefärbt in Hämatoxylin nach Heidenhain und Bordeaux-R. Lota vulgaris. Zeiss, homog. Immers. 1/12; Zeichenokular von Leitz. Fig. 10. Das Neurokeratinnetz einer markhaltigen Nervenfaser. ax = Achsenzylinder; n = Kern einer sog. Zelle der Schwannschen Scheide. le = dickere Scheidewände des Neurokeratinnetzes. Längsschnitt durch eine markhaltige, in Chromessigsäure fixierte und in Hämatoxylin nach Heidenhain und Bordeaux-R. gefärbte Nervenfaser von Lota vulgaris. Zeiss, homog. Immers 1/12; Okular 4, Kamera lucida von Abbé. Fig. 11. Eine markhaltige, in Osmiumsäure gefärbte Nervenfaser. Optischer Längsschnitt. ax = Achsenzylinder; m = durch Osmiumsäure geschwärztes Mark; le = dickere Scheidewände des protoplasmatischen Skelettes in Osmiumsäure nicht geschwärzt; pr = Ranvierscher Schnürring. Lota vulgaris. Zeiss' homog. Immers. 1/12; Zeichenokular von Leitz. Nemiloff, A. (1908) Einige Beobachtungen über den Bau des Nervengewebes bei Ganoïden und Knochenfischen. Teil II. Der Bau der Nervenfasern. *Arch. Mikrosk. Anat. Entwicklungsgesch.* 72, 575–606 [Plate 30, Figures 5, 7–11].

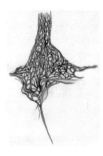

### FIGURE 181.

Rossi, 1909. Ganglion cell of the anterior horn of the spinal cord.

Ganglienzelle des Vorderhorns des Rückenmarks: Verdickung der intracellulären Fibrillen, die stellenweise zu kompakten schwarzen Fäden verschmolzen. Verwirrung des Faserwerks. Cajals Silberimprägnationsmethode. Vergrößerung: 1640 mal. Rossi, O. (1909) Üeber die neurotoxischen Sera und die dadurch im Zentralnervensystem verursachten Veränderungen. *J. Psychol. Neurol.* 14, 188–201 [Figure 5].

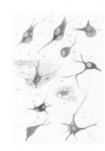

### FIGURE 182.

Da Fano, 1909. The optic thalamus in psychoses, I.

FIG. 43. Doppelkernige Nervenzelle des Nucl. lateralis (in zwei Einstellungsebenen gezeichnet). Dementia paralytica

(Fall 3, Sektion 3 Stunden nach dem Tode). *Bielschowskys* Methode (ohne Vergoldung). FIG. 44. Desgleichen, nach *R. y Cajals* Methode. FIG.45. Ziemlich gut erhaltene Ganglienzelle des Nucl. lateralis. Vermehrung der Gliazellen. Kleine Faseranschwellungen. Dementia paralytica (Fall 4, Sektion 12 Stunden nach dem Tode). *R. y Cajals* Methode. FIG. 46. Etwas stärker veränderte Ganglienzelle des Nucl. lateralis desselben Falles. Pigmentanhäufung mit Verkleinerung der Maschen. *Bielschowskys* Methode. FIG. 47. Ziemlich gut erhaltene Ganglienzellen aus demselben Kern. Ohne Pigmentanhäufung. Verkleinerung der Maschen. Zerbröcklung einiger Fortsatzfibrillen. Dementia paralytica (Fall 5, Sektion 18 Stunden nach dem Tode). Meth. wie Fig. 46. FIG. 48. Ganglienzelle aus dem Nucl. lateralis. Pigmentanhäufung. Verkleinerung der Maschen. Zerbröcklung einiger Fortsatzfibrillen. Kleine knotenförmige Anschwellungen am Achsenzylinder. Dementia paralytica (Fall 1, Sektion 6 Stunden nach dem Tode). Meth. wie Fig. 46. FIG. 49. Pigmentanhäufung in der oberflächlichen Schicht einer Ganglienzelle aus dem Nucl. lateralis desselben Falles. Verklebung und stellenweise Zerbröcklung der Zellleibfibrillen. Meth. wie Fig. 46. FIG. 50. Einfache Atrophie einer Ganglienzelle des Nucl. medialis. Dementia paralytica (Fall 3, Sektion 3 Stunden nach dem Tode). *R. y Cajals* Methode. FIG. 51. Zelle aus dem Nucl. lateralis desselben Falles; dieselbe ist in ihrer äusseren Form gut erhalten, zeigt aber totalen Schwund des Maschenwerkes und stellenweise Zerbröcklung der übrig gebliebenen Fibrillen. *Bielschowsky* Methode. Da Fano, C. (1909) Studien über die Veränderungen im Thalamus opticus bei Defektpsychosen. *Monatsschr. Psychiatr. Neurol.* 26, 4–36 [Figures 43–45, 47–51].

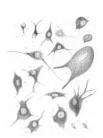

**FIGURE 183.**

Da Fano, 1909. The optic thalamus in psychoses, II.

FIG. 8. Zellen aus dem medialen Abschnitt des Ganglion habenulae des erwachsenen Hundes nach *Bielschowskys* Methode. Obj. 3 mm. Zeiss Oc. 6 comp. Fig. 9. Zelle aus dem lateralen Abschnitt des Ganglion habenulae des erwachsenen Hundes. Meth. und Vergr. wie Fig. 8. Fig. 10. Zelle aus dem Nucl. ant. *a* des erwachsenen Hundes. Meth. und Vergr. wie Fig. 8. Fig. 11. Zellen aus dem Nucl. ant. *c* des erwachsenen Hundes. Nach *Nissl* Methode. Vergr. wie Fig. 8. Fig. 12. Kleinere Zelle aus dem Nucl. lateralis *a* des erwachsenen Hundes nach *Bielschowskys* Methode. Vergr. wie Fig. 8. Fig. 13. Zelle aus

demselben Kern. Meth. wie oben. Obj. 3 mm. Z. Oc. 18 comp. Fig. 14. Zelle aus dem Nucl. lat. *b* eines 4 Wochen alten Hundes nach *Cajals* Methode (mit Vergoldung des Präparates). Obj. 3 mm. Z. Oc. 6 comp. Fig. 15. Zelle aus den Nuclei zonales des erwachsenen Hundes nach *Bielschowskys* Methode. Vergr. wie Fig. 14. Fig. 16. Zelle aus dem Nucl. triqueter des erwachsenen Hundes nach *Nissls* Methode. Vergr. wie Fig. 14. Fig. 17. Zelle aus dem Nucl. rotundus des erwachsenen Hundes. Meth. und Vergr. Wie oben. Fig. 18. Zelle aus dem Nucl. med. *c* des erwachsenen Hundes nach *Bielschowskys* Methode. Vergr. wie Fig. 14. Fig. 19. Zelle aus dem Nucl. med. a¹ des erwachsenen Hundes. Meth. und Vergr. wie Fig. 18. Fig. 20. Zelle des Nucl. med. *c* des erwachsenen Hundes nach *Nissls* Methode. Vergr. wie oben. Fig. 21. Kleine Zelle aus dem Nucl. *"y"* des erwachsenen Hundes *(v. Monakow).* Meth. und Vergr. wie oben. Fig. 22. Zelle aus dem Nucl. ventralis des erwachsenen Hundes. Meth. und Vergr. wie oben. Da Fano, C. (1909) Studien über die Veränderungen im Thalamus opticus bei Defektpsychosen. *Monatsschr. Psychiatr. Neurol.* 26, 4–36 [Figures 8–22].

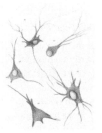

**FIGURE 184.**

Da Fano, 1909. The optic thalamus in psychoses, III.

FIG. 31. Zelle aus dem Nucl. medialis des Menschen . *R. y Cajals* Methode. Obj. 3 mm. Z. Oc. 6 comp. FIG. 32. Kleine Zelle aus dem Nucl. lateralis des Menschen. Vergr. wie oben. *Bielschowskys* Methode. FIG. 33. Mittelgrosse Zelle aus demselben Kern. Meth. und Vergr. wie oben. FIG. 34. Desgleichen, nach *R. y Cajals* Methode. FIG. 35. Grosse Zelle aus demselben Kern. *Bielschowskys* Methode. Vergr. wie oben. Da Fano, C. (1909) Studien über die Veränderungen im Thalamus opticus bei Defektpsychosen. *Monatsschr. Psychiatr. Neurol.* 26, 4–36 [Figures 31–35].

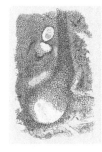

**FIGURE 185.**

Besta, 1910. Peripheral reticulum of the nerve cell, I.

Tutte le figure rappresentano elementi ad uno stesso ingrandimento ( 1/15 semiapocromatico Koristka, Oculare 4 compensatore) e disegnate in tutti i particolari col sussidio

dell'apparato Abbe-Apáthy, tenendo il foglio del disegno alla stessa altezza del tavolino del microscopio. L'ingrandimento è perciò per tutte le figure perfettamente uguale e approssimativamente di 600 diametri. La diversità di ampiezza delle maglie è in rapporto esclusivamente con differenze strutturali. Tutte le figure rappresentano cellule di cane adulto e sano. Eccettuate le figure 6 e 26, che sono tratte da preparati fatti con una modificazione al metodo fotografico del Cajal, tutte sono tratte da preparati fatti colla terza delle mie modalità (formalina più aldeide acetica); è da notare che le figure 14, 15, 16, 17,18, rappresentanti diversi tipi di cellule corticali, sono disegnate da preparati sottoposti, prima del differenziamento, al mordenzaggio con soluzione di molibdato di ammonio al 4%: da ciò il colore violetto dei nuclei e la non evidenza delle zolle del Nissl. FIG. 1. Cellule delle corna anteriori. Besta, C. (1910) Sul reticolo periferico della cellula nervosa nei mammiferi. *Int. Monatsschr. Anat. Physiol.* 27, 402–446 [Figure 1].

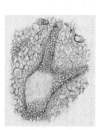

**FIGURE 186.**

Besta, 1910. Peripheral reticulum of the nerve cell, II.

Tutte le figure rappresentano elementi ad uno stesso ingrandimento ( 1/15 semiapocromatico Koristka, Oculare 4 compensatore) e disegnate in tutti i particolari col sussidio dell'apparato Abbe-Apáthy, tenendo il foglio del disegno alla stessa altezza del tavolino del microscopio. L'ingrandimento è perciò per tutte le figure perfettamente uguale e approssimativamente di 600 diametri. La diversità di ampiezza delle maglie è in rapporto esclusivamente con differenze strutturali. Tutte le figure rappresentano cellule di cane adulto e sano. Eccettuate le figure 6 e 26, che sono tratte da preparati fatti con una modificazione al metodo fotografico del Cajal, tutte sono tratte da preparati fatti colla terza delle mie modalità (formalina più aldeide acetica); è da notare che le figure 14, 15, 16, 17,18, rappresentanti diversi tipi di cellule corticali, sono disegnate da preparati sottoposti, prima del differenziamento, al mordenzaggio con soluzione di molibdato di ammonio al 4%: da ciò il colore violetto dei nuclei e la non evidenza delle zolle del Nissl. FIG. 5. Cellule del nucleo del Deiters. Besta, C. (1910) Sul reticolo periferico della cellula nervosa nei mammiferi. *Int. Monatsschr. Anat. Physiol.* 27, 402–446 [Figure 5].

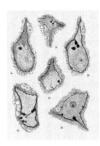

**FIGURE 187.**

Besta, 1910. Peripheral reticulum of the nerve cell, III.

Tutte le figure rappresentano elementi ad uno stesso ingrandimento ( 1/15 semiapocromatico Koristka, Oculare 4 compensatore) e disegnate in tutti i particolari col sussidio dell'apparato Abbe-Apáthy, tenendo il foglio del disegno alla stessa altezza del tavolino del microscopio. L'ingrandimento è perciò per tutte le figure perfettamente uguale e approssimativamente di 600 diametri. La diversità di ampiezza delle maglie è in rapporto esclusivamente con differenze strutturali. Tutte le figure rappresentano cellule di cane adulto e sano. Eccettuate le figure 6 e 26, che sono tratte da preparati fatti con una modificazione al metodo fotografico del Cajal, tutte sono tratte da preparati fatti colla terza delle mie modalità (formalina più aldeide acetica); è da notare che le figure 14, 15, 16, 17,18, rappresentanti diversi tipi di cellule corticali, sono disegnate da preparati sottoposti, prima del differenziamento, al mordenzaggio con soluzione di molibdato di ammonio al 4%: da ciò il colore violetto dei nuclei e la non evidenza delle zolle del Nissl. FIG. 19. Cellula del nucleo dentato con propaggini endocellulari. FIG. 20. Cellula del nucleo motore del pneumogastrico con propaggini endocellulari. FIG. 21 a 26. Cellule del nucleo rosso con propaggini di diverso tipo: le fig. 24 e 25 rappresentano la stessa cellula in due piani diversi, la fig. 26 una cellula ottenuta col metodo fotografico modificato. La spiegazione più dettagliata delle figure si trova nel testo.  Besta, C. (1910) Sul reticolo periferico della cellula nervosa nei mammiferi. *Int. Monatsschr. Anat. Physiol.* 27, 402–446 [Figures 19–21, 23–25].

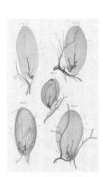

**FIGURE 188.**

Dogiel, 1910. Vater-Pacinian corpuscles.

Sämtliche Figuren sind vermittelst des Zeichenapparates von Abbe angefertigt. FIG. 9A, B, C, D und E. Vater-Pacinische Körperchen in toto mit injizierten Gefäßen. Mesenterium einer erwachsenen Katze. Reichert, Obj. 3, Ok. 3.  Dogiel, A. S. (1910) Zur Frage über den Bau der Kapscln der Vater-Pacinischen und Herbstschen Köperchen und über das Verhalten der Blutgetäße zu denselben. *Folia Neurobiol.* 4, 218–241 [Figures 9 A–D].

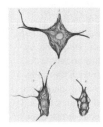

**FIGURE 189.**

Mattioli, 1910. Neurofibrillar alterations, I.

Sezioni dello spessore di 5μ, colorate col metodo Besta. L'esame'è stato fatto con obbiettivo Koristka a imm. omog. 1/12 e con l'ocul. 4, comp. FIG. 3 Cellula delle corna anter. del rigonf. lombare; da midollo di coniglio morto dopo 4 g; FIG. 7 Cellula delle corna anter. del rigonf. lombare; da midollo di coniglio morto dopo 11 g; FIG. 8 Cellula delle corna anter. del rigonf. lombare; da midollo di coniglio morto dopo 12 g.  Mattioli, L. (1910) Effetti dell'azione combinata del digiuno e del freddo sul reticolo neurofibrillare della cellula nervosa. *Riv. Patol. Nerv. Ment.* 15, 649–656 [Figures 3, 7, 8].

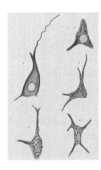

**FIGURE 190.**

Mattioli, 1910. Neurofibrillar alterations, II.

Sezioni dello spessore di 5μ, colorate col metodo Besta. L'esame'è stato fatto con obbiettivo Koristka a imm. omog. 1/12 e con l'ocul. 4, comp. FIG. 1 - Cellula delle corna anter. del rigonf. cervicale; da midollo di coniglio morto dopo 2 g; FIG. 2 - Cellula delle corna anter. del rigonf. lombare; da midollo di coniglio morto dopo 3 g; FIG. 4 - Cellula delle corna anter. del rigonf. lombare; da midollo di coniglio morto dopo 4 g. FIG. 5 - Cellula delle corna anter. del rigonf. lombare; da midollo di coniglio morto dopo 5 g. FIG. 6 - Cellula delle corna anter. del rigonf. lombare; da midollo di coniglio morto dopo 6 g.  Mattioli, L. (1910) Effetti dell'azione combinata del digiuno e del freddo sul reticolo neurofibrillare della cellula nervosa. *Riv. Patol. Nerv. Ment.* 15, 649–656 [Figures 1, 2, 4–6].

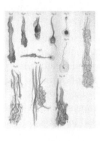

**FIGURE 191.**

Sala and Cortese, 1910. Alterations of the spinal cord, I.

Fig. 1 u. 2. Fasern der Vorderhörner, infolge der Ausreißung in ihrer Kontinuität unterbrochen. Durcheinander verwickelte Neurofibrillen und Auftreten von ringförmigen Gebilden und kleinen Bolas. - 3 Tage nach der Läsion (junges Kätzchen) Cajals Methode. Fig.1. Okul. 6, Komp.-Obj. 2 mm Zeiß. Fig.2. Okul. 3, Obj. E. Zeiß. Fig.3. Faser der Vorderhörner, infolge der Ausreißung in ihrer Kontinuität unterbrochen. Eiförmige Anschwellung von fibrillärer Struktur, von welcher zahlreiche sich vielfach teilende Fibrillen abgehen, die zur Bildung von verschieden gestalteten Anschwellungen Anlaß geben. 3 Tage nach der Läsion (junges Kätzchen) Cajals Methode. Okul. 6, Komp.-Obj. 2 mm Zeiß. Fig.4. Faser, die mit einem knopfartigen Gebilde endigt. - Vom verdickten Anteil gehen dünne Fasern ab. 5 Tage nach der Läsion (Hund) Cajals Methode. Okul. 3, Obj. E. Zeiß. Fig.5, 6, 22, 23, 24. Degenerationserscheinungen an den Nervenfasern (graue Substanz der Vorderhörner). Fig.5, 6, 24: 5 Tage nach der Läsion (Hund) Cajals Methode. Okul. 6, Komp.-Obj. 2 mm Zeiß. Fig. 22, 23: 2 Tage nach der Läsion (Kätzchen) Cajals Methode. Okul. 4, Komp.-Obj. 2 mm Zeiß. Fig.7. Nervenfaser der Vorderhörner. - Fehlgeschlagener Versuch einer Regeneration. 3 Tage nach der Läsion (Kätzchen) Cajals Methode. Okul. 6, Obj. 2 mm Zeiß. Fig.8, 9, 10. Charakteristische Gebilde, die sowohl in der grauen Substanz der Vorderhörner als auch längs des intramedullären Verlaufes der Vorderwurzeln anzutreffen sind. 14 Tage nach der Läsion (Kätzchen) Cajals Methode. Fig 8 u.9: Okul. 4, Komp.-Obj. 2 mm Zeiß. Fig. 10: Okul. 3, Obj. E. Zeiß. Fig. 11. Art von ziemlich kompliziertem helikordalen Apparate. 5 Tage nach der Läsion (Hund) Cajals Methode. Okul. 4, Komp.-Obj. 2 mm Zeiß. Sämtliche Figuren wurden direkt nach den Präparaten vermittelst der Hellkammer (Modell Apáthy) abgebildet.  Sala, G. and Cortese, G. (1910) Über die im Rückenmark nach Ausreißung der Wurzeln eintretenden Erscheinungen. *Folia Neurobiol.* 4, 63–75 [Figures 1–11].

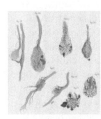

**FIGURE 192.**

Sala and Cortese, 1910. Alterations of the spinal cord, II.

Fig. 12. Rundliche Anschwellung von rein fibrillärer Struktur, von welcher dünne Fasern abgehen. - Beginn von Faserteilungen. 5 Tage nach der Läsion (Hund) Cajals Methode. Okul. 4, Komp.-Obj. 2 mm Zeiß. Fig.13, 14, 18, 20, 21. Charakteristische, mehr oder weniger komplizierte Knäuelbildungen in der grauen Substanz der Vorderhörner und im intramedullären Abschnitt der Vorderwurzeln. Fig.13, 14, 21: 5 Tage nach der Läsion (Hund) Cajals Methode. Fig. 13 u. 21. Okul. 4, Komp.-Obj. 2 mm Zeiß. Fig. 14. Okul. 6, Obj. 2 mm Zeiß. Fig. 18: 14 Tage nach der Läsion (Kätzchen) Cajals Methode. Okul. 3, Obj. E. Zeiß. Fig. 20: 14 Tage nach der Läsion (Kätzchen) Cajals Methode. Okul. 4, Komp.-Obj. 2 mm Zeiß. Fig.15 u. 19. Anteil von Knäuelbildungen, wie sie im Inneren der grauen Substanz der Vorderhörner angetroffen werden. 14 Tage nach der Läsion (Kätzchen) Cajals Methode. Okul. 6, Kom.-Obj. 2 mm Zeiß. Fig.16 u. 17. Weiterteilungen und Zerfaserang der Hauptfaser. - Um diese letztere (Fig.17) sowie um eine Weiterteilung (16) finden sich besondere Knäuelbildungen. Fig.16: 14 Tage nach der Läsion (Kätzchen) Cajals Methode . Okul. 4, Momp.Obj. 2 mm Zeiß. Fig. 17: 5 Tage nach der Läsion (Hund) Cajals Methode. Okul. 4, Komp.-Obj. 2 mm Zeiß. Sämtliche Figuren wurden direkt nach den Präparaten vermittelst der Hellkammer (Modell Apáthy) abgebildet. Sala, G. and Cortese, G. (1910) Über die im Rückenmark nach Ausreißung der Wurzeln eintretenden Erscheinungen. *Folia Neurobiol.* 4, 63–75 [Figures 12–19].

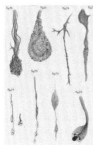

**FIGURE 193.**

Sala and Cortese, 1910. Alterations of the spinal cord, III.

Fig. 13, 14, 18, 20, 21. Charakteristische, mehr oder weniger komplizierte Knäuelbildungen in der grauen Substanz der Vorderhörner und im intramedullären Abschnitt der Vorderwurzeln. Fig.13, 14, 21: 5 Tage nach der Läsion (Hund) Cajals Methode. Fig. 13 u. 21. Okul. 4, Komp.-Obj. 2 mm Zeiß. Fig. 25. Nicht sehr bäufig vorkommende Varietät einer Knäuelbildung. - Graue Substanz der Vorderhörner in der Nähe der Wurzeln. 3 Tage nach der Läsion (Kätzchen) Cajals Methode. Okul. 4, Komp.-Obj. 2 mm Zeiß. Fig.26 u. 29. Zellen der Vorderhörner. - Dünne, aus dem angeschwollenen Anteil des Axenzylinders hervorspringende Verzweigungen. 14 Tage nach der Läsion (Kätzchen) Cajals Methode. Okul. 3, Obj. DD. Zeiß (Reduktion auf 2/3). Sämtliche Figuren wurden direkt nach den Präparaten vermittelst der Hellkammer (Modell Apáthy) abgebildet. Sala, G. and Cortese, G. (1910) Über die im Rückenmark nach Ausreißung der Wurzeln eintretenden Erscheinungen. *Folia Neurobiol.* 4, 63–75 [Figures 20–27].

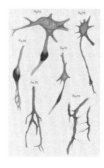

**FIGURE 194.**

Sala and Cortese, 1910. Alterations of the spinal cord, IV.

FIG. 28. Zelle der Vorderhörner - Eigentümliches Verhalten des in einer gewissen Entfernung vom Zellkörper in seiner Kontinuität unterbrochenen Nervenfortsatzes. Bildung der (keulenförmigen) Anschwellung . 2 Tage nach der Läsion (Kätzchen) Cajals Methode. Okul. 4, Komp.-Obj. 2 mm Zeiß (Reduktion auf 2/3 vermittelst der Reduktionsmaschine für Lithographie). Fig. 30. Der unter der keulenförmigen Anschwellung gelegene Faseranteil ist in Entartung begriffen; es gelangen schon Vakuolisationserscheinungen zur Beobachtung. 2 Tage nach der Läsion (Kätzchen) Cajals Methode. Okul. 4, Komp.-Obj. 2mm Zeiß (Reduktion auf 2/3). Fig. 31. Zelle der Vorderhörner. - Etwas langgestreckte keulenförmige Anschwellung von fibrillärer Struktur. 2 Tage nach der Läsion (Kätzchen) Cajals Methode. Okul. 4, Komp.-Obj. 2 mm Zeiß (Reduktion auf 2/3). Fig.26 u. 29. Zellen der Vorderhörner. - Dünne, aus dem angeschwollenen Anteil des Axenzylinders hervorspringende Verzweigungen. 14 Tage nach der Läsion (Kätzchen) Cajals Methode. Okul. 3, Obj. DD. Zeiß (Reduktion auf 2/3). Fig. 27. Zelle der Vorderhörner. - Merkwürdiges Aussehen des verdickten Anteils des Axenzylinders. Bemerkenswerte aber dünne, mehrmalige Spiralwindungen um den Axenzylinder vollziehende Faser. 5 Tage nach der Läsion (Hund) Cajals Methode. Okul. 3, Obj. E. Zeiß (Reduktion auf 2/3). Fig. 32 u. 33. Teilungen und Weiterteilungen von Fasern, die sowohl längs des intramedullären Verlaufes der Vorderwurzeln als auch im Inneren der grauen Substanz der Vorderhörner angetroffen werden. Fig.32: 14 Tage nach der Läsion (Kätzchen) Cajals Methode. Okul. 4, Obj. 2 mm Zeiß (Reduktion auf 2/3), Fig.33: 5 Tage nach der Läsion (Hund) Cajals Methode. Okul. 3, Obj. E. Zeiß (Reduktion auf 2/3). Sämtliche Figuren wurden direkt nach den Präparaten vermittelst der Hellkammer (Modell Apáthy) abgebildet. Sala, G. and Cortese, G. (1910) Über die im Rückenmark nach Ausreißung der Wurzeln eintretenden Erscheinungen. *Folia Neurobiol.* 4, 63–75 [Figures 28–33].

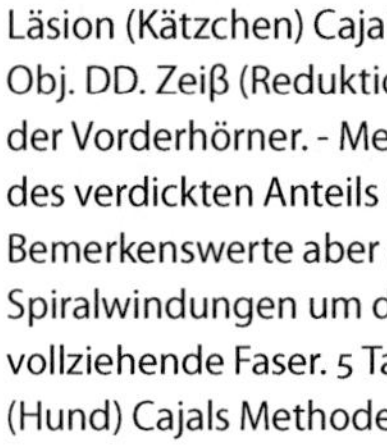

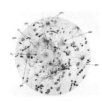

**FIGURE 195.**

Alzheimer, 1911. Neuritic plaque.

Gliabeizege-frierschnitte.

Weigertsche Gliafaserfärbung. Homogen. Inmers. Zeiß 1/13. Fig. 1 mit 140 Tubuslänge, Fig. 2 mit 160 Tubuslänge, Kompensationsokular 4 gezeichnet. *gaz.* Ganglienzelle, *glz.* Gliazelle. *P* zentraler Teil (Kern) der Plaque, $P_2$ peripherer Teil, Hof der Plaque. Fig. 1: Verhältnis der faserbildenden Gliazellen zu einer Plaque. Oberes Scheitelläppchen rechts. Im Kern der Plaque ein ganz kleiner, offenbar durch das Jod dunkelbraun gefärbter zentraler Teil, um den sich ein dunkler und dann hellerer Ring anschließen. Der periphere Teil ist von außerordentlich zahlreichen, ungemein feinen Gliafäserchen durchzogen, welche von den großen, am Rande des Hofes gelegenen faserbildenden Gliazellen herstammen. Alzheimer, A. (1911) Über eigenartige Krankheitsfälle des späteren Alters. *Z. gesamte Neurol. Psychiatr.* 4, 356–385 [Plate 4, Figure 1].

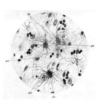

**FIGURE 196.**

Alzheimer, 1911. Hypertrophic glial cells.

Gliabeizege-frierschnitte. Weigertsche Gliafaserfärbung. Homogen. Inmers. Zeiß 1/13. Fig. 1 mit 140 Tubuslänge, Fig. 2 mit 160 Tubuslänge, Kompensationsokular 4 gezeichnet. *gaz.* Ganglienzelle, *glz.* Gliazelle. *P* zentraler Teil (Kern) der Plaque, $P_2$ peripherer Teil, Hof der Plaque. Fig. 2: Mächtige faserbildende Gliazellen aus der tieferen Schicht der Hirnrinde des oberen Scheitelläppchens rechts, vielfach benachbarte Ganglienzellen umfassend. Alzheimer, A. (1911) Über eigenartige Krankheitsfälle des späteren Alters. *Z. gesamte Neurol. Psychiatr.* 4, 356–385 [Plate 4, Figure 2].

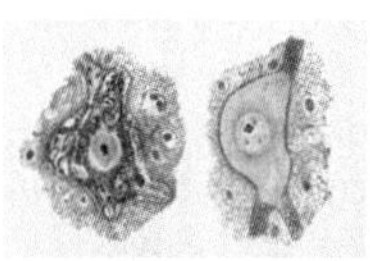

**FIGURE 197.**

Besta, 1911. Alterations of the peripheral reticulum of neurons.

Tutte le figure sono state disegnate col sussidio dell' apparato Abbe- Apathy, tenendo il foglio del disegno alla stessa altezza del tavolo del microscopio. L'ingrandimento è quello dato dal semiapocromatico $^{1}/_{15}$-Koristka e dall'oculare compensatore 4 (ad un dipresso 600 diametri). La spiegazione delle figure è nel testo. Besta, C. (1911) Sul modo di comportarsi del reticolo pericellulare in alcuni processi patologici del tessuto nervoso. *Int. Monatsschr. Anat. Physiol.* 27, 604–620 [Figures 15, left; 16, right].

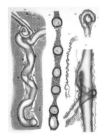

**FIGURE 198.**

Cerletti, 1911.
Cerebral vessels, I.

FIG. 65, 66, 70, 73, 74 stammen aus in Alkohol, Fig. 67, 68, 69, 71, 72 aus in WEIGERTscher Gliabeize fixiertem Material (resp. aus Zelloidin- und Gefrierschnitten). Phosphormolybdänsäurebeizung. Färbung mit dem MANNschen Gemisch. Fig. 65. Leitz' Imm. 1/12, Ok. 1. Sehr erweiterte und geschlangelte Präkapillare der Lamina pyramidalis einer Parietalwindung bei einem 97 jährigen Greise. In c ein Kollateralast, der eine vollständige Schlinge bildet. Beim Spielen der Mikrometerschraube sieht man, daß die große Präkapillare eine echte spiralartige Schlängelung darbietet. In der Krümmungsstellen sieht man scharfe, tief gefärbte Falten. In der Konkavität jeder Knickung, große Ansammlungen von Pigmentkugeln in der Adventitia. (Großer Teil der Fettstoffe ist wegen der Alkoholfixierung gelöst!) Dicke des Schnittes 25 μ. Fig. 66. Leitz' Obj. 5, Ok. 1. Reihe von sechs Schnitten eines und desselben regelmäßig geschlängelten Gefäßes (Vene) der weißen Substanz einer stark atrophischen Parietalwindung (unmittelbar unten und parallel an der Lamina multiformis) von einem Fall von progressiver Paralyse. In diesen Präparaten findet man ähnliche Luminareihen, die 10–15 aufeinanderfolgende Gefäßschnitte darstellen. Die einzelnen Gefäßschnitte sind durch zahlreiche, mit Plasmazellen, Lymphozyten, Pigmentschollen usw. überfüllte Adventitialfaserbündel unter sich verbunden. Vgl. eine ähnliche, von der Seite gesehene Anordnung in der unteren Hälfte des Gefäßes in Fig. 65. Fig. 67. Aus der weißen Substanz einer Frontalwindung eines 6ojährigen Mannes. Leitz' Imm. 1/12, Ok. 1. Bindegewebsfaserbündel, das zwei benachbarte Kapillare wie eine Brücke verbindet. Man achte auf die Kontinuität der diesem Bündel gehörenden Fasern mit den adventitiellen Fasern der beiden Gefäße. Fig. 68. Leitz' Imm. 1/12, Ok. 1. Quergeschnittenes, vom Kollateralast k ringsumgebenes Gefäß g, ("Bischofsstab") in der Lamina magnopyramidalis der linken vorderen Zentralwindung bei einem 94jährigen Greise. Solche Bilder stellen horizontale Schnitte von Kollateralastumwindungen dar, welche in Längsschnitte bei Fig. 69, 71, 72, 73 zu sehen sind. Fig.71. Leitz' Imm. 1/12, Ok.1. Durch Lamina granularis interna einer Parietalwindung verlaufende Arteriole bei einem 90 jährigen Greise. Der Kollateralast k macht eine vollständige Umdrehung

ringsum die Stammarteriole. Kein Zeichen von Erwürgung des Stammgefäßes. Dicke des Schnittes 25 μ. Cerletti, U. (1911) Die Gefäßvermehrung im Zentralnervensystem. In *Histologische und histopathologische Arbeiten über die Grosshirnrinde*, eds. F. Nissl and A. Alzheimer, vol. 4, 1–168. Jena: Gustav Fischer [Figures 65–68, 71].

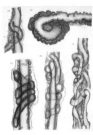

**FIGURE 199.**

Cerletti, 1911.
Cerebral vessels, II.

FIG. 65, 66, 70, 73, 74 stammen aus in Alkohol, Fig. 67, 68, 69, 71, 72 aus in WEIGERTscher Gliabeize fixiertem Material (resp. aus Zelloidin- und Gefrierschnitten). Phosphormolybdänsäurebeizung. Färbung mit dem MANNschen Gemisch. Fig. 69. Ähnliche Bildung, wie bei Fig. 68. Hier ist aber das Hauptgefäß längsgeschnitten. Aus der weißen Substanz einer Frontalwindung, unmittelbar unter der Lamina multiformis, bei einem 91 jährigen Greise. Die Stammarteriole erscheint von dem rings herumgehenden Kollateralast k beträchtlich verengt. k' ein zweiter quergeschnittener Kollateralast. Leitz' Imm. 1/12, Ok. 1. Fig.70. Leitz' Obj. 5, Ok. 3. Vollständige Schlinge einer Arteriole der weißen Substanz der Hirnwindungen bei einem 97 jährigen Greise. Man achte auf die Unregelmäßigkeiten des Gefäßkalibers, die mächtige Wucherung des Adventitialbindegewebes. Dieses kolossale Bindegewebige Bündel verläuft spiralartig um die Arteriole. Im Zentrum der Schlinge sieht man eine dichte Ansammlung von Fettkörnchenzellen. Dicke des Schnittes 35 μ. Fig. 72. Leitz' Imm. 1/12, Ok. 1. Dreimalige Umwindung durch ein (oder zwei) Kollateraläste einer Arteriole der Lamina multiformis einer hinteren Zentralwindung bei einem 79 jährigen Presbyophreniker. Hier erscheint die Stammarteriole durch den umgeschlungenen Kollateralast etwas eingeschnürt. Fig. 73. Leitz' Imm. 1/12, Ok. 1. Mehrmalige Umwindung einer Arteriole durch ein (oder zwei?) Gefäße. Aus der Lamina multiformis einer Parietalwindung bei einem 89 jährigen Presbyophreniker. Wegen der relativen Dünnheit des Schnittes ist es unmöglich, den ganzen Verlauf der eingerollten Gefäße zu verfolgen. Dicke des Schnittes 25 μ. Fig. 74. Gefäßkonvolut in der Lamina magnopyramidalis einer hinteren Zentralwindung bei einem 97 jährigen Greise. Leitz' Imm. 1/12, Ok. 1. Die Längsachse des Konvolutes verläuft parallel der Gehirnoberfläche. Man achte auf die häufige Erweiterung des Gefäßkalibers und auf die große Pigmentkugelhäufungen zwischen

den Gefäßrohren. Dicke des Schnittes 40 μ. Cerletti, U. (1911) Die Gefäßvermehrung im Zentralnervensystem. In *Histologische und histopathologische Arbeiten über die Grosshirnrinde*, eds. F. Nissl and A. Alzheimer, vol. 4, 1–168. Jena: Gustav Fischer [Figures 69, 70, 72–74].

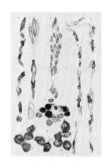

**FIGURE 200.**

Cerletti, 1911. Mast cells in the olfactory bulb.

FIG. 1. Kapillare der zentralen weissen Substanz des Bulbus olfactorius eines jungen normalen Hundes. Zahlreiche rundliche und langgestrekte Mastzellen längs der Gefässwand. Alkoholfixierung. Toluidinblaufärbung. Leitz hom. imm. 1/12 komp. Ok. 6. Fig. 2. Grosse langgestreckte auf einer Kapillare gelagerte Mastzelle. Oben eine Endothelzelle (rechts) und eine längliche Adventitialzelle (links). Aus der um die Ventrikularspalte des Bulbus olfactorius liegenden Zone. Alkoholfixierung. Toluidinblaufärbung. Leitz hom. Imm. 1/12. komp. Ok. 12. Fig. 3. Reihe von Mastzellen längs einer Präkapillare in der zentralen weissen Substanz: des Bulbus olfactorius eines normalen erwachsenen Hundes. Alkoholfixierung. Unna-Pappenheimsche Färbung. Durch diese Methode werden zwischen den Orange gefärbten, spärliche intensiv-braun gefärbte Körnchen dargestellt, deren Natur noch umbestimmt erscheint. Leitz hom. Imm. 1/12. komp. Ok. 6. Zwecks Vereinfachung der lith. Reproduktion wurden die Zellkerne statt blau-grün einfach blau wiedergegeben. Fig. 4. Eine grosse Präkapillare der zentralen weissen Substanz des Bulbus olfactorius eines erwachsenen normalen Hundes. Zahlreiche Mastzellen liegen in der adventitiellen Lymphscheide. Alkoholfixierung. Ehrlich-Westphalsche Färbung zur Darstellung der Mastzellengranula. Leitz hom. Imm. 1/12. komp. Ok. 6. Fig. 5. Gruppierung von 5 Mastzellen um eine dünne Kapillare des Bulbus olfactorius eines erwachsenen normalen Hundes. Die "nackten" blauen Kerne gehören den Gliazellen des umliegenden Gewebes. Alkoholfixierung. Weigertsche Resorcin-Fuch-sinfärbung. Toluidinblau. Leitz hom. Imm. 1/12. Komp. Ok. 12. Fig. 6. Anhäufung zahlreicher Mastzellen, die anscheinend frei im nervösen Gewebe des Bulbus olfactorius eines jungen normalen Hundes lagen. (s. Text). Alkoholfixierung. Ehrlich – Westphalsche Färbung zur Darstellung der Mastzellengranula. Leitz hom. Imm. 1/12. Komp. Ok. 12. Cerletti, U. (1911) Die Mastzellen als regelmässiger Befund im Bulbus olfactorius des normalen Hundes. *Folia Neurobiol.* 5, 718–722 [Figures 1–6].

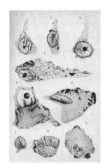

**FIGURE 201.**

Cerletti, 1911. Pathology of ganglion cells.

Alle Abbildungen stammen aus Toluidinblaupräparaten (Alkoholfixierung) und wurden mit dem Abbéschem Apparat, Leitz Komp Ok. 12, homog. Imm. 1/12 gezeichnet. Zur Vereinfachung der Bilder wurden die Kernkörperchen so gezeichnet als ob sie in der Ebene der Kernoberfläche lägen. Fig. 1, 2, 3, 7 Pyramidenzellen mit starker Kernrunzelung aus äusserrt atrophischen Windungen von Fällen sehr chronisch verlaufender Paralyse. Von der chromophilen Substanz sind nur spärliche Spuren zu sehen. Man beachte die beträchtliche Verkleinerung des Zellleibes im Vergleich zu den Kernen, welche, trotz ihrer Schrumpfung, im Verhältnis zum Zellleib gross erscheinen. Bei den Zellen 1 und 3 zeigen die Pigmentschollen eine kaum wahrnehmbare gelbliche Farbe. Fig. 4, 5, 6, 8, 9. Zellen des Nucleus dorsalis tegmenti und des Nucleus lateralis aquaeducti bei einem an Wernickescher Polienzephalitis gestorbenen chronischen Alkoholisten. Es wurden verschiedene Stadien der Kernrunzelung dargestellt. Die chromophile Substanz ist meist fast vollständing verschwunden. Die schwersten Kernveränderungen sind an den Zellen zu beobachten, welche eine tiefe Umgestaltung des Zellleibes zeigen. Cerletti, U. (1911) Zur Pathologie der Ganglienzellenkerne. *Folia Neurobiol.* 5, 861–868 [Figures 1–9].

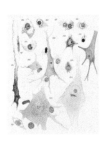

**FIGURE 202.**

Cerletti, 1911. Histopathology of cerebral malaria.

Mit Ausnahme der Fig. 239-257, welche mit Ok. 5 gezeichnet sind, wurden alle Abbildungen mit Imm. 1/12, Ok. 3 (Leitz) gezeichnet. Fig. 194. Große Pyramidenzelle der vorderen Zentralwindung. Alkoholfixierung, Toluidinblaufärbung. Schrumpfung des Zelleibes. Körniger Zerfall der chromophilen Substanz. Apikaler Zellfortsatz abnorm färbbar. Hochgradige Schrumpfung und abnorm intensive Färbung

des Kernes. Schwellung des Kernkörperchen. Fig. 195. Spindelformige Nervenzelle aus der Lamina multiformis einer Frontalwindung. Alkoholfixierung, Toluidinblaufärbung. Zellschrumpfung. Pigmentäre Umwandlung des Zytoplasmas. Schwere Formveränderung des Kernes. Fig. 196. Große Pyramidenzelle einer hinteren Zentralwindung bei einem besonders schweren Fall. Alkoholfixierung, Toluidinblaufärbung. NISSLsche "schwere Zellerkrankung". Bläschenbildung im Zellkern. Fig. 197. Fall, Färbung usw. wie Fig. 196. Pyramidenzelle. Beträchtliche Schrumpfung des Kernes mit Verdickung der Chromatinkörnchen. Kernvakuole. Breiter perinukleärer Hof. Fig. 198. Pyramidenzelle wie bei Fig. 196, bei der eine hypertrophische Gliazelle dicht anliegt. Fig. 199. Fall usw. wie bei Fig. 196. Regelmäßige Verkleinerung des Zellkernes bei einer von der schweren Zellerkrankung NISSLS betroffenen Pyramidenzelle. Zahlreiche große Chromatinkörnchen im Kern. Fig. 207. Pyramidenzelle aus der Lamina magnopyramidalis der vorderen Zentralwindung. Alkoholfixierung, Toluidinblaufärbung. NISSLsche "schwere Erkrankung". Man achte auf das bruchbildende Bläschen im Kern. Vollständiger Verlust der Zellform. Fig.208. Pyramidenzelle aus einer Parietalwindung. Alkoholfixierung, Toluidinblaufärbung. (63 jähriges Individuum.) Totale pigmentäre Umwandlung des Zelleibes. Schrumpfung und Schlängelung der Zellfortsätze. Kernablassung. Fig. 209. Große Pyramidenzelle aus einer Frontalwindung bei einem sehr akuten Fall. Alkoholfixierung, Toluidinblaufärbung. Akute Zellerkrankung. Veränderung der Kernform. Kernverkleinerung. In der Basis der Zelle eine eigentümlich blaßgelbe Pigmentanhäufung. In den Zelleibern der umliegenden Gliazellen zahlreiche blasse, dicht angehäufte Pigmentschollen. Fig. 210. Grobkörnige, äußerst intensiv gefärbte Einlagerungen (Inkrustation?) in einer Pyramidenzelle der hinteren Zentralwindung. Alkoholfixierung, Toluidinblaufärbung. Schrumpfung und abnorm intensive Färbung des Kernes. Verschiebung des angeschwollenen Kernkörperchen. Fig. 211. Pyramidenzelle aus einer Frontalwindung. Alkoholfixierung, Toluidinblaufärbung. Terminales Stadium der in Fig. 197, 199-201 dargestellten Kernveränderung. Die zahlreichen verdickten Chromatinkörnchen liegen dicht nebeneinander, eine rundliche brombeerenähnliche kleine Anhäufung bildend. Fig. 222. Pyramidenzelle aus einer Frontalwindung bei einem besonders schweren Fall. Alkoholfixierung, Toluidinblaufärbung. Vorgeschrittenes Stadium der NISSLschen

schweren Zellerkrankung. Erhaltene Kernform. Im Karyoplasma sind zwei Kernkörperchen, wovon das eine angeschwollen und vaknolisiert ist. Fig. 223. BETZsche Riesenpyramidenzelle bei einem sehr akuten Fall. Alkoholfixierung, Toluidinblaufärbung. NISSLche akute Zellerkrankung. Man achte auf die Kernveränderungen und auf die eigentümliche Vermehrung der Chromatinkörnchen in den umliegenden hypertrophischen Gliakernen. Fig. 224. Pyramidenzelle einer Parietalwindung bei einem besonders schweren Fall. Alkoholfixierung, Toluidinblanfärbung (s. Fig. 199). Fig. 225. BETZsche Riesenpyramidenzelle. Alkoholfixierung, Toluidinblaufärbung. Akute Zellveränderung. Unter dem Kern spärliche Reste chromophiler Schollen. Mächtige Vergrößerung des Kernkörperchens und gleichmäßige Vakuolisierung desselben. Umwandlung eines Teiles des Zelleibes in eine homogene, fein punktierte Substanz. Cerletti, U. (1911) Die histopathologichen Veränderungen der Hirnrinde bei Malaria perniciosa. (Beiträge zur Kenntnis der akuten Rindenerkrankungen) In *Histologische und histopathologische Arbeiten über die Grosshirnrinde*, eds. F. Nissl and A. Alzheimer, vol. 4, 169–266. Jena: Gustav Fischer [Figures 194–199, 207–211, 222–225].

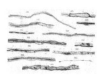

**FIGURE 203.**

Doinikow, 1911. Peripheral nerve histology and histopathology, I.

Bielschowskysche Neurofibrillenfärbung. Fig. 136. Meerschweinchen. Bleineuritis. Vergiftungsdauer 70 Tage. Aus einem Stamm des Plex. brachiális. Zupfpräparat. Zeiss' homog. Imm. 1/12, Ok. 2. Markhaltige Nervenfaser mit gut erhaltenem Achsenzylinder und einer Menge von dünnen sich vielfach teilenden und Geflechte bildenden neugebildeten Axonen. *ax* Achsenzylinder. *er* Endringe. *ms* Markscheide. Fig. 137. Huhn. Reisneuritis. Längsschnitt aus dem Nerv. ischiadicus. Zeiss' homog. Imm. 1/12, Ok. 4. *ax* Achsenzylinder. *ax'* Zwei Teilungsäste desselben. *a* Endkolbe mit kurzem Stiel. *b* Kolbige Anschwellungen. Fig. 138. Vom selben Objekt. Zeiss' homog.Imm. 1/12, Ok. 6. Netzartiger Auswuchs des Achsenzylinders. Fig. 139. Meerschweinchen. Bleineuritis. Vergiftungsdauer 60 Tage. Längsschnitt aus dem N. ischiadicus. Zeiss' homog. Imm. 1/12, Ok. 6. *ax* Achsenzylinder. *ax'* Neugebildete in spiralen Schlingen ziehende Axone. *a* Varikositäten in ihrem Verlauf. *ms* Markscheide. *mb* Markballen. Bei *x* ist der Achsenzylinder wahrscheinlich angeschnitten, bei *y* ein neugebildeter Axon angeschnitten. Fig. 140. Kaninchen. Bleineuritis. Vergiftungsdauer 10 Wochen. Längsschnitt aus dem N. ischiadicus. Zeiss' homog. Imm. 1/12, Ok. 4. *a* Körnige Ballen (an der Stelle der Lantermannschen Einkerbungen). Fig. 141. Meerschweinchen. Bleineuritis. Vergiftungsdauer 60 Tage. Längsschnitt aus dem N. ischiadicus. Zeiss' homog. Imm. 1/12, Ok. 8. *ax* Achsenzylinder. *ax'* Neugebildete Axone mit Endringen *(er)*. *a* Schwarze Körnchen (wahrscheinlich Zerfallsprodukte des Achsenzylinders). *ms* Markscheide. Fig. 142. Meerschweinchen. Bleineuritis. Vergiftungsdauer 4 Wochen. Längsschnitt aus einem Nervenstamm des Plex. brachialis. Zeiss' homog. Imm. 1/12,' Ok. 6. *ax* Achsenzylinder. *ms* Markscheide. *ax'* Neugebildete Axone. *a* Varikositäten. *r* Ringelchen. Fig. 143. Meerschweinchen. Bleineuritis. Vergiftungsdauer 6 Wochen. Längsschnitt aus dem N. ischiadicus. Zeiss' homog. Imm. 1/12, Ok. 6. *ax* Achsenzylinder. *ax'* Neugebildeter Achsenzylindersproß. *a* Degenerierte große Endkolbe. *ms* Markscheide. Fig. 144. Meerschweinchen. Bleineuritis. Vergiftungsdauer 70 Tage. Längsschnitt aus dem N. ischiadicus. Zeiss' homog. Imm. 1/12,' Ok. 6. *a* Polypöse Exkreszenzen. *ax* Achsenzylinder. *ax'* Neugebildete Achsenzylindersprossen. *b* Anschwellungen des Achsenzylinders. *mb* Markballen, die den Achsenzylinder zur Seite drängen. *ms* Markscheide, durchweg alteriert. *schwz* Kern der Schwannschen Zelle. Fig. 145. Huhn. Reisneuritis. Längsschnitt aus dem N. ischiadicus. Zeiss' homog. Imm. 1/12, Ok. 6. Das Lumen der Faser von Markballen *(mb)* und Achsenzylinderfragmenten *(a)* angefüllt. *b* Brückenartige Auffaserung eines neuge-bildeten Achsenzylinders *(ax)*. Fig. 146. Vom selben Objekt. Zeiss' homog. Imm. 1/12, Ok. 8. *a* Polypöse Exkreszenzen des Achsenzylinders. Fig. 147. Meerschweinchen. Bleineuritis. Vergiftungsdauer 4 Wochen. Zeiss' homog. Imm. 1/12, Ok. 6. Junger Achsenzylindersproß. *e* Endkeule. *a* Varikositäten. Fig. 148. Huhn. Reisneuritis. Längsschnitt aus dem N. ischiadicus. Zeiss' homog. Imm. 1/12, Ok. 8. Auffaserung des Achsenzylinders und Sprossenbildung. *a* Zerfallsprodukte des Achsenzylinders. *ax'* Aufgefaserter Achsenzylinder an der Peripherie der Faser. *er* Endringe. *k* Zellkerne. Doinikow, B. (1911) Beiträge zur Histologie und Histopathologie des peripheren Nerven. In *Histologische und Histopathologische Arbeiten über die Grosshirnrinde*, eds. F. Nissl and A. Alzheimer, vol. 4, 445–630. Jena: Gustav Fischer [Plate 28].

**FIGURE 204.**
Doinikow, 1911. Peripheral nerve histology and histopathology, II.

*Meerschweinchen.* Fig. 104-109 Methode VIII. Fig. 110-111 Methode I. Fig. 104. Bleineuritis. Vergiftungsdauer 70 Tage. Zeiss' homog. Imm. 1/12, Ok. 4. Zupfpräparat aus dem N. ischiadi-cus. *mls* Marklose Strecken der Nervenfaser. *abp* Abbauprodukte der Markscheide. *mb* rot gefärbte Markballen. *ax* Achsenzylinder. *ax'* Komprimierte intensiver gefärbte Strecke des Achsenzylinders. *ms* Markscheide; innere Teile stellenweise gut erhalten. *schwz* Stark vermehrte Schwannsche Zellen. Fig. 105. Bleineuritis. Vergiftungsdauer 60 Tage. Zupfpräparat aus dem N. ischiadicus. Zeiss' homog. Imm. 1/12, Ok. 6. *schwz* Schwannsche Zelle mit Zerfallsprodukten *(abp)* beladen. *ms* Junge, noch dünne Markscheide mit sehr feinem Wabenwerk. *ax* Achsenzylinder. *schws* Schwannsche Scheide. *x* Erweiterter Raum unter der alten Schwannsche Scheide. Fig. 106. Bleineuritis. Zupfpräparat aus dem N. ischiadicus. Vergiftungsdauer 45 Tage. Zeiss' homog. Imm. 1/12, Ok. 4. *abp* Abbauprodukte. *ax* Achsenzylinder. *ax'* Verengte, intensiver gefärbte Abschnitte des Achsenzylinders. *mls* Marklose Strecke der Nervenfaser. *nnf* Normale Strecke der Nervenfaser. *schwz* Gewucherte Schwannsche Zelle. *schwz'* Kleine Schwannsche Zelle in einer ovoiden Auftreibung, mit Abbauprodukten beladen. Fig. 107. Bleineuritis. Vergiftungsdauer 30 Tage. Längsschnitt aus einem Nervenstamm des Plex. brachialis. Zeiss' homog. Imm. 1/12' Ok. 2. *ax* Achsenzylinder. *elzk* Elzholzsche Körperchen. *mb* Größere, gelblich gefärbte Markballen. *ms* Markscheide. *schwz* Kern der Schwannsche Zelle. Fig. 108. 12 Tage nach Einspritzung von Diphtherietoxin. Längsschnitt aus dem N. ischiadicus. Methode VIII ohne Osmierung. Zeiss' homog. Imm. 1/12, Ok. 2. *schwz* Kern der Schwannsche Zelle. *schpl* stark gewuchertes Plasma der Schwannsche Zelle. Fig. 109. Bleineuritis. Vergiftungsdauer 70 Tage. Längsschnitt aus dem N. radialis. Markhaltige Faser mit stark geschwellten Protoplasmastrukturen der Schwannsche Zelle. Methode VIII ohne Osmierung. *schwz* Kern der Schwannschen Zelle. *schpl* Plasma. der Schwannschen Zelle. *ax* Achsenzylinder. *ax'* Achsenzylinderauswuchs. *mb* Markballen. *ms* Markscheide. Fig. 110. Bleineuritis. Vergiftungsdauer 60 Tage. Zupfpräparat aus dem N. ischiadicus. Zeiss' homog. Imm. 1/12, Ok. 2. *schwz* Schwannsche Zellen mit schaumartigem, das Mark durchwachsenden Plasma. *ax* Achsenzylinder. *ms* Markscheide, sehr blaß gefärbt. Man beachte die auch

in weiterer Entfernung von den Zellkernen deutlich sichtbaren Protoplasmastrukturen. Fig. 111. Bleineuritis. Vergiftungsdauer 70 Tage. Zupfpräparat aus dem N. ischiadicus. Zeiss' homog. Imm. 1/12, Ok. 2. *schwz* Schwannsche Zelle mit stark gewuchertem Plasma. *abp* Abbauprodukte (basophile Körnchen, wie in Fig. 57-59). *mdz* Mesodermale Elemente (das Plasma ragt über die Grenzen der Nervenfaser hinaus). Doinikow, B. (1911) Beiträge zur Histologie und Histopathologie des peripheren Nerven. In *Histologische und histopathologische Arbeiten über die Grosshirnrinde*, eds. F. Nissl and A. Alzheimer, vol. 4, 445–630. Jena: Gustav Fischer [Plate 25].

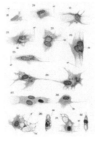

**FIGURE 205.**
Doinikow, 1911. Peripheral nerve histology and histopathology, III.

*Kaninchen.* Zeigt die mesodermalen Elemente der periph-eren Nerven. Sämtliche Figuren, mit Ausnahme von Fig. 36, 39, 40, Alkoholfixierung, Unnas pol. Methylenblau. Sämtliche Figuren, falls nicht bezeichnet, mit Zeiss' homog. Imm. 1/12, Ok. 6, geze-ichnet. Fig. 19-30. Fixe Bindegewebszellen aus dem Endoneurium. In den Fig. 19, 20, 21, 22, 24, 25, 27 sind auch die Umrisse der anliegenden Nervenfaser gezeichnet, um die gegenseitige Lage zu zeigen. Man beachte die Zellfortsätze und die zackigen Zellumrisse. Fig. 19. Aus dem N. ischiadicus eines gesunden Kaninchens. Fig. 20, 21. 3 Tage nach Nervendurchschneidung. Aus dem N. tibialis. Fig. 22. 8 Tage nach Durchschneidung des Nerven. *hh* Heller Plasmahof. Fig. 24. 8 Tage nach Nervendurchschneidung. Zelle mit zwei Kernen. Fig. 25. 6 Tage nach Nervendurchschneidung. Fig. 23, 26. Bleineuritis. Vergiftungsdauer 6 Wochen. Stark gewucherte Exemplare aus dem N. peroneus. Fig. 27. 42 Tage nach Nervendurchschneidung. Mehrkerniges Exemplar. Fig. 28. 14 Tage nach Nervendurchneidung. Aus dem N. tibialis. In Abrundung begriffene Zelle, die noch dünne fadenförmige Fortsätze behält. Mit Ausnahme des kleinen hellen Hofes *hh*, Gitterstruktur des gesamten Zelleibes. Fig. 29. Vom selben Objekt. Zweikerniges Exemplar. Blasenzellenbildung. *K'* Winziger degeneri-erender Zellkern. *vk'* Große blasenförmige Vakuolen. Die Zellfortsätze sind noch gut erhalten. Fig. 30. Bleineuritis. Vergiftungsdauer 10 Wochen. Eine in eine "Blasenzelle" sich umwandelnde fixe Bindegewebszelle. Bei *hh* der gut ausgeprägte differenzierte Plasmahof.

Zeiss' homog. Imm. 1/12, Ok.4. Fig.31. 8 Tage nach Nervendurchschneidung. Eine vakuolisierte Zelle aus dem Endoneurium. Übergang zur Blasenzellenform. (Wahrscheinlich eine in Abrundung begriffene fixe Bindegewebszelle.) Fig. 32. Vom selben Objekt. Zelle aus dem Endoneurium, deren Abstammung nicht näher zu bestimmen ist. Fig. 33. 2 Tage nach Nervendurchschneidung. Zur differentiellen Diagnose zwischen wuchernden Bindegewebszellen und SCHWANNschen Zellen. *schwz* Wuchernde SCHWANNschen Zelle. Man beachte das grobwabige Plasma. *rwz* Ruhende Wanderzelle (Klasmatozyt). Fig. 34, 35. Ruhende Wanderzellen (Klasmatozyten) aus dem Endoneurium des normalen Nerven. Fig. 36. Mastzelle aus dem Epineurium des N. ischiadicus eines gesunden Kaninchens. Fixierung in absol. Alkohol, Färbung in gesättigter 50 proz. alkoholischer Thioninlösung (MICHAELIS). Fig. 37. Flächenschnitt durch das Perineurium eines gesunden Nerven (N. ischiadicus). *e* Endothelzellen; die Zellgrenzen sind nicht sichtbar. *fbl* Fixe Bindegewebszelle. *rwz* Ruhende Wanderzelle. Fig. 38. Bleineuritis. Vergiftungsdauer 5 Wochen. Endoneurales Gefäß. Zeiss' homog. Imm. 1/12, Ok. 4. *lmz* In Emigration begriffene Lymphozyten. *ez* Endothelzellen. *l* Gefäßlumen. *adv* Adventitia. Fig. 39, 40. Bleineuritis. Vergiftungsdauer 5 Wochen. Methode I. Zeiss' homog. Imm. 1/12, Ok. 8. Mobile Elemente aus dem endoneuralen Gewebe des N. peroneus. Fig. 39 wahrscheinlich Leukozyt, Fig. 40 Polyblast. Fig. 41. 8 Tage nach Durchschneidung des Nerven. Polyblast aus dem endoneuralen Gewebe des N. tibialis. Fig. 42. Bleineuritis. Vergiftungsdauer 5 Wochen. Zwei Polyblasten aus dem endoneuralen Gewebe des N. peroneus. Fig. 43. 5 Tage nach Nervendurchschneidung. Polyblast mit Gitterstruktur des Zelleibes (Fett). Aus dem endoneuralen Gewebe des N. tibialis. Fig. 44. Bleineuritis. Vergiftungsdauer 6 Wochen. Zeiss' homog. Imm. 1/12, Ok. 8. Zerschnürung des Zellkerns eines Polyblasten. Fig. 45-48. Bleineuritis. Vergiftungsdauer 6-8 Wochen. Verwandlung von Polyblasten zu Blasenzellen. Zeiss' homog. Imm. 1/12, Ok.8. Fig. 45, 46. Vakuolisierung des Zelleibes. Fig. 47. Einkernige Blasenzelle. Fig. 48. Zweikernige Blasenzelle. Fig. 49. 8 Tage nach Nervendurchschneidung. Körnchenzelle aus einem endoneuralen Lymphraum. Zeiss' homog. Imm. 1/12, Ok. 8. Fig. 50. 21 Tage nach Durchschneidung des Nerven. Flächenschnitt durch das Perineurium des N. peroneus. *e* Endotbelzellen. Doinikow, B. (1911) Beiträge zur Histologie und Histopathologie des peripheren Nerven. In *Histologische und histopathologische Arbeiten über die Grosshirnrinde*, eds. F. Nissl and A. Alzheimer, vol. 4, 445–630. Jena: Gustav Fischer [Plate 21].

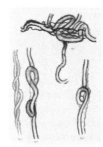

**FIGURE 206.**

Lafora, 1911. Histopathology of the spinal cord, I.

FIG. 1. Dementia senilis: Schr coomplicierte Gefässpakete ader Gefässknänel (modif. Mannsche Methode). Fig. 5. Dementia senilis: Gefässpakete (Alkohol, Resorcin, Fuchsin und Toluidin). Fig. 6. Dementia senilis: Gefässknoten (modif. Mannsche Methode). Fig. 8. Dementia senilis: Gefässknoten (modif. Mannsche Methode). Lafora, G. R. (1911) Beitrag zur Histopathologie des Rückenmarkes bei der Dementia arteriosclerotica und senilis. *Monatsschr. Psychiatr. Neurol.* 39, 1–32 [Figures 1, 5, 6, 8].

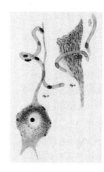

**FIGURE 207.**

Lafora, 1911. Histopathology of the spinal cord, II.

FIG. 3. Dem. arteriosclerotica: Vorderhornzelle von einer kapillare umgeben (Alkohol, Resorcin-Fuchsin u, Toluidin). Fig. 4. Dem. arteriosclerotica: Dasselbe. Lafora, G. R. (1911) Beitrag zur Histopathologie des Rückenmarkes bei der Dementia arteriosclerotica und senilis. *Monatsschr. Psychiatr. Neurol.* 39, 1–32 [Figures 3, 4].

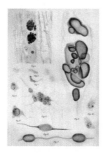

**FIGURE 208.**

Lafora, 1911. Histopathology of the spinal cord, III.

FIG. 1. Dementia senilis: Longitudinal-Schnitt, Maulheerbildungen in einem Achsenzylinder ( ?), vielleicht von amyloider Natur (Rankesehe Methode). Fig. 2. Dementia senilis: Longit. Schnitt; Markfaserdegeneration (amyloider Natur?) (Hankesche Methode). Fig. 3. Dementia arteriosclerotica: Regressiv veränderte Gliazellen (ohne Chromatin) (Alkohol, Thionin]. Fig. 4. Dementia arteriosclerotica:Stäbchenäbnliche Gliazelle (Alkohol, Thionin). Fig. 5. Dementia arteriosclerotica: Mittelgrosse Satellitzelle (Alkohol, Thionin). Fig. 6. Dementia arteriosclerotica: Grosse-Satellitzello (Alkohol, Thionin). Fig. 7. Dementia arteriosclerotica: Gliarasen im Hinterhorn (Alkohol, Thionin). Fig. 8. Dementia senilis: Markfaser mit einer Anschwellung (amyloid ?) [modif. Mannsche Methode}. Fig. 9. Dementia senilis: Dieselbe Faser wie in Fig. 2. Fig. 10. Dementia arteriosclerotica: Gliazellen mit Vakuolen (Alkohol , Thionin). Lafora, G. R. (1911) Beitrag zur Histopathologie des Rückenmarkes bei der Dementia arteriosclerotica und senilis. *Monatsschr. Psychiatr. Neurol.* 39, 1–32 [Figures 1–10].

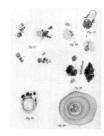

**FIGURE 209.**

Lafora, 1911. Histopathology of the spinal cord, IV.

FIG. 13. Dementia senilis: Gliazellen mit Fettröpichen (Fischer-Herxheimersche Methode). Fig. 15. Dementia arteriosclerotica: Kleine Gefässe mit Fett in dem adventitiellen Lymphraum (Fischer- Herxheimersche Methode). Fig. 17. Dem. Senilis:Körnchenzelle von endothelialer Herkumft (Fischer-Herxheimersche Methode). Fig. 18. Dem. Arteriosclerotica: Cliogene Körnchenzellen (Triacid-Färbung). Fig. 19. Dementia arteriosclerotica: Körnchenzellen mit Fett in der Umge bung eines Gefässchens (Pappenheimsche Färbung). Fig. 20. Dementia arteriosclerotica: Hyaline Degeneration eines kleinen Gefässes (Alkohol, Resorcin-Fuchsin und Toluidin). Lafora, G. R. (1911) Beitrag zur Histopathologie des Rückenmarkes bei der Dementia arteriosclerotica und senilis. *Monatsschr. Psychiatr. Neurol.* 39, 1–32 [Figures 13, 15, 17–20].

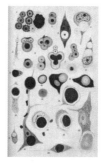

**FIGURE 210.**

Lafora, 1911. Amyloid desposits inside neurons.

FIG. 1. stellt eine große Ganglienzelle aus derOblongata dar, mit. 8 Amyloidkörpern ( einige mit konzentrischer Schichtung und zahnartigen, radiären, äußeren Streifungen) (Hämatoxylin-Eosin). Fig. 2. Kleine Ganglienzelle aus der Lamina granuıaris interna (okzipital Kortex ), von einem ziemlich großen Amyloidköper belegen (Heidenhainsche Methode).

Fig. 3. Ganglienzelle aus dem Ammonshorn, mit einem sehr blassem Amyloidkörper, welcher im Innern einen dreieckigen Kristall zeigt (Heidenhainsche Methode). Fig. 4. Pyramidenzelle aus der frontalen Kortex, mit einem blassen Amyloidkörper und Pigment (schwarz gefärbt) (Heidenhainsche Methode). Fig. 5. Kleine und atrophische Ganglienzelle aus dem Ammonshorn, die einen kleinen Amyloidkörper in ihrer Protoplasmafortsetzung enthält (Toluidin). Fig. 6. Isolierte und gruppierte Amyloidkörperchen, die von Gliazellen umgeben sind (Heidenhainsche Methode). Fig. 7. stellt die Ausammlung der Amyloidkörperchen, und ihre Zusammenschmelzung dar. Ein Amyloidkörper zeigt im Zentrum sehr deutlich gefärbte Kristalle (Heindenhainsches Hämatoxylin). Fig. 8. stellt dar eine Pyramidenzelle aus der Gehirncortex mit zwei blassen Amyloidkörperchen, un die herum man Pigmentgranula (schwarz gefärbt) sehen kann (Heidenhainsche Methode). Fig. 9. Kleine Ganglienzelle aus dem posterioren Horn des dorsalen Bückenmarks, verhältnismäßig große Amyloidkörper enthaltend (Hämatoxylin-Eosin). Fig. 10. Zwei amyloidkörperchen aus dem Pons, mit der Mannschen Methode gefärbt. Kleine cosinophile Kristalle in dem Zentrum. Fig. 11. Ganglienzellen aus der Tuber-quadrigemina posterior, mit Amyloidkörperchen, dessen Zentrum einige eosinophile Kristalle enthält (Mannsche Methode). Fig. 12. Ganglienzelle aus der Oblongata, mit einem Amyloidkörper, mitten in das Zellpigment hineingelegt (Toluidin). Fig. 13. Amyloidkörper mit Bestscher Methode gefärbt. Fig. 14. stellt eine Ganglienzelle aus der Oblongata dar in deren Innerem sich ein großer Amyloidkörper gebildet hat (Toluidin). Fig. 15. Kleine Ganglienzelle aus dem Ammonshorn mit einem Amyloidkörper (Toluidin). Fig. 16. Ganglienzelle aus dem lumbalen Rückenmark (Seitenhorn), mit zwei Amyloidkörpern (Hämatoxylin- Eosin). Fig. 17. Ganglienzelle aus dem Pons, dessen Kern durch die Amyloidkörper deformiert ist (Hämatoxylin- Eosin). Fig. 18. stellt eine Ganglienzelle aus der Oblongata dar, mit einem großen amyloidkörperchen, das zwei ganz kontrastierende Schichten zeigt (Toluidin). Fig. 19. Ganglienzelle aus der Oblongata, mit einem dicken Amyloidkörper (Toluidin). Fig. 20. Kleine Ganglienzelle aus der Oblongata, mit einem dicken Amyloidkörperchen zwischen dem Zellpigment (Toluidin). Lafora, G. R. (1911) Über das Vorkommen amyloider Körperchen im Innern der ganglienzellen; zugleich Ein beitrag zum Studium der amyloiden Substanz im Nervensystem. *Virchows Archiv. Path. Anat.* 205, 295–303 [Plate 6].

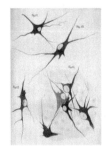

**FIGURE 211.**

Marcora, 1911. Histogenesis and the internal structure of neurons.

FIG. 12. Nervenzelle. Hühnerembryo am 12. Tag der Bebrütung. Cajalsche Meth. Ö1. imm. Comp. Oc. 8. Fig. 13. Nervenzelle. Hühnerembryo am 12. Tag der Bebrütung. Cajalsche Meth. Ö1. imm. 1/15. Comp. Oc.8. Fig. 14. Nervenzelle. Hühnerembryo am 15. Tag der Bebrütung. Cajalsche Meth. Ö1. imm. 1/15., Comp. Oc. 8. Fig. 15. Gruppe von Nervenzellen. Hühnerembryo am 12. Tag der Bebrütung. Cajalsche Meth. Ö1. imm. 1/15. Comp. Oc. 8. Marcora, F. (1911) Ueber die Histogenese des Zentralnervensystems mit besonderer Rücksicht auf die innere Struktur der Nervenelemente. *Folia Neurobiol.* 5, 928–960 [Figures 12–15].

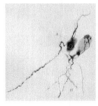

**FIGURE 212.**

Michailow, 1911. The regeneration of the neuron, I.

*A* = Zelle des IV. Typus, einer von deren Dendriten endet mit einem Endapparat auf der benachbarten Zelle. Pferd. Reichert 7a. Michailow, S. (1911) Die Regeneration des Neurons. Nervenzellen, Wachstumskugeln oder Nervenendapparate? *J. Psychol. Neurol.* 18, 247–273 [Figure 17].

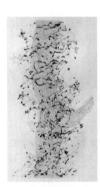

**FIGURE 213.**

Michailow, 1911. The regeneration of the neuron, II.

Nervenstämmchen, aus dem eine große Anzahl markloser Nervenfasern heraustritt und hierselbst bei dem Nervenstämmchen mit Keulen, Knöpfen und Platten endigen; *a* = komplizierter Apparat; derselbe ist auf Fig. II bei starker Vergrößerung abgebildet. Pferd. Leitz 3. Michailow, S. (1911) Die Regeneration des Neurons. Nervenzellen, Wachstumskugeln oder Nervenendapparate? *J. Psychol. Neurol.* 18, 247–273 [Figure 18].

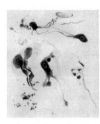

**FIGURE 214.**

Michailow, 1911. The regeneration of the neuron, III.

P = gelbes Pigment. Fig.9. Kleines Ganglion. *A* = Zelle des III. Typus: einer von ihren Dendriten *(d)* endigt bei der Zelle C mit einer Platte, wobei er sie zuerst umflicht; Nervenfortsatz *(n)* geht in den Achsenzylinder der markhaltigen Faser über. E = Kapsel der Zelle, die Pigment enthält und auf der drei Endknöpfe liegen. Pferd. Zeiß. Apochr. 4,0 mm. Apert. 0,95. Fig. 10. Ein Teil der Fig. 9. die mit E bezeichnet ist und mit Reicherts; Objektiv 186, homog. Immersion 1/12 abgebildet ist. Fig. 11. Nervenendapparat in Form einer komplizierten Platte. Ein Teil der Fig. 18. Pferd. Leitz 7. Fig. 12. Sympathische Zelle vom V. Typus. Ganglion stellatum. Pferd. Leitz. Ok.2, Obj. 3. Fig. 13. Plattenförmige Endigungen der marklosen und markhaltigen Nervenfaser an der Kapsel einer Nervenzelle. Ganglion coeliacum. Pferd. Leitz. Ok. 4, Obj. 7. Michailow, S. (1911) Die Regeneration des Neurons. Nervenzellen, Wachstumskugeln oder Nervenendapparate? *J. Psychol. Neurol.* 18, 247–273 [Figures 9–13].

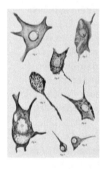

**FIGURE 215.**

Modena and Cavara, 1911. Cytological alterations in polyneuritis and poliomyelitis.

FIG.1. Zelle aus der Medulla lumbalis, anterolaterale Gruppe, des Menschen. Der Bau des Netzes nähert sich normalen Verhältnissen. Färbung nach Donaggio 3. Oc. 6. Obj. 1/15. Koristka. (Alle folgenden Abbildungen beziehen sich auf den beschriebenen Fall.) Fig.2. Zelle aus dem Vorderhorn der Medulla lumbalis. Durcheinanderwerfung und "Wirbel"bildung der Fibrillen. Oc. 6. Obj. 1/15 Koristka. Fig. 3. Zelle aus der vorderen inneren Gruppe der Medulla lumbalis. Bündelung der Fibrillen, die längs einer einzigen Zellachse verlaufen. Oc. 6. Obj. 1/15. Koristka. Fig.4. Zelle aus dem anterolateralen Abschnitt des Vorderhornes der Medulla cervicalis. Lücken und Rarefizierung des Netzes, Destruktion desperinuklearen Ringes (Cercine perinucleare). Oc. 6. Obj. 1/15 K. Fig. 5. Zelle aus der Cervikalregion, äussere Vordergruppe. Konglutination des Fibrillennetzes. Fig. 6.

Zelle aus der Lumbalregion, Vordergruppe. Beginnende Konglutination der langen Fibrillen. Fig.7. Atrophische Zelle aus der Vordergruppe des Vorderhorns der Medulla dorsalis (11. Segment). Oc.6. Obj. 1/15 K. Fig.8. Desgl. aus dem 11. Segment. In diesen beiden Zellen sieht man, wie ungeachtet der beträchtlichen Atrophie der Zellelemente noch ein deutliches Fibrillen-Netz vorhanden ist. Modena, G., and Cavara, V. (1911) Polyneuritis und Poliomyelitis. Klinisch-anatomische Studie. *Monatsschr. Psychiatr. Neurol.* 29, 129–146 [Figures 1–8].

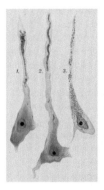

### FIGURE 216.

Simchowicz, 1911. Neuronal changes in senile dementia, I.

FIG. 1–4, 7–10 Scharlachrotfärbung nach Herxheimer, Fig. 5, 6, 11 bis 15 Methylblau-Eosinfärbung nach Alzheimer. Zeiss' homog. Immersion 2 mm, Apert. 1,30, Fig. 1, 2, 4, 7, 8 Okul. 8, die übrigen Okul. 4. FIG. 1, 2. Ganglienzellen aus dem Ammonshorn eines 22jährigen Pferdes. Die lipoiden Körnchen finden sich fast ausschließlich im Spitzenfortsatz in einer zusammenliegenden Reihe angehäuft. FIG. 3. Ganglienzelle aus dem Ammonshorn einer Dementia senilis. Die lipoiden Körnchen liegen im Zelleib und in der ganzen Ausdehnung des sichtbaren Spitzenfortsatzes. Simchowicz, T. (1911) Histologische studien über die senile Demenz. In *Histologische und histopathologische Arbeiten über die Grosshirnrinde*, eds. F. Nissl and A. Alzheimer, vol. 4, 267–444. Jena: Gustav Fischer [Plate 14, Figures 1–3].

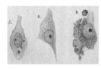

### FIGURE 217.

Simchowicz, 1911. Neuronal changes in senile dementia, II.

FIG. 1–4, 7–10 Scharlachrotfärbung nach Herxheimer, Fig. 5, 6, 11 bis 15 Methylblau-Eosinfärbung nach Alzheimer. Zeiss' homog. Immersion 2 rnm, Apert. 1,30, Fig. 1, 2, 4, 7, 8 Okul. 8, die übrigen Okul. 4. FIG. 4. Pyramidenzelle aus dem Ammonshorn einer Dementia senilis, von drei Trabantzellen umlagert. Es ist hier schwer zu entscheiden, ob die in der Nachbarschaft der basalen Gliazellen gelegenen lipoiden Körnchen zu der Ganglienzelle oder zu den Gliazellen gehören. FIGS. 5, 6. Zwei Ganglienzellen aus dem Ammonshorn einer Dementia senilis mit der grobkörnigen Degeneration. Im

Zelleib eine Reihe von Vakuolen, in denen große blaue Körner liegen (vgl. Tafel XII, Fig. 15; Tafel XVII, Fig. 5). Simchowicz, T. (1911) Histologische studien über die senile Demenz. In *Histologische und histopathologische Arbeiten über die Grosshirnrinde*, eds. F. Nissl and A. Alzheimer, vol. 4, 267–444. Jena: Gustav Fischer [Plate 14, Figures 4–6].

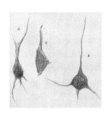

### FIGURE 218.

Simchowicz, 1911. Neuronal changes in senile dementia, III.

FIG. 5. Die Fibrillen sind fast nur noch in den Fortsätzen erhalten. Im Zellkörper zahlreiche argentophile Körner von verschiedener Größe, die größeren meistens in einer hellen Vakuole gelegen. FIG. 6. Die Fortsätze haben noch eine deutliche fibrilläre Struktur. Im eigenen Zelleib zeigen die noch erhaltenen Fibrillen eine ganz ungewöhnliche, vielfach verschlungene Anordnung. In den einzelnen Schlingen liegen zahlreiche argentophile Körnchen. FIG. 7. Eine Pyramide des ersten Blattes des Ammonshorns einer senilen Demenz, die aus Bündeln feiner entarteter Fibrillen besteht, welche noch die äußere Form der Ganglienzelle wiedergeben. Der Kern und das Plasma sind zugrunde gegangen. Simchowicz, T. (1911) Histologische Studien über die senile Demenz. In *Histologische und histopathologische Arbeiten über die Grosshirnrinde*, eds. F. Nissl and A. Alzheimer, vol. 4, 267–444. Jena: Gustav Fischer [Plate 17, Figures 5–7].

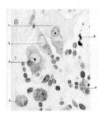

### FIGURE 219.

Von Hoesslin and Alzheimer, 1912. Seudosclerosis of Westphal-Strümpell (dentate nucleus).

Alle Figuren sind nach Präparaten, die nach Alkoholhärtung mit Toluidinblau gefärbt sind, mit Zeiß' homogener Immersion 1/13, Okular 6 gezeichnet. Fig. 4. Schnitt aus dem Nucleus dentatus des Kleinhirns. *a, b* Ganglienzellen; *c* eine diesen ähnliche Gliazelle, als solche besonders durch den 2. kleinen Kern erkennbar; *d* Anhäufung basophiler Körnchen; *e* mit grünlichen lipoiden Abbaustoffen beladene Gliazellen. Von Hoesslin, C., and Alzheimer, A. (1912) Ein Beitrag zur Klinik und pathologischen Anatomie der Westphal-Strümpellschen Pseudosklerose. *Zeitschr. ges. Neurol. Psych.* 8, 183–209 [Figure 4].

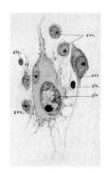

### FIGURE 220.

Von Hoesslin and Alzheimer, 1912. Seudosclerosis of Westphal-Strümpell (corpus striatum).

Alle Figuren sind nach Präparaten, die nach Alkoholhärtung mit Toluidinblau gefärbt sind, mit Zeiß' homogener Immersion 1/13, Okular 6 gezeihnet. Fig. 5. Schnitt aus dem Corpus striatum. *glz.* riesige Gliazelle mit 2 Kernen. *gaz.* größere Ganglienzelle; *gaz.1* kleinere Ganglienzellen; *glz.1* kleine Gliazellen. Von Hoesslin, C., and Alzheimer, A. (1912) Ein Beitrag zur Klinik und pathologischen Anatomie der Westphal-Strümpellschen Pseudosklerose. *Zeitschr. ges. Neurol. Psych.* 8, 183–209 [Figure 5].

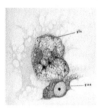

### FIGURE 221.

Von Hoesslin and Alzheimer, 1912. Seudosclerosis of Westphal-Strümpell (insular cortex).

Alle Figuren sind nach Präparaten, die nach Alkoholhärtung mit Toluidinblau gefärbt sind, mit Zeiß' homogener Immersion 1/13, Okular 6 gezeihnet. Fig. 1. Riesengliazelle (*glz*) einer Ganglienzelle (*gaz.*) anliegend. Aus der 3. Schichte der Inselrinde. Von Hoesslin, C., and Alzheimer, A. (1912) Ein Beitrag zur Klinik und pathologischen Anatomie der Westphal-Strümpellschen Pseudosklerose. *Zeitschr. ges. Neurol. Psych.* 8, 183–209 [Figure 1].

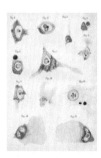

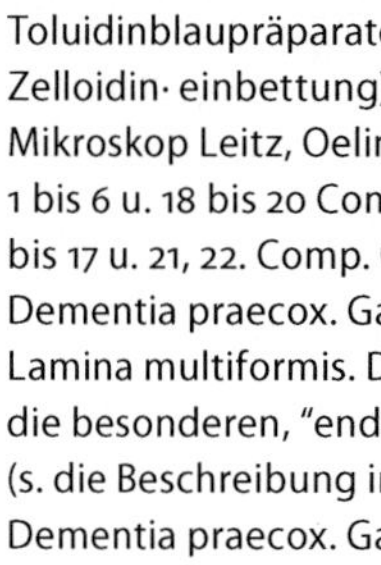

### FIGURE 222.

Bonfiglio, 1912. Alterations of ganglion cells.

Alle Abbildungen, ausser Abb. 17, die einem Unna-Pappenheimschen Präparat entnommen ist, stammen aus Toluidinblaupräparaten (Alkoholfixierung, Zelloidin· einbettung). Für alle Abbildungen Mikroskop Leitz, Oelimmersion 1/12. Fig. 1 bis 6 u. 18 bis 20 Compens. Ok. 6. Fig. 7 bis 17 u. 21, 22. Comp. Ok. 4. Fig. 1, 2, 3, 4. Dementia praecox. Ganglienzellen aus der Lamina multiformis. Die Kerne enthalten die besonderen, "endonukleären Ballen" (s. die Beschreibung im Text). Fig. 5, 6. Dementia praecox. Ganglienzellen aus der

Lamina multiformis. Die Kerne enthalten je zwei "endonukleäre Ballen." Fig. 7, 8. Angiosarkom. Ganglienzellen aus den Umgebungen des Tumors. Im Kern sieht man anstatt des normalen Kernkörperchens ein viel grösseres poligonal gestaltetes Gebilde und zwei kleine metachromatische Granula (s. Beschreibung im Text). Fig. 9, 10, 11, 12, 13, 14, 15, 16, 17. Angiosarkom. Stark gewucherte Gliazellen aus den Umgebungen des Tumors. Man beachte die starke Vergrösserung der Protoplasmaleiber; kleine regressiv veränderte Kerne sind in Vakuolen des Protoplasmaleibes bei Fig. 9, 14 enthalten. Im Kerne aller dieser Gliazellen liegen besondere, rundliche oder unregelmässige, metachromatisch gefärbte, zum Teil mit einer blauen Membran versehene Gebilde, die bis 2/3 der Kerngrösse erreichen (siehe die nähere Beschreibung im Text). Fig. 18, 19, 20. Angiosarkom. Stark gewucherte Gliazellen. Man beachte die ausserordentliche starke Vermehrung der metachromatischen Bestandteile des Kernes. Fig. 21, 22. Angiosarkom. Stark gewucherte Gliazellen. Die metachromatischen Granula des Kernes sind in einem Häufchen stark zusammengedrückt (Nähere Beschreibung im Text). Bonfiglio, F. (1912) Ueber besondere Veränderungen der Ganglienund Gliazellenkerne. *Folia Neurobiol.* 6, 442–451 [Figures 1–8, 16, 18, 19, 21].

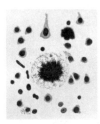

**FIGURE 223.**

Fischer, 1912. Senile plaques, I.

Sphaerotichiebildungen gefärbt mit Carbol-Methylenblau-Methylenviolett. Fig. 1. Alkoholfixierung und Celloidineinbettung. Fischer, O. (1912) Ein weiterer Beitrag zur Klinik und Pathologie der presbyophrenen Demenz. *Z. gesamte Neurol. Psychiatr.* 12, 99–134 [Figure 1].

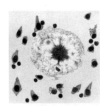

**FIGURE 224.**

Fischer, 1912. Senile plaques, II.

Sphaerotichiebildungen gefärbt mit Carbol-Methylenblau-Methylenviolett. Fig. 2. Formolfixierung und Paraffineinbettung. Fischer, O. (1912) Ein weiterer Beitrag zur Klinik und Pathologie der presbyophrenen Demenz. *Z. gesamte Neurol. Psychiatr.* 12, 99–134 [Figure 2].

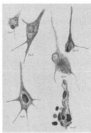

**FIGURE 225.**

Krause, 1912. Histopathology of encephalic cystocercosis, I.

FIG. 17. Kleine pyramidenförmige Zelle, in der Schicht der Riesenpyramiden (1. v. C. W.) belegen (cysticerkenfreie Gegend). Der Zelleib ist kollabiert und von kleinen Vakuolen durchsetzt, die Fortsätze sind atrophisch und im Schwinden begriffen. Thioninfärbung. *Zeiß* Oc. IV, I/12 Immersion (Fall 1). Sämtliche nachfolgenden nach *Bielschowsky* gefärbten Zellen stammen aus cysticerkenfreien Rindenstücken. Fig.18. Zelle aus der 3. Schicht (Lamina pyramidalis Br.) der r. 2. St. W. Die Fibrillen im Zelleib sind zerfallen, die Körnchen sind größtenteils geschwunden. Im Zelleib ist ein protoplasmatisches Netz mit verdickten Knotenpunkten sichtbar, in dessen Maschen z. T. gelblich tingierte Körnchen liegen. Aufhellung in der Umgebung des Kerns. Die Fibrillen in den Fortsätzen sind erhalten. *Leitz,* Oc. IV, I/12 Oel-Immersion (Fall 1). Fig.19. Mittelgroße Pyramide aus der 5. Schicht der r. h. C. W. Die Zelle ist leicht aufgeschwollen, der Kern ist randständig, das Kernkörperchen geschwunden. Im Zellkörper ist keine Spur von Fibrillen mehr vorhanden. Der Zellkörper ist angefüllt von größeren und kleineren lipoiden Kugeln, die ungeordnet zusammengehäuft liegen. Die Fortsätze sind atrophisch, ihre Fibrillen sind z. T. verschwunden. *Leitz* Oc. IV, 1/12 Oel-Immersion (Fall 1). Fig. 20. Kleine pyramidenförmige Zelle aus der 3. Schicht der e. 3. St. W. Die Zelle erscheint etwas geschrumpft, die Fibrillen im Zelleib sind zerfallen, der Zelleib zeigt Andeutung eines wabigen Baus. Die Fibrillen des Spitzenfortsatzes sind verdickt und verklumpt. Der Kern ist dunkel. Der basale Fortsatz ist atrophisch und verläuft geschlängelt. *Leitz* Oc. IV, I/12 Oel-Immersion (Fall 1). Fig. 21. Multipolare Ganglienzelle aus der 3. Schicht der. 1. St. W. Körniger Zerfall der Fibrillen in Zelleib und Fortsätzen. Andeutung eines Retikulums im Zellplasma. Kern sehr deutlich begrenzt, dunkel gefärbt. In seiner Peripherie ist der Zerfall der Fibrillen und die Aufhellung des Plasmas am weitesten vorgeschritten. *Leitz* Oc. IV, 1/12 Oel-Immersion (Fall 1). Fig.22. Zelle aus der 3. Schicht der r. h. C. W. Die Zelle befindet sich in vollem Zerfall. Der Kern ist verschwunden, die Fortsätze sind verschwunden. In den zerfallenden Zellkörper dringen zahlreiche Gliazellen ein. (Neuronophagie.) *Leitz* Oc. IV, I/12 Oel-Immersion. (Fall 1). Krause, K. (1912) Zur Histopathologie der Gehirncysticerkose.

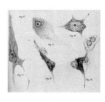

*Monatsschr. Psychiatr. Neurol.* 31, 429–462; 513–545 [Figures 17–22].

**FIGURE 226.**

Krause, 1912. Histopathology of encephalic cystocercosis, II.

FIG. 9. Uebergang einer Cysticerkenkapsel auf die Hirnrinde, deren 1. und 2. Schicht bereits verschwunden ist. In der Randschicht der Kapsel spindelförmige Zellen *mit* metachromatisch gefärbtem Leib, die wohl als komprimierte Plasmazellen aufzufassen sind, weiter nach außen liegen Bindegewebszellen. Zwischen der Kapselgrenze und den Ganglienzellen liegen einige Gliazellen. Der Leib der Ganglienzellen ist mit z. T. gelblich tingierten hellen Körnchen angefüllt, die in den Maschen eines plasmatischen Netzes liegen, das bei einer Anzahl von Zellen bereits zerfallen ist. Neben diesem Wabenwerk sind an einer Zelle noch verklumpte Massen färbbarer Substanz zu sehen, die andern Zellen enthalten nur noch einzelne Körnchen färbbarer Substanz. Toluidinfärbung. *Zeiß,* Oc. II,1/12 Immersion (Fall 1). Fig. 13. Unipolare Ganglienzelle 1. v. C. W., 3. Schicht, cysticerkenfreie Partie. unterhalb der pachymeningitischen Membran gelegen. Anschwellung der Zelle und ihres Fortsatzes. Kern an die Peripherie gerückt, eckig. Die färbbare Substanz ist in feine Stäubchen zerfallen, ein feines Netzwerk ist in dem Zellkörper sichtbar. Spitzenfortsatz hellhomogen. {Akute Veränderung kombiniert mit chronischer.) Toluidinblaufärbung. *Leitz* Oc. IV, Oel-Immersion 1/12 (Fall 2). Fig. 14. Mittelgroße sternförmige Zelle aus der 3. Schicht der 1. 1. St. W. (cysticerkenfreie Gegend). Diffuser Zerfall der färbbaren Substanz in Körnchen, zwischen diesen helle Flecken mit Andeutung eines Reticulums. Die Zellmembran ist größtenteils verschwunden, der Kern erscheint dadurch gebläht. Die Fortsätze sind stark abgeblaßt und im Schwinden. Thioninfärbung. *Zeiß* Oc. IV, 1/12 Immersion (Fall I). Fig. 15. Kleine pyramidenförmige Zelle aus der' 2. (äußeren Körner-) Schicht der 1. v. C. W. Cysticerkenfreie Gegend. Die Zelle ist geschrumpft, die nicht färbbare Substanz ist größtenteils gefärbt, die färbbare Substanz atrophisch. Der Kern ist dunkel gefärbt. Im Zelleib tritt Wabenbildung hervor. Thioninfärbung. *Zeiß* Oc. IV, I/12 Immersion (Fall 1). Fig. 16. Sklerotische, in ganz ähnlicher Weise wie die Zelle der Fig. 15 veränderte Zelle aus der 4. (inneren Körner-) Schicht der 1. v. C. W. (cysticerkenfreie Gegend) mit andrängenden Gliazellen. Thioninfärbung. *Zeiß* Oc. IV, 1/12 Immersion (Fall I). Krause, K. (1912) Zur Histopathologie der Gehirncysticerkose.

*Monatsschr. Psychiatr. Neurol.* 31, 429–462; 513–545 [Figures 9, 13–16].

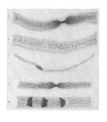

**FIGURE 227.**

Maccabruni, 1912. Fine structure of the nerve fibers, I.

FIG. 5–6 = Nervenfaser des Ischiadicus eines Hundes, behandelt mit: Natriumphosphit (18 Stunden), Silbernitrat, Hydrochinon, plus Natriumsulfit; Zerzupfung in Glyzerin. Im Niveau des Achsenzylinders bemerkt man die fadenartig ausgezogenen Stäbchen. Fig. 7 = Zarte makhaltige Nervenfaser des Ischiadicus eines Hundes, wie oben behandelt. Die Stäbchen sind kurz. Fig. 8 = Nervenfaser des Ischiadicus vom Frosch - Behandlung mit Kalium- phosphit (20 Stunden im Bruthafen). Silbernitrat, Hydrochinon plus Natriumsulfit; Zerzupfung in Glyzerin. Die Stäbchen bleiben von einander unabhängig, selbst im Niveau der Ranvierschen Einschnürungen. Fig. 9 = Nervenfasern des Ischiadicus vom Frosch, behandelt mit: Kaliumtelurit (12 Stunden), Silbernitrat, Hydrochinon plus Natriumsulfit; Zerzupfung in Glyzerin. Maccabruni, F. (1912) Zur feineren Struktur der Nervenfasern. *Folia Neurobiol.* 6, 17–23 [Figures 5–9].

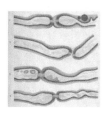

**FIGURE 228.**

Maccabruni, 1912. Fine structure of the nerve fibers, II.

FIG. 1-2-3. Markhaltige Nervenfaser der Cauda equina vom Kaninchen, nach der von Veratti modifizierten Golgischen Methode behandelt. Die periaxialen Spiralen sind im Niveau der Ranvierschen Einschnürungen unterbrochen. Fig. 4. Nervenfaser der Cauda equina eines Kaninchens behandelt wie oben. Die periaxiale Spirale erweist sich als eine kontinuierliche, insofern als sie den Achsenzylinder auch im Niveau der Einschnürung begleitet. Maccabruni, F. (1912) Zur feineren Struktur der Nervenfasern. *Folia Neurobiol.* 6, 17–23 [Figures 1–4].

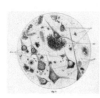

**FIGURE 229.**

Marinesco and Minea, 1912. Senile plaques, I.

Die Fig. 1–14 stammen von dem ersten, 15–30 von dem zweiten Falle. Fig.1. Aus einem Präparate nach der modifizierten Cajalschen Methode. Elektive Imprägnierung der in den senilen Plaques abgelagerten Substanz. I.F. isolierte Fädchen; St. Sternchenbildungen; E. P. erwachsene Plaques; M.st. morgensternähnliche Bildungen *Fischers.* Marinesco, G., and Minea, J. (1912). Untersuchungen über die "senilen Plaques." *Monatsschr. Psychiatr. Neurol.* 31, 79–133. [Figure 1].

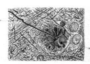

**FIGURE 230.**

Marinesco and Minea, 1912. Senile plaques, II.

Die Fig. 1–14 stammen von dem ersten, 15–30 von dem zweiten Falle. Fig. 6. Dasselbe Verfahren. Man sieht hier verschiedene Endformationen der Nervenfasern, die an der Peripherie der Plaque radiär gestellt sind. K. Kern der Einlagerung. Marinesco, G., and Minea, J. (1912). Untersuchungen über die "senilen Plaques." *Monatsschr. Psychiatr. Neurol.* 31, 79–133 [Figure 6].

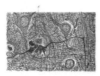

**FIGURE 231.**

Marinesco and Minea, 1912. Senile plaques, III.

Die Fig. 1–14 stammen von dem ersten, 15-30 von dem zweiten Falle. Fig. 7. Aus einem mit Aether vorbehandelten Bielschowskypräparat. Man sieht den Ursprung einer durch die Plaque unterbrochenen Faser. Die eingelagerte Substanz ist größtenteils aufgelöst, nur ein blasser Kern ist noch sichtbar (K). Marinesco, G., and Minea, J. (1912). Untersuchungen über die "senilen Plaques." *Monatsschr. Psychiatr. Neurol.* 31, 79–133 [Figure 7].

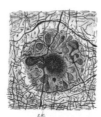

**FIGURE 232.**

Marinesco and Minea, 1912. Senile plaques, IV.

Die Fig. 1–14 stammen von dem ersten, 15–30 von dem zweiten Falle. Fig. 9. Mit Aceton behandelter Schnitt. Z. k. stark imprägniertes,von zahlreichen nervösen Endanschwellungen umgebenes Zentralkörperchen mit radiär gestreifter Peripherie. Marinesco, G., and Minea, J. (1912). Untersuchungen über die "senilen Plaques." *Monatsschr. Psychiatr. Neurol.* 31, 79–133 [Figure 9].

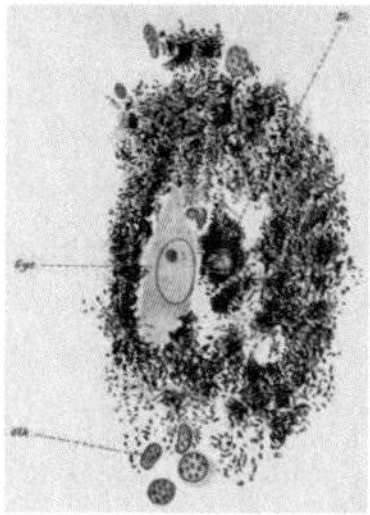

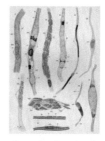

**FIGURE 233.**

Marinesco and Minea, 1912. Senile plaques, V.

Die Fig. 1–14 stammen von dem ersten, 15–30 von dem zweiten Falle. Fig. 13. Ganglienzelle, die gänzlich innerhalb einer Plaque liegt (Ggz). Zk. Zentralkörperchen; Glk. Gliakerne. Nach einem mit Thionin gefärbten *Cajalschen* Formolpräparate. Marinesco, G., and Minea, J. (1912). Untersuchungen über die "senilen Plaques." *Monatsschr. Psychiatr. Neurol.* 31, 79–133 [Figure 13].

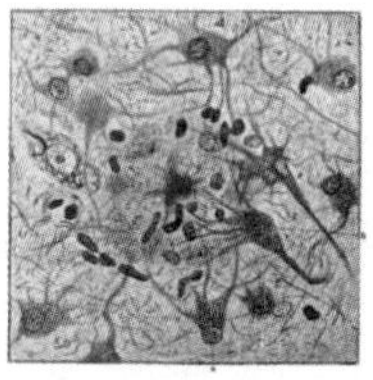

**FIGURE 234.**

Marinesco and Minea, 1912. Senile plaques, VI.

Die Fig. 1–14 stammen von dem ersten, 15–30 von dem zweiten Falle. Fig. 15. Plasmareiche Gliazellenwucherung um eine alte Plaque. Die meisten Fortsätze durchziehen die Plaque. Die mit a und b bezeichneten Körperchen sind besonders bemerkenswert. Marinesco, G., and Minea, J. (1912). Untersuchungen über die "senilen Plaques." *Monatsschr. Psychiatr. Neurol.* 31, 79–133 [Figure 15].

**FIGURE 235.**

Rachmanow, 1912. Structure of peripheral nerve fibers, I.

FIG. I, Fall 17. N. Radialis. Längsschnitt. Eine Markfaser. Färbung nach Mann. *ax* = Achsen-zylinder. *vk* = Vakuole. *pl* = Plasma der Schwannschen Zelle. Fig. 2, Fall 17. N. Radialis. Längsschnitt. Eine Markfaser. Färbung nach Mann. *ax* = Achsenzylinder. *plh* = stark entwickelter perinucleärer Plasmahof. Fig. 3, Fall I. N. Peroneus. Längsschnitt. Eine Markfaser. Färbung nach Unna. *pl* = zartes Plasmareticulum. Der blattförmige Kern der Schwannschen Zelle liegt der Faser dicht an. Fig. 4, Fall I. N. Peroneus. Zupfpräparat. Eine Markfaser. Färbung nach Unna. Bezeichnungen wie auf Fig. 3. Fig. 5, 6, 7 und 8. Verschiedene Stadien der mitotischen Teilung des Kerns der Schwannschen Zelle. Fig. 5. Fall 10. N. Peroneus. Zupfpräparat. Eine Markfaser.

Färbung nach Unna. *k* = ruhender Kern der Schwannschen Zelle. K¹ = eben geteilter Kern der Schwannschen Zelle. *plh* = Perinucleärer Plasmahof. π = π -Granula. Fig. 6, Fall 12. N. Femoralis. Längsschnitt. Färbung nach Unna. Eine Markfaser. *k* = Mitose des Schwannschen Kerns. *pl* = Plasmareticulum. Fig. 7, Fall 14. N. Peroneus. Längsschnitt. Eine Markfaser. Thionin. Kanadabalsam. *k* = Mitose des Schwannschen Kerns. *pl* = Plasmareticulum. Fig. 8. Fall 10. N. Peroneus. Zupfpräparat. Färbung nach Unna. Kanadabalsam. Eine Mark-faser. Bezeichnungen wie auf Fig. 7. Fig. 9, Fall 17. N. Femoralis. Längsschnitt. Färbung nach Unna. Markfaser mit zwei Kernen, die grobe Chromatinpartikelchen enthalten. Fig. 10, Fall 23. N. Plantaris. Zupfpräparat. Sudan-Hämatox. Eine Bandfaser ohne Einlagerungen. Fig. 11, Fall 23. N. Femoralis. Längsschnitt. Thionin. Kanadabalsam. Eine dicke Markfaser. *ms* = Markscheide. *Rs* = Ranvierscher Schnürring. *msz* = zwei anliegende Mesodermazellen. *x* = Gebilde, die innerhalb der Faser liegen. Fig. 12, Fall 23. N. Femoralis. Zupfpräparat. Thionin. Kanadabalsam. Sehr dünne markhaltige Faser. π = π -Granula. Fig. 13, Fall 3. N. Peroneus. Zupfpräparat. Thionin. Kanadabalsam. Markhaltige Faser. *plh* π = Schwach entwickelter perinucleärer Plasmahof mit spärlichen π -granula. *ms* = Markscheide. Fig. 14, Fall 24. N. Peroneus. Zupfpräparat. Thionin. Kanadabalsam. Dicke markhaltige Faser. *Elz* = Elzholsches Körperchen. π = π -granula, die im perinucle-ären Plasmahof liegen; bei *a* eine Anhäufung von π -granula, die eine Einkerbung im Kern bildet. π¹ = π -granula, die in größerer Entfernung vom Kern liegen. *ms* = Markscheide. Fig. 15. Fall 17. N. Peroneus. Zupfpräparat. Sudan. Thionin. Glycerin. Faser mit zwei Kernen. π = π -granula. *mb* = Markballen. Fig. 16. Fall 17. N. Femoralis. Zupfpräparat. Thionin. Glycerin. *k* = zwei Schwannsche Kerne. k¹ = Pyknotischer Kern. *pl* = Plasma mit Einlagerungen. π = π -granula. *mb* = Markballen. Fig. 17. Fall 17. N. Femoralis. Zupfpräparat. Sudan-Thionin. Glycerin. Faser mit 2 Kernen und einer großen Menge von Abbauprodukten. *mb* = Markballen. π = π -granula. Fig. 18, Fall 17. N. Peroneus. Längsschnitt. Thionin. Kanadabalsam. Faser in Wallerscher Degeneration. *k* = Schwannscher Kern. π = π -granula. *vk* = Vakuolen. k¹ = Dunkel gefärbter Kern. Fig. 19, Fall 23. N. Plantaris. Zupfpräparat. Sudan-Hämatoxylin. Glycerin. Bandfasern. *k* = Kerne. *mb* = Markballen. Fig. 20, Fall 24. N. Plantaris. Zupfpräparat. Sudan-Thionin. Bandfaser. *mr* = in der Einbuchtung des Kerns liegende Markreste. Fig. 21, Fall 17. N. Femoralis. Zupfpräparat. Thionin. Glycerin.

Faser mit ovoider Auftreibung. Fig. 22, Fall 9. N. Plantaris. Zupfpräparat. Sudan-Thionin. Dünne markhaltige Faser. *ms* = Markscheide. *mb* = Markballen. Fig. 23, Fall 19. N. Plantaris. Längsschnitt. Thionin. Kanadabalsam. Anhäufung von Endoneuralzellen in der Nähe einer Kapillare. *mstz* = Mastzellen. *krz* = Zellen mit π -granula. *mdz* = Mesodermalzellen. Fig. 24, Fall 17. N. Femoralis. Zupfpräparat. Sudan-Thionin. Dünne markhaltige Faser. *plh* = stark entwickelter perinucleärer Plasmahof. *pl* = Plasmaanhäufung. π – π - granula. *ms* = Markscheide. Fig. 25, Fall 17. N. Peroneus. Längsschnitt. Thionin. Kanadabalsam. *mb* = Markballen. Fig. 26, Fall 20. N. Plantaris. Längsschnitt. Scharlach. Bandfasel-R. *mb* = Markballen. Fig. 27, Fall 7. N. Femoralis. Längsschnitt. Marchi. Mastzelle. *f* = schwarz gefärbte Lipoidtröpfchen; Körnelung durch Safranin rot gefärbt. Fig. 28, Fall 7. N. Plantaris. Längsschnitt. Marchi. Idem. Fig. 29, Fall 7. N. Plantaris. Längsschnitt. Thionin. Kanadabalsam. Mastzelle. *vk* = Vakuolen, die negative Bilder von Lipoidtröpfchen darstellen. Fig. 30, Fall 7. N. Femoralis. Längsschnitt. Thionin. Kanadabalsam. Mastzelle.   Rachmanow, A. (1912) Zur normalen und pathologischen Histologie der peripheren Nerven des Menschen. *J. Psychol. Neurol.* 18, 522–545 [Plate 49].

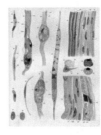

**FIGURE 236.**
Rachmanow, 1912. Structure of peripheral nerve fibers, II.

FIG. 31, Fall 5. N. Plantaris. Zupfpräparat. Sudan. Hämatoxylin. Dicke markhaltige Faser mit schwach angedeuteter wabiger Struktur. *plh* = Perinucleärer Plasmahof mit π - granula. Fig. 32, Fall 4. N. Peroneus. Zupfpräparat. Sudan-Hämatoxylin. Markhaltige Faser. Die Markscheide sieht homagen aus. *Schk* = Dicht an der Markscheide liegen-der Kern der Schwannschen Zelle. Fig. 33, Fall 5. N. Plantaris. Zupfpräparat. Sudan-Hämatoxylin. Dünne markhaltige Faser mit gut ausgeprägtem perinucleären Plasmahof = *plh*. Fig. 34, Fall 21. N. Peroneus. Längsschnitt. Sudan-Hämatoxylin. Dicke markhaltige Faser, welche ein rundes diffus mit Hämatoxylin gefärbtes Gebilde enthält. Fig. 35, Fall 21. N. Plantaris. Zupfpräparat. Sudan-Hämatoxylin. Dicke markhaltige Faser, deren Kern in einem gut entwickelten perinucleären Plasmahof liegt. π. = π -grallula. *pl* = Deutlich ausgeprägte Plasmaschicht, die stellenweise Anhäufungen bildet. *ax* = Achsenzylinder. *mb* = Markballen. Fig. 36, Fall

15. N. Plantaris. Zupfpräparat. Sudan-Thionin. Dicke markhaltige Faser. *Rs* = Ranvierscher Schnürring. *k* = Kerne von mesodermalen Zellen. *Elz* = Elzholzsches Körperchen. Fig. 37, Fall 19. N. Peroneus. Zupfpräparat. Sudan-Hämatoxylin. *Rs* = Ranvierscher Schnürring. *Schk* = Schwannscher Kern. *pl* = Plasma der Schwannschen Zelle. *mdz* = Mesodermalzellen. Fig. 38, Fall 15. N. Plantaris. Längsschnitt. Sudan-Hämatoxylin. *mb* = Markballen. Fig. 39, Fall 23. N. Femoralis. Zupfpräparat. Sudan-Hämatoxylim. Dicke markhaltige Faser, dicht daneben lieg-ende Bandfasern = *bf;* einige der letzteren Lipoidtropfen -*f*- enthaltend. Fig. 40, Fall 3. N. Peroneus. Längsschnitt. Sudan-Hämatoxylin. Bandfaser. *mb* = Markballen *k* = Kerne. Fig. 41, Fall 22. N. Peroneus. Zupfpräparat. Sudan-Hämatoxylin. Dünne markhaltige Faser, deren Kern in einem deutlich ausgeprägten perinucleären Plasmahof *(plh)* liegt, in welchem π -granula und Lipoidtröpfchen *(f)* abgelagert sind. Fig. 42, Fall 7. N. Plantaris. Längsschnitt. Sudan-Hämatoxylin. Dicke markhaltige Faser. *ax* = Achsenzylinder. *plh* = Perinucleärer Plasmahof mit Lipoidtropfen *(f)* einige von diesen sind halbmondförmig. Fig. 43, Fall 2. N. Peroneus. Längsschnitt. Sudan-Hämatoxylin. Mastzellen mit rot gefärbten Lipoidtröpfchen. Fig. 44. Fall 7. N. Femoralis. Längsschnitt. Sudan-Hämatoxylin. Mastzelle. *f* = Lipoidtropfen. Fig. 45, Fall 7. N. Plantaris. Längsschnitt. Sudan-Hämatoxylin. Idem. Fig. 46, Fall 9. N. Suralis. Zupfpräparat. Sudan-Hämatoxylin. *Schk* = Schwannscher Kern. *plh* = Perinucleärer Plasmahof. *k* = Körnchenzellen. *ms* = Markscheide. *mb* = Markballen. *f* = Lipoidtröpfchen. Fig. 47. Fall 23. N. Plantaris. Zupfpräparat. Sudan-Hämatoxylin. Bandfaser. *f*= Lipoidtröpfchen. Fig. 48, Fall 9. N. Suralis. Zupfpräparat. Sudan-Hämatoxylin. Faser mit ovoider Auftreibung. *pl* = Plasma. *f* = Lipoidtröpfchen. *mr* = Markreste. Fig. 49, Fall 9. N. Plantaris. Zupfpräparat. Sudan-Hämatoxylin. *mb* undms = Markballen. *k* = Durch Markballen deformierter Kern. *f* = Lipoidtröpfchen. Fig. 50, Fall 17. N. Femoralis. Längsschnitt. Sudan-Hämatoxylin. Faser mit Markballen *(mb)* und Lipoidtröpfchen *(f)*. Im Plasma *(plπ)* blau gefärbte π-granula. Die Kernmenbran ist gefältelt. Fig. 51, Fall 22. N. Plantaris. Längsschnitt. Sudan-Hämaloxylin. *pn* = Perineurium. *nf* = markhaltige Fasern. *bf* = Bandfasern. *f*= Lipoidtröpfchen. Fig. 52, Fall 24. N. Cutaneus brachii. Längsschnitt. Sudan-Hämatoxylin. *erz* = rote Blutkörperchen. *krz* = Zelle mit π-granula und Lipoid. Fig. 53, Fall 25. N. Plantaris. Längsschnitt. Sudan-Hämatoxylin. Körnchenzelle. *f* = Lipoidtröpfchen. Fig. 54, Fall 25. N. Plantaris. Längsschnitt. Thionin. Kanadabalsam. Gitterzelle. *vk* = Vakuolen.

Fig. 55. Fall 9. N. Plantaris. Längsschnitt. Sudan-Hämatoxylin. Teil eines stark veränderten Nerven. *nf* = dünne markhaltige Faser. *bnf* = Faser in Wallerscher Degeneration. *bf* = Bandfaser. *blf* = ovoide Auftreibung. *f* = Lipoidtröpfchen. *mdz* = mit Lipoidtröpfchen vollgepfropfte Mesodermalzelle. *mb* = Markballen. Rachmanow, A. (1912) Zur normalen und pathologischen Histologie der peripheren Nerven des Menschen. *J. Psychol. Neurol.* 18, 522–545 [Plate 50].

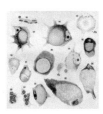

### FIGURE 237.

Rezza, 1912. Pellagra and histopathology of the nervous system, I.

Alle Figuren wurden mit dem Abbeschen Apparat gezeichnet. Mikroskop Leitz. Obj. 1/12 homog. Imm. Tubus 160. Ok. 4 comp. Die Figuren 1–5, 7–8, 13–14, 19–20, 33–34 Nisslsche Methode, Färbung mit Ludwigshafener Toluidinblau. Die Figuren 6,11–12,21–23,35–36 Herxheimersche Methode. Die Fig. 9–10, 17–18 Alzheimersche Methode IX. Die Fig.15-16 Unna- Pappenheimsche Methode. Die Fig. 24–25, 37–46 Alzheimersche Methode IV. Fig. 10. Längs der Gefäßwand, fast in einer Reibe, große Tropfen, in deren Mitte man etwas wie eine kleine helle Vakuole sieht (id. id.). Fig. 13. Große Pyramidenzelle. (Rolandosche Zone.) Der Kern ist an die Basis eines der Fortsätze gedrängt und wie ein Dreieck geformt. Das Pigment ist an die Peripherie der Zelle verlagert. Fig. 14. Betzsche Zelle (ansteigende frontale Windung). Dieselben Veränderungen wie bei der vorigen Zelle. In dem sehr vergrößerten Kernkörperchen sieht man zahlreiche Vakuolen. Fig. 15. Zelle der Vorderhörner des dorsalen Markes. Keine Spur von einem Kernkörperchen. In der hellen zentralen Zone bemerkt man eine feingranulöse Struktur. pg = Pigment. Fig. 16. Große Pyramidenzelle. (Rolandosche Zone.) Vakuolen im Kernkörperchen. Das Pigment (pg) ist in einer Art von Tasche enthalten, die sich aus der Zellwand vorstülpt. Fig. 17. Zelle aus dem Vorderhorn des Halsmarks. In dem geschwollenen Teile der Zellen liegen zahlreiche lipoide Granulationen. Fig. 18. Große Pyramidenzelle (Occipitalhirn). Die lipoiden Granulationen nehmen die ganze geschwollene zentrale Zone ein. Fig. 19. und 20. Elemente der Schicht der polymorphen Zellen (Frontalhim). Schwere chronische Veränderungen der Nervenzellen. An sie lehnen sich zahlreiche Gliazellen an, von denen einige Nisslsche Gliarasen bilden. Fig. 21. Große Pyramidenzelle (Rolandosche Zone). An der Peripherie der Zelle sieht

man spärliche Fetttropfen. Fig. 22. Zelle aus dem Vorderhorn des Halsmarks. Die helle zentrale Zone ist wie von einem aus Fetttropfen gebildeten Ring umgeben. Im übrigen Protoplasma unterscheidet man vom Hämatoxilin intensiver gefärbte Massen. Fig. 23. Zelle aus dem Vorderhorn des Lendenmarks. In der zu einem großen Teil von den Fetttröpfchen umgebenen zentralen Zone ist eine fein granuläre Struktur mit mehr oder minder großen Vakuolen deutlich zu erkennen. In dem übrigen Teil des Protoplasmas sind die vom Hämatoxilin gefärbten Massen augenfälliger. Auch im peripher gelegenen Kern sieht man intensiv gefärbte Körnchen. Im Kernkörperchen zahlreiche Vakuolen. Fig. 24. Zelle aus dem Vorderhorn des dorsalen Markes. In der degenerierten zentralen Zone ist eine vakuoläre, granuläre Struktur sichtbar. So weit die Struktur alveolar ist, befindet sich in den Alveolen ein gelber Inhalt (Fett). Rezza, A. (1912) Beitrag zur pathologischen Anatomie der Pellagrapsychosen. *Z. Gesamte Neurol. Psychiatr.* 12, 31–98 [Figures 10, 13–24].

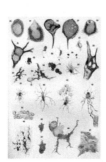

### FIGURE 238.

Rezza, 1912. Pellagra and histopathology of the nervous system, II.

Alle Figuren wurden mit dem Abbeschen Apparat gezeichnet. Mikroskop Leitz. Obj. 1/12 homog. Imm. Tubus 160. Ok. 4 comp. Die Figuren 1–5, 7–8, 13–14, 19–20, 33–34 Nisslsche Methode, Färbung mit Ludwigshafener Toluidinblau. Die Figuren 6, 11-12, 21–23, 35–36 Herxheimersche Methode. Die Fig. 24–25, 37–46 Alzheimersche Methode IV. Die Fig. 26–27 Alzheimersche Methode III. Die Fig. 28–32 Bielschowskysche Methode. Die Fig. 48–50 Alzheimersche Methode V. Fig. 26. Zelle aus dem Vorderhorn des Halsmarks. Die zentrale Zone fein granulär und wie von einem Ring von blau gefärbten, deutlich unterschiedenen Granulationen umgeben. (Färbung mit 1 proz. wässeriger Lösung von Toluidinblau Ludwigshafen.) Fig. 27. Wie bei der vorigen Figur. (Färbung mit May - Grünwaldscher Farblösung.) Fig. 28. Große Pyramidenzelle (Frontalhirn). In der zentralen Zone zahlreiche sehr feine schwarze Granulationen. Das spärliche Pigment ist nur enthalten in der kleinen peripheren Zone mit großmaschigem Netz. Fig. 29. Zelle aus dem Vorderhorn des dorsalen Marks. In der zentralen Zone ist die vakuoläre, granuläre Struktur sehr augenfällig. An der Peripherie

der Zelle sind die Fibrillen zerbröckelt, verflochten. Im schmalen hellen Rand rechts ist das spärliche Pigment enthalten. Fig. 30. Zelle aus dem Vorderhorn des Halsmarks. Der Kern ist noch gut erkennbar. In der zentralen Zone vakuoläre Struktur. Seitwärts auf beiden Seiten ein dichtes Geflecht von zerbröckelten Fibrillen; jenseits von ihnen die gewöhnliche alveoläre Struktur, in der das Fett enthalten ist. Fig. 31. Große Pyramidenzelle (Frontalhirn). Am Rand der Zelle sind noch die aus den Fortsätzen kommenden langen Fibrillen zu verfolgen. In der zentralen Zone ist keine Struktur erkennbar. Fig. 32. Betzsche Zelle (ansteigende frontale Windung). In der zentralen Zone vakuoläre Struktur in Form sehr großer farbloser Vakuolen. Auch der zentrale Teil eines der Fortsätze, der wie angeschwollen aussieht, erscheint farblos. Fig. 33. a, b, Glia-Stäbchenzelle. (Schicht der großen Pyramidenzellen. Frontalhirn.) Fig. 34. a, b, Degenerierte, pyknotische Gliakerne. (id. id.) Fig. 35. Gliazelle mit zahlreichen, in Form einer Traube angeordneten Fetttropfen. (Schicht der polymorphen Zellen. Rolandosche Zone.) Fig. 36. Gliakerne mit großen Fetttropfen, an deren Rand man viel intensiver gefärbte kleinere Tröpfchen sieht. Die drei Kerne des oberen Teiles der Figur sind in einen einzigen Protoplasmasaum eingeschlossen (op) und stellen vielleicht einen Gliarasen dar. Fig. 37 und 38. Amöboide Gliazellen (weiße Substanz des Frontalhirns). Fig. 39 und 40. Amöboide Gliazellen (Ränder der Vorderhörner des dorsalen Marks). Das Protoplasma dieser Elemente besteht aus sehr dichten, intensiv vom Hämatoxilin gefärbten Körnchen. In ihm sieht man kleine Vakuolen mit gelbem Inhalt und eine größere leere Vakuole, die den Kern (n) darstellt - (vs) transversal geschnittenes Blutgefäß, an welchem einer der Fortsätze inseriert. Fig.41.Astrocyt (weiße Substanz der Rolandoschen Zone). In den zahlreichen Fortsätzen Knoten und Schleifer. Kleine Vakuolen im Kern, größere im Protoplasma mit gelblichem Inhalt. Zwischen den Fortsätzen zahlreiche runde Zellen. Fig. 42. Glia-Stäbchenzelle (weiße Substanz des Occipitalhirns). In den Fortsätzen zahlreiche Knötchen. Vakuolen im Kern und im Protoplasma. Fig. 43. Astrocyt (weiße Substanz des Occipitalhirns). Im Kern eine starke Vakuole, die sich von der Kernwand nach außen vorstülpt. Fig. 44. Starker Astrocyt (weiße Substanz des Frontalhirns). In den Fortsätzen sehr zahlreiche Knötchen. Einige Fortsätze inserieren an den Wänden eines Gefäßes. Im Protoplasma zahlreiche Vakuolen mit gelblichem Inhalt. Fig. 45. Blutgefäß (weiße Substanz. Occipitalhirn). An die eine Wand lehnen sich zahlreiche runde Gliazellen an. Fig. 46. Randzone eines der Vorderhörner des Halsmarks. Neben einer amöboiden Gliazelle sieht man Teile der Fortsätze anderer in den Schnitt nicht einbezogener Elemente. Zahlreiche, intensiv vom Hämatoxilin gefärbte Granulationen sind auch im übrigen Gewebe zerstreut. Fig. 47. Randzone wie oben. Zahlreiche amöboide Gliazellen mit spärlicher "Methylblaugranula" im Protoplasma. In der Zwischensubstanz blau gefärbte Granula. Fig.48. Große Gliazelle (amöboide?). Vorderhorn des Lendenmarks. Die Fortsätze lösen sich in große blaue Körnchen auf. Neben dem Kern eine große farblose Vakuole (v). Einer der Fortsätze scheint ein kleines Gefäß (v s) zu umfassen. Fig. 49 und 50. Amoböide Gliazellen (Vorderhorn des Halsmarks). Große "Methylblaugranula." Rezza, A. (1912) Beitrag zur pathologischen Anatomie der Pellagrapsychosen. *Z. Gesamte Neurol. Psychiatr.* 12, 31–98 [Figure 26–50].

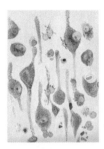

### FIGURE 239.

Schob, 1912. Histopathology of juvenile amaurotic idiocy.

Fig. 2. Scharlachrot-Hämatoxylin. Hirnrinde. Einlagerung lipoider Massen in den geblähten Zellen und Fortsätzen; letztere erscheinen teilweise außer Zusammenhang mit ihren Zellen. Auch in den, teilweise gewucherten, Gliazellen Einlagerung lipoider Körner. Schob, F. (1912) Zur pathologischen Anatomie der juvenilen Form der amaurotischen Idiotie. *Z. gesamte Neurol. Psychiatr.* 10, 303–324 [Figure 2].

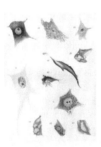

### FIGURE 240.

Trzebinski, 1912. Spinal cord histopathology, I.

Sämtliche Präparate gezeichnet bei Oel Immers. 1/12. Ocular 2 Reichert. Zeich. App. Abbé. Fig. 1. Kontrolpräparat Hund. Fig. 2. 0.9% Na Cl Lösung + Chloroform 2 Tage Hund. Fig. 3. Isoton (Δ-073) Na Cl Lösung: *a* 1 Tag, *b* u. *c* 4 Tage; Kaninchen. Fig. 4. Isoton Na Cl Lösung + 0.2% acid acet *a b c* 3 Tage Kaninchen. Fig. 5. Hyperton Na Cl (2% ) 7 Tage Kaninchen. Fig. 6. Destill. Wasser *a, b, c* 1 Tag Kaninchen. Trzebinski, S. (1912) Beitrag zur Morphologie der Nervenzellen bei der Autolyse des Rückenmarks. *Folia Neurobiol.* 6, 166–181 [Figures 1–6].

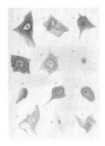

### FIGURE 241.

Trzebinski, 1912. Spinal cord histopathology, II.

Sämtliche Präparate gezeichnet bei Oel Immers. 1/12. Ocular 2 Reichert. Zeich. App. Abbé. Fig. 7. Agar *a, b*, 5 Tage; *c* 7 Tage; Hund. Fig. 8. Ohne Medium in zugeschmolzener Röhre *a* u. *b* 3 Tage, *c* 4 Tage - Kaninchen. Fig. 9. *a, b, c* In Agar 15 Minuten lang auf 100° C. erhitzt, darauf 21 Tage lang bei 37° C. aufbewahrt (Hund). Fig. 9, *d, e, f* ohne vorhergehendes Erhitzen 21 Tage lang im Thermostat auf be wahrt. (Hund). Trzebinski, S. (1912) Beitrag zur Morphologie der Nervenzellen bei der Autolyse des Rückenmarks. *Folia Neurobiol.* 6, 166–181 [Figures 7–9].

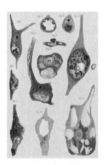

### FIGURE 242.

Rezza, 1913. Changes in neurons of the medulla oblongata in a case of dementia precox.

Tutte le figure furono disegnate a luce artificiale con apparecchio di Abbe, microscopio Leitz, obb. 1/12 imm. om., oculare comp. 4 (le figg. 4 e 11 furono disegnate con oc. Comp. 6). Fig. 1–4. Metodo Mann-Alzheimer. Fig. 5–6. Metodo Alzheimer-Mallory. Fig. 7. Metodo Bielschowscky. Fig. 8–9. Metodo Weigert per la nevroglia. Fig. 10–11. Metodo Daddi-Herxheimer. La spiegazione dettagliata delle figure si trova nel testo. Rezza, A. (1913) Alterazioni delle cellule gangliari del bulbo in un caso di demenza precoce con morte improvvisa. *Riv. Patol. Nerv. Ment.* 18, 426–429 [Figures 1–11].

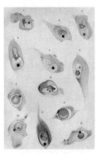

### FIGURE 243.

Achúcarro, 1913. Alterations of ganglion cells.

Sämtliche Figuren stellen Ganglienzellen aus der Geschwulst dar. Viele Kerne enthalten die endonukleären Kugeln. Andere zeigen die Vorgänge von Kernfaltung und Kernrunzelung mit Häufung von chromatischer Substanz am Pol wo die Runzelung am stärksten hervortritt. Toluidinblaupräparat. Zeiss Hom. Imm. 1, 30. Comp. Ok. 6. 1. Ganglienzelle von amöboider Gestalt, welche die Runzelung des Kerns an einem Pol deutlich sehen lässt. Wie bei 4 und 3, ist eine stärkere Färbung am Zusammenkommen der Falten zu erkennen. 2, 5. Einfache Faltung der Kernmembran nebst Einbuchtung des Kernes an der betreffenden Seite. Bei 2, 6, 7, 8, 9,10,11,12, verschiedene Formen der Kerneinschlüsse. Bei 8 ist der Zusammenhang des Kerneinschlusses mit dem Protoplasma deutlich zu sehen. Bei 7, 9, 11. 10 12 sieht man das Kernkörperchen an der Wand der Kernmembran gelagert. Bei 9 ist das Kernkörperchen vom kugeligen Kerneinschluss gedrängt und gedrückt, wobei eine Veränderung der Gestalt desselben hervorgerufen wird. An verschiedenen Zellen (1, 4, 5, 6, 10 und 12) sieht man, obwohl spärliche, unverkennbare Nissschollen. An der Fig. 7 gibt es eine Andeutung der Vakuolenbildung des kugeligen Einschlusses. Bei 10 sieht man auch die Zeichen einer Struktur. Achúcarro, N. (1913) Ganglioneurom des Zentranervensystems. *Folia Neurobiol.* 7, 524–538 [Plate 6].

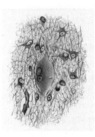

### FIGURE 244.

Bielschowsky and Gallus, 1913. Histopathology and tuberous sclerosis.

Tafel II (bezieht sich auf Fall II). Fig. I. Protoplasmatisches Gliareticulum mit eingestreuten Gliafasern, Astrocyten und einer zweikernigen "großen" Zelle. (Gliafärbung nach Held in eigner Modif.) Bielschowsky, M. and Gallus, K. (1913) Über tuberöse Sklerose. *J. Psychol. Neurol.* 20, 1–88 [Plate 2, Figure 1].

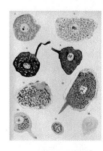

### FIGURE 245.

Cowdry, 1913. Spinal ganglion cells and mitochondria, I.

All the illustrations have been drawn from preparations of spinal ganglion cells of the pigeon. Camera lucida, Zeiss apochromatic objective 1·5 mm, and compensating ocular 6 were employed for all except figures 15 and 18 (vide infra). They were reduced by one-third in reproduction giving a magnification of

1,067 diameters as they now appear on the plates. This magnification does not, however, obtain for figures 15 and 18. Unless stated to the contrary, all the sections were cut 4 μm in thickness. Fig. 3. Fixed in Meves' fluid and stained with iron hematoxylin according to his directions. Mitochondria black and Nissl substance gray (p. 481). Fig. 4. Fixed and stained by Benda's method. Mitochondria blue, Nissl substance reddish brown and the canals as clear uncolored spaces (p. 481). Fig. 8. Fixed in Carnoy's 6: 3: 1 fluid, impregnated with silver after Cajal, toned with gold chloride, counterstained in a saturated aqueous solution of safranin, and differentiated in 95% alcohol. Neurofibrils blue-black, canals as clear space, and the ground substance red (p. 497). Fig. 9. Same, counterstained in 1% aqueous solution of toluidin blue and differentiated in 95% alcohol. Neurofibrils, dark blue; Nissl substance, light blue (p. 497). Fig. 11. Fixed in chrome-sublimate at 40°C, and stained by Bensley's neutral safranin method. Mitochondria and neurosomes of Held type I bluish green, and the Nissl substance red with a tinge of purple (p. 485). Fig. 12. Fixed in Carnoy's 6: 3: 1 fluid and stained by Held's erythrosin-methylene blue method, i. e., his first method for neurosomes. Neurosomes type I red, Nissl substance blue (p. 477). Fig. 16. Prepared by Kopsch's method. Shows excentric type of blackened canalicular apparatus. Section 5 μm (p. 493). Fig. 17. Same. Shows circumnuclear type of blackened canalicular apparatus. Section 6 μm (p. 493). Fig. 18. Stained intravitam with a l : 10,000 solution of Janus green in 75% sodium chloride solution. Mitochondria bluish green. Zeiss apochromatic objective 3 mm, compensating ocular 4, and camera lucida. Magnification 380 diameters (p. 481). Cowdry, E. V. (1913) The relations of mitochondria and other cytoplasmic constituents in spinal ganglion cells of the pigeon. *Int. Monatsschr. Anat. Physiol.* 29, 473–504 [Figures 3, 4, 8, 9, 11, 12, 16–18].

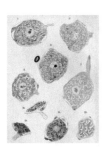

**FIGURE 246.**

Cowdry, 1913. Spinal ganglion cells and mitochondria, II.

All the illustrations have been drawn from preparations of spinal ganglion cells of the pigeon. Camera lucida, Zeiss apochromatic objective 1·5 mm, and compensating ocular 6 were employed for all except figures 15 and 18 (vide infra). They were reduced by one-third in reproduction giving a magnification of 1,067 diameters as

they now appear on the plates. This magnification does not however obtain for figures 15 and 18. Unless stated to the contrary, all the sections were cut 4 μm in thickness. Fig. 1. Fixed in acetic-osmic-bichromate and stained by Bensley's acid fuchsintoluidin blue method. Mitochondria red, Nissl substance slaty blue, canals as clear clefts, and neurofibrils in the axone brown. Note the orientation of the mitochondria parallel to the neurofibrils (p. 484). Fig. 2. Fixed in a cold saturated aqueous solution of potassium bichromate, stained with iron hematoxylin, and counterstained in a 1% aqueous solution of erythrosin. Mitochondria black, Nissl substance pinkish gray, and neurofibrils in the axone black. Held's third method for neurosomes (p. 478). Fig. 5. Altmann's osmic-bichromate fixation, stained with acid fuchsin and differentiated in alcoholic picric acid. Mitochondria red, Nissl substance yellow, and neurofibrils in the axone light brown. Held's second method for neurosomes (p. 481). Fig. 6. Kingsbury's modification of the Weigert hematoxylin method for mitochondria. Mitochondria blue-black, and the Nissl substance brown. The myelin sheath and the mitochondria within it are stained the same blue-black color (p. 486). Fig. 7. Fixed in Altmann's osmic-bichromate mixture and stained by Bensley's copper-chrome-hematoxylin method. Mitochondria blue, Nissl substance very pale yellow, and the canals as clear uncolored spaces. A few neurofibrils are visible in the axone hillock stained blue (p. 483). Fig. 10. Fixed in chrome-sublimate at 40°C, stained with iron hematoxylin, and counterstained by the application of Held's erythrosin-methylene blue method (i.e., his first method for neurosomes). Mitochondria black, neurosomes of Held type I red and the Nissl substance red with a tinge of purple. Section 3 μm (p. 488). Fig. 13. Same, axone hillock showing neurosomes and neurofibrils together (p. 5). Fig. 14. Prepared by Kopsch method, followed by staining in a saturated aqueous solution of safranin and differentiation in 95% alcohol. Canalicular apparatus black and Nissl substance red (p. 493). Fig. 15. Stained intravitam with a 1:1000 solution of pyronin in 0.75% sodium chloride solution. The canalicular apparatus appears as a network of clear, uncolored, continuous spaces winding in and out in a highly granular red-stained cytoplasm. Zeiss apochromatic objective 3 mm and compensating ocular 4. Magnification of about 404 diameters (p. 490). Cowdry, E. V. (1913) The relations of mitochondria and other cytoplasmic constituents in spinal ganglion cells of the pigeon. *Int. Monatsschr. Anat. Physiol.* 29, 473–504 [Figures 1, 2, 5–7, 10, 13–15].

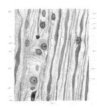

**FIGURE 247.**

Jakob, 1913. Nerve fiber degeneration.

Enthält Zeichnungen aus Präparaten, welche mit Methode I gewonnen sind (mit Ausnahme von Fig. 12 Alkohol-Toluidinblau). Zeiss homogene Immersion 1/12. Okular 6 außer Fig.13 mit Okular 8. Tubus-Länge 160. Fig. 1 und 2 stellen die normalen Strukturverhältnisse der weißen Substanz des Rückenmarks beim Kaninchen dar: Fig. 1. Längsschnitt zeigt die drei Formen der Gliazelle mit ihren Beziehungen zu den Nervenfasern und in ihrer gegenseitigen Lagerung; r RANVIERscher Schnürring; r' ähnliche Erscheinung mit Gliazelle. e ELZHOLZsches Körperchen.

Allgemein angewendete Abkürzungen: *ax* = Achsenzylinder; *ax'* = degenerierter Achsenzy linder; *msch* = Markscheide; *msch'* = Marchischolle; *dmsch* = degenerierte Markscheide; *dmsch'* = zerfallene Marchischolle; *msch''* = ausgelauchte Marchischolle; *e* = physiologisches ELZHOLZsches Körperchen; *e'* = pathologisches ELZHOLZsches Körperchen; *(d)glz* = (degenerierte) Gliazelle; *(d)glz'* = degenerierte protoplasmareiche Gliazelle; *(d)glz''* = degenerierte protoplasmaarme Gliazelle; *(d)glz'''* = degenerierte protoplasmaärmste Gliazelle; *gglz* = gewucherte Gliazelle; *(g) gtst* =( gewucherte ) protoplasmatische Gliastruktur; *glpl* = Protoplasma der Gliazelle; *glfs* = protoplasmatischer Fortsatz der Gliazelle; *mkl* = Myeloklast; *(d)mph* = (degenerierter) Myelophage; *kz a* = Körnchen- oder Gitterzellen *a;* β= Körnchen oder Gitterzellen β; γ = Körnchen- oder Gitterzellen γ; *adv(z)* = Adventitia(l)zelle; *ez* = Endothelzelle; *g* = Blutgefäβ; *blz* = Blutzelle. Jakob, A. (1913) Über die feinere Histologie der sekundären Faserdegeneration in der weiβen Substanz des Rückenmarks (mit besonderer Berücksichtigung der Abbauvorgänge). In *Histologische und histopathologische Arbeiten über die Grosshirnrinde*, eds. F. Nissl and A. Alzheimer, vol. 5, 1–35. Jena: Gustav Fischer [Figure 1].

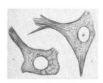

**FIGURE 248.**

Rigotti, 1913. Alteration of the endocellular fibrillary reticulum, I.

Le figure 3 ( fissazione in formalina cloridrica) e 4 (fissazione in alcool nitrico) mostrato appunto come si presentano i reperti : il confronto colle figure 1 e 2 [see Figure 249], che raffigurano le corrispondenti cellule normali, fa vedere quanto profonda e grave sia stata l'alterazione indotta sul reticolo endocellulare dall'ipertermia sperimentale. Rigotti, L. (1913) Indagini sulle alterazioni del reticolo endocellulare degli elementi nervosi nell'ipertermia sperimentale. *Riv. Patol. Nerv. Ment.* 18, 388–394 [Figures 3, 4].

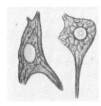

**FIGURE 249.**

Rigotti, 1913. Alteration of the endocellular fibrillary reticulum, II.

Le figure 3 (fissazione in formalina cloridrica) e 4 (fissazione in alcool nitrico) mostrato appunto come si presentano i reperti : il confronto colle figure 1 e 2 [see Figure 248], che raffigurano le corrispondenti cellule normali, fa vedere quanto profonda e grave sia stata l'alterazione indotta sul reticolo endocellulare dall'ipertermia sperimentale. Rigotti, L. (1913) Indagini sulle alterazioni del reticolo endocellulare degli elementi nervosi nell'ipertermia sperimentale. *Riv. Patol. Nerv. Ment.* 18, 388–394 [Figures 1, 2].

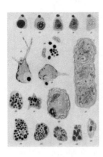

**FIGURE 250.**

Rossi, 1913. Histopathology and pellagra.

Vorbemerkungen. Fig. 1, 2, 3, 7, 8, 10. Ok. 6, Zeiß Apochromat 1,5 n. A. 1,3. Fig. 5, 9. Ok. 12, Obj. wie oben. Fig.6, 11, 12, 13, 14, 15,16, 20, 21, 23, 24, 25, 26, 27. Ok. 8, Obj. wie oben, alle mit Zeiß Prisma nachgezeichnet; Papier an der Höhe des Mikroskoptischleins. Fig.4, 17, 18. Ok.4, Obj. wie oben. Fig. 19 u. 22. Ok.4, Obj. 1/12 Imm. hom. Koristka, Leitz' Zeichenokular. Fig. l, 2, 3, 4, 7, 19, 24. Cajal trichromische Färbung nach Flemmings Fixierung. Fig. 16, 17. 18. Toluidinblau nach Alkoholfixierung. Fig.10, 11, 12, 13, 14, 15. Bestsche Glykogenmethode. Fig. 5, 6, 9. Pappenheims Pyronin-Methylgrünfärbung. Fig. 22. Mallorys Bindegewebsverfahren nach Flemmings Fixierung. Fig. 8. Mannsche Methode nach Zenker Fixierung. Fig.20 u. 23. Flemmings Fixierung, leichte Färbung mit Charmoalaun. Fig. 25. Gefrierschnitt, intensive Färbung mit B-Fuchsin. Differenzierung in Weinsteinsäurelösung. Fig. 26. Herxheimersche Fettfärbung. Fig. 21. Alzheimers Methode VI. Fig. 27. Färbung mit Sudan III nach Ciaccios Verfahren. Fig. 1. Neurogliazellen der Rückenmarkshinterstränge mit großen plumpen Ausläufern Amyloydkörper umgebend. Fig. 2. Neurogliazellen der Zirbeldrüse; der Zelleib enthält Körner, geschwärzt von Osmiumsäure und andere von Fuchsin gerötet. Fig. 3. Hauptzelle einer Langérhansschen Insel. Fig. 4. Vorderhornzelle des Rückenmarks mit Körnchen von Os.o⁴ bräunlich gefärbt und fuchsinophilen Körnchen. Fig. 5. Kern einer Vorderhornganglienzelle: Homogenisierung des Kerns. Schwund der Kernbasichromatin. Vakuolisierung des Kernkörperchens. Fig. 6. Neurogliaelemente b) der grauen Substanz des Rückenmarks. Fig. 7. Zweikernige Pankreaszellen mit Sekretionserscheinungen und Homogenisierung eines Kerns. Fig. 8. Zelle der Marksubstanz der Nebennieren mit eosinophilen und basophil-eosinophilen Körpern. Fig. 9. Kern einer Strangzelle des Rückenmarks, in welchem die Basichromatin fadenförmig erscheint. Fig. 10. Kapillar der Hirnrinde; Adventitialzelle mit Körper und Körnchen rot gefärbt von Bestscher Färbung. Fig. 11, 12, 13, 14, 15. Gliazellen der grauen Substanz des Rückenmarks, welche amyloide Körper einziehen und bearbeiten. Fig. 16. Adventitialzelle eines Kapillargefäßes der Hirnrinde mit grünen Körperchen. Fig. 17, 18. Radikuläre Ganglienzellen des Vorderhorns des Rückenmarks; Wanderung des Kerns an die Peripherie, Homogenisierung des Kerns, Chromatolyse. Fig. 22. Sympathische Ganglienzelle des Plexus von Meißner. Die Zelle enthält Fettkörnchen; Vermehrung der Begleitzellen; Körnchenzelle mit sog. Lipoidecystchen. Fig. 19. Sympathische Ganglienzellen des Auerbachschen Plexus. Die Zellen zeigen ausgerissene Konturen; enthalten Fettkörnchen und rotgefärbte Körnchen. Vermehrung der Begleitzellen. Fig. 20, 21, 23, 24, 25, 26, 27 siehe Erklärung im Text. Rossi, O. (1913) Klinischer und anatomo-pathologischer Beitrag zur Kenntnis des sogen. Pellagratyphus. *J. Psychol. Neurol.* 20, 1–23 [Plate 1].

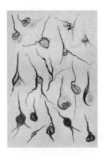

**FIGURE 251.**

Sala, 1913. Histopathology and dementia, I.

Alle Figuren wurden direkt aus den Präparaten mittels der Hellkammer Mod. Apàthy gezeichnet. Die Präparate wurden mit der (leicht modifizierten) Bielschowskyschen Methode angefertigt. Die Beschreibung der Figuren befindet sich im Text der Arbeit. Für die Vergrösserung halte man sich gegenwärtig, dass : die Figuren 1, 2, 3, 7, 8, 10, 12, 20, 21 durch Gebrauch einer Ok. 6 comp. und eines Ob. 2 mm. Zeiss gezeichnet wurden, die Figuren 4, 5 ,6 ,9, 11, 13, l4, 15, 16, 17, 18, 19, 22, 23, 24, 25, 26, 27, 28, 29, 30, 31, 32, 33, 34, 35, 36, 37, 38 durch Gebrauch einer Ok. 4 comp. und eines Ob, 2 mm. Zeiss, die Figur 39 durch Gebrauch einer Ok. 4 comp. und eines Ob. C. Zeiss [see Figure 252]. Sala, G. (1913) Über einen Fall von präseniler Demenz mit Herdsymptomen. *Folia Neurobiol.* 7, 512–521 [Figures 1–18].

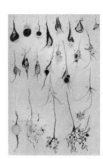

**FIGURE 252.**

Sala, 1913. Histopathology and dementia, II.

Alle Figuren wurden direkt aus den Präparaten mittels der Hellkammer Mod. Apàthy gezeichnet. Die Präparate wurden mit der (leicht modifizierten) Bielschowskyschen Methode angefertigt. Die Beschreibung der Figuren befindet sich im Text der Arbeit. Für die Vergrösserung halte man sich gegenwärtig, dass : die Figuren 1, 2, 3, 7, 8, 10, 12, 20, 21 durch Gebrauch einer Ok. 6 comp. und eines Ob. 2 mm. Zeiss gezeichnet wurden, die Figuren 4, 5 ,6 ,9, 11, 13, l4, 15, 16, 17, 18, 19, 22, 23, 24, 25, 26, 27, 28, 29, 30, 31, 32, 33, 34, 35, 36, 37, 38 durch Gebrauch einer Ok. 4 comp. und eines Ob, 2 mm. Zeiss, die Figur 39 durch Gebrauch einer Ok. 4 comp. und eines Ob. C. Zeiss [see Figure 251]. Sala, G. (1913) Über einen Fall von präseniler Demenz mit Herdsymptomen. *Folia Neurobiol.* 7, 512–521 [Figures 19–39].

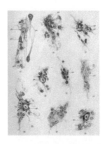

**FIGURE 253.**

Jakob, 1914. Histopathology and epilepsy.

Sämtliche Figuren sind gezeichnet mit Öl-Immersion, Oc. 6, Tub.-Länge 150. Sie stellen Ganglienzell- und Gliazellveränderungen von Fall II dar. Fig. 17. Atypische große Ganglienzelle *(ga)* aus der Lamina ganglionaris des Temporalhirns; *ga'* normal große aber chronisch degenerierte Ganglienzellen mit relativ großem Kern in unregelmäßiger Lagerung. *gl* gewucherte Gliazellen der Umgebung. Fig. 18. Zellkomplex aus der Lamina pyramidalis des Temporalhirns. Umlagerung einer schwer veränderten Ganglienzelle von zahlreichen gewucherten Gliazellen. Fig. 19, 20,21. Von gewucherten Gliazellen in charakteristischer Weise umlagerten Ganglienzellen (ga), die Gliazellen schmiegen sich dem Zelleib enge an und lassen sich oft von ihm nicht abgrenzen. Tiefste Schicht der Temporal- und Frontalrinde. Fig. 19 ga' Ganglienzellkern mit zwei Kernkörperchen. Fig. 22. Ganglienzelle aus dem subcorticalen Mark des Temporalhirns mit zwei Kernkörperchen, von zahlreichen Gliazellen umlagert. Fig.23. Zellkomplex aus dem subcorticalen Mark von $F_2$. Atypische Ganglienzelle (ga), umlagert von zahlreichen, in charakteristischer Weise gewucherten Gliazellen. Fig. 24. Gruppe gewucherter Gliazellen aus dem Herd im Parietalhirn (vgl. Text- fig. 18). Fig. 25. Aus dem gleichen Herd im Situationsbild einer mit keulenartig aufgetriebenen Ausläufern versehenen Ganglienzelle, umgeben von zahlreichen gewucherten Gliazellen. Jakob, A. (1914) Zur Pathologie der Epilepsie. *Z. gesamte Neurol. Psychiatr.* 23, 1–65 [Plate 3].

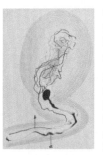

## FIGURE 254.

Martynoff, 1914. Encapsulated endings, I.

Körperchen von Golgi-Mazzoni im Stratum reticulare der Brustwarze einer Kuh; a - dicke, markhaltige Nervenfaser; b - dünne markhaltige Nervenfaser. Zeiss, Obj. C.; Oc. III. Martynoff, W. (1914) Nervenendapparate in der Brustwarze der Frau und von Säugetierweibchen. *Folia Neurobiol.* 8, 249–263 [Figure 4].

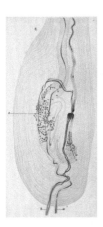

## FIGURE 255.

Martynoff, 1914. Encapsulated endings, II.

Ein Vater-Pacinisches Körperchen aus der Tela subcutanea der Brustwarze einer Frau; a - dicke, markhaltige Nervenfaser; b - dünne; markhaltige Nervenfaser, die baumförmige Verzweigungen - e an der Peripherie des Innenkolbens bildet. Zeiss, Obj. C.; Oc. II. Martynoff, W. (1914) Nervenendapparate in der Brustwarze der Frau und von Säugetierweibchen. *Folia Neurobiol.* 8, 249–263 [Figure 8].

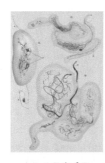

## FIGURE 256.

Martynoff, 1914. Encapsulated endings, III.

Fig. 12. Ein modifiziertes Körperchen von Golgi-Mazzoni, aus dessen der Eintrittstelle der Nerven entgegengesetztem Pole feine marklose Fasern - a austreten; b - dicke markhaltige Nervenfaser, die in weiter Entfernung vom Körperchen die Markscheide verlóren hat; c - plättchenförmige Verdickung. Brustwarze der Kuh. Zeiss. Obj. C.; Oc III. Fig. 13. Ein modifiziertes Körperchen von Golgi-Mazzoni, aus dem Stratum reticulare der Brustwarze einer Kuh; a - dicke markhaltige Nervenfaser; b - dünne markhaltige Nervenfaser. Zeiss. Obj. C.; Oc. III. Martynoff, W. (1914) Nervenendapparate in der Brustwarze der Frau und von Säugetierweibchen. *Folia Neurobiol.* 8, 249–263 [Figures 12, 13, 15].

## FIGURE 257.

De Nunno, 1914. Nervous system infection due to *Micrococcus melitensis.*

Coniglio, A. Metodo Cajal. Zeiss, oc. 3 obb. F. De Nunno, R. (1914) L'azione del micrococco di Bruce (melitense) e delle sue tossine sul sistema nervoso centrale e periferico. *Riv. Patol. Nerv. Ment.* 19, 351–372 [Figure 2].

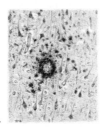

## FIGURE 258.

Cowe, 1915. Senile plaque, I.

Levaditisches Präparat: Ausgebildete Plaques. Cowe, A. (1915) Der gliöse Anteil der senilen Plaques. *Z. gesamte Neurol. Psychiatr.* 29, 92–96 [Plate 1, Figure 1].

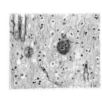

## FIGURE 259.

Cowe, 1915. Senile plaque, II.

Levaditi - Merzbachersches Präparat: zeigt die Anfangsstadien und einen ausgebildeten Plaque. Keine besondere Beziehung zwischen der Glia und den Plaques zu konstatieren. Faserring bläulich gefärbt.

Silbersalzablagerung. Cowe, A. (1915) Der gliöse Anteil der senilen Plaques. *Z. gesamte Neurol. Psychiatr.* 29, 92–96 [Plate 2, Figure 2].

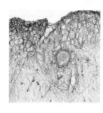

## FIGURE 260.

Cowe, 1915. Senile plaque, III.

Plaque aus den oberen Rindenpartien. Auseinanderdrängung der Gliafasern. Cowe, A. (1915) Der gliöse Anteil der senilen Plaques. *Z. gesamte Neurol. Psychiatr.* 29, 92–96 [Plate 3, Figure 1].

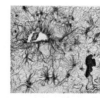

## FIGURE 261.

Cowe, 1915. Senile plaque, IV.

Plaque aus der Tiefe der Rinde; in seiner Umgebung gewucherte Glia. Cowe, A. (1915) Der gliöse Anteil der senilen Plaques. *Z. gesamte Neurol. Psychiatr.* 29, 92–96 [Plate 3, Figure 2].

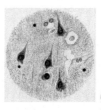

## FIGURE 262.

Papadia, 1916. Histopathology of the cerebral cortex.

Da un preparato di corteccia cerebrale. Fissazione nel liquido di Müller (10 giorni), inclusione in paraffina e colorazione colla miscela di Mann. Si vedono tre corpi ialoidi intensamente colorati in rosso. Micr. Koristka: obb. ad imm. 1/15, oc. comp. 4. Papadia, G. (1916) Su alcune formazioni ialoidi del sistema nervoso centrale. *Riv. Patol. Nerv. Ment.* 21, 129–134 [Figure 1].

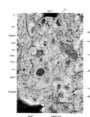

## FIGURE 263.

Lotmar, 1918. Histological alterations in acute myelitis and encephalitis, I.

Degeneration feiner nervöser Strukturen (Achsenzylinder, eventuell feine Dendriten) in Randpartie eines Vorderhornherdes (Längsschnitt). *cap* Kapillare; *ax* Achsenzylinder, *deg ax* degenerierender Achsenzylinder (eosinfarbig), *deg ax'*, *deg ax"* desgleichen mit einem eosingefärbten Tropfen als Zerfallsprodukt. *varic ax* varikös gequollener Achsenzylinder, degenerierend. *gaz* Ganglienzellen. *gaz'* (etwas links unten von der Mitte) Querschnitt durch den einen Pol einer solchen. *glz* kleinere Gliazellen.

*Glz* stark gewucherte Gliazellen. *tr* tropfiges Degenerationsprodukt (leuchtend eosinfarbig) im gittrigen Plasma einer gewucherten Gliazelle. *tr'* ebensolche Tröpfchen. *Den* Dendrit von *gaz'*. Grundgewebe im ganzen aufgelockert, feinmaschig, plasmatisches Glianetzwerk gewuchert, in das perinukleäre Plasma der Gliazellen übergehend. Markscheiden infolge starker Differenzierung fast ganz entfärbt. Tier 9 (16. Tag). ZEISS (hier wie überall), Imm. 1/12. Komp. Ok. 6. MANN. S. auch S. 318 ff. Lotmar, F. (1918) Beiträge zur Histologie der akuten Myelitis und Encephalitis, sowie verwandter Prozesse. In *Histologische und histopathologische Arbeiten über die Grosshirnrinde*, eds. F. Nissl and A. Alzheimer, vol. 6, 245–432. Jena: Gustav Fischer [Figure 1].

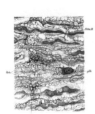

**FIGURE 264.**

Lotmar, 1918. Histological alterations in acute myelitis and encephalitis, II.

Quellung des Gliaretikulum *(Ret)* in der weißen Substanz (in einer leichter geschädigten Partie des Seitenstranges). *glk* Gliazellkern. *Schn R* Schnürringe. Achsenzylinder zum Teil mehr oder weniger stark gequollen. Zusammenhang des Gliaretikulum mit dem Plasma der Gliazelle erkennbar. Tier 49 (2. Tag). Rückenmarklängsschnitt. Imm. 1/12. *Komp.* Ok. 6. MANN. Lotmar, F. (1918) Beiträge zur Histologie der akuten Myelitis und Encephalitis, sowie verwandter Prozesse. In *Histologische und histopathologische Arbeiten über die Grosshirnrinde*, eds. F. Nissl and A. Alzheimer, vol. 6, 245–432. Jena: Gustav Fischer [Figure 3].

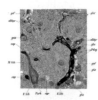

**FIGURE 265.**

Lotmar, 1918. Histological alterations in acute myelitis and encephalitis, III.

Kleinhirnrinde. Unten Beginn der Körnerschicht *(Ksch)*, *Msch* Molekularschicht. *Purk* denegerierte PURKINJEsche Zelle. *Pdeg* denegerierte Protoplasmafortsätze PURKINJEscher Zellen. *rar* Auflockerung des Gewebes und Quellung des Gliaretikulum in der Schicht der PURKINJEschen Zellen. *gef* Gefäße, in deren Umgebung sich methylblau- und eosinfarbige Abbauprodukte ansammeln *(abbpr)*, zum Teil in erkennbaren Beziehungen zum Plasma von Gliazellen *(glz)*. Die Gliazelle *glz'* enthält Pigmentschollen (eisenhaltig). *gaz* Ganglienzelle. *cap* Kapillaren. Tier 7 (3. Tag).

Imm. 1/12. Komp. Ok. 4. MANN. Lotmar, F. (1918) Beiträge zur Histologie der akuten Myelitis und Encephalitis, sowie verwandter Prozesse. In *Histologische und histopathologische Arbeiten über die Grosshirnrinde*, eds. F. Nissl and A. Alzheimer, vol. 6, 245–432. Jena: Gustav Fischer [Figure 42].

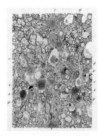

**FIGURE 266.**

Lotmar, 1918. Histological alterations in acute myelitis and encephalitis, IV.

Achsenzylinderquellung, Übersichtsbild aus Querschnitt durch Randpartie eines Herdes in der weißen Substanz des Rückenmarkes. (Die Verweiselinie *c* müßte bis zu dem in der Mitte der Figur gelegenen, von einer großen Lichtung umgebenen unregelmäßigen Achsenzylinderquerschnitt weitergeführt sein.) *gl* Gliazellen. Übrige Erklärungen S. 333 Kleindruck. Tier II (8. Tag). Imm. *1/12.* Ok. 2. Fuchsinlichtgrün. Lotmar, F. (1918) Beiträge zur Histologie der akuten Myelitis und Encephalitis, sowie verwandter Prozesse. In *Histologische und histopathologische Arbeiten über die Grosshirnrinde*, eds. F. Nissl and A. Alzheimer, vol. 6, 245–432. Jena: Gustav Fischer [Figure 49].

**FIGURE 267.**

Lotmar, 1918. Histological alterations in acute myelitis and encephalitis, V.

Längsschnitt eines Gefäßes und seiner Umgebung aus der Nachbarschaft eines Verflüssigungsherdes des Vorderhorns. Ansammlung von fuchsinophilen und Lichtgrüntropfen *(li)* und -tröpfchen bzw. -granula innerhalb der limitans *(lim)*. Übergang in osmierte (bräunliche) Tröpfchen nach Aufnahme in Adventitialzellen *(advz', advz")* zwei solche mit stark vergrößertem Plasmaleib). *glz'* Gliazellen des Gliakammerraumes *(glk* Gliakammern). Die gröberen grünen Balken sind Fibrinausscheidungen *(fibr)*, die feineren Züge gehören überwiegend der Glia an. *gefw* Gefäßwand. *geflum* Gefäßlumen. *adv lr* adventitieller Lymphraum. *Gr* graue Substanz. Tier 22 (3. Tag). Vorderhornlängsschnitt. Imm. 1/12. Komp. Ok. 6. Fuchsinlichtgrün. Lotmar, F. (1918) Beiträge zur Histologie der akuten Myelitis und Encephalitis, sowie verwandter Prozesse.

In *Histologische und histopathologische Arbeiten über die Grosshirnrinde*, eds. F. Nissl and A. Alzheimer, vol. 6, 245–432. Jena: Gustav Fischer [Figure 44].

**FIGURE 268.**

Lotmar, 1918. Histological alterations in acute myelitis and encephalitis, VI.

FIG. 47. Gefäß aus Nachbarschaft eines Verflüssigungsherdes im Vorderhorn mit fuchsin- und lichtgrünfarbigen Abbauprodukten. *mglz* marginale Gliazellen. *lim* limitans gliae. *glk* Gliakammern. *fibr* Fibringerinnsel. *gefwz* Gefäßwandzellen. Tier 18 (7. Tag). Imm. 1/12. Komp. Ok. 6. Fuchsinlichtgrün. FIG. 50. Herd des Nucleus caudatus. Zwei Gliazellen des Parenchyms *(gaz* Ganglienzelle), die eine *(glk')* enthält reichlich mit Lichtgrün gefärbte Produkte *li*, eine größere fuchsinophile Scholle (mit schon leicht bräunlichem Schimmer) *fph*, mehrere gebräunte lipoide Produkte *lp. gr* Grau der Umgebung. Tier 7 (3. Tag). Imm. 1/₁₂. Ok. 4. Fuchsinlichtgrün. FIG. 51. *gaz* schwer veränderte Ganglienzelle mit geschrumpftem dunklem Kern. Daneben Gliazelle, deren Kern nicht getroffen ist, mit großen fuchsinophilen Abbautropfen. Tier 7 (3. Tag), gleiche Gegend wie Fig. 50. Imm. 1/12. Ok. 4. Fuchsinlichtgrün. FIG. 52. Dasselbe neben einer nicht merklich veränderten Ganglienzelle *(gaz)*. *glz* Trabantgliazelle mit fuchsinophilen Abbauprodukten. Herd im Nucl. caudatus. Tier 7 (3. Tag). Imm *1/12*. Ok. 4. Fuchsinlichtgrün. FIG. 53. Querschnitt eines gequollenen Achsenzylinders aus Herd der weißen Substanz. *a, b,c* axophagische Gliazellen. Die Zelle *a* mit sehr vergrößertem körnigem Plasmaleib sich in den Achsenzylinder hineinschiebend. *v* Vakuole im Achsenzylinder, enthält ein fuchsinfarbiges Degenerationsprodukt. Tier II (8. Tag). Imm. *1/12*. Komp. Ok. 6. Fuchsinlichtgrün. Lotmar, F. (1918) Beiträge zur Histologie der akuten Myelitis und Encephalitis, sowie verwandter Prozesse. In *Histologische und histopathologische Arbeiten über die Grosshirnrinde*, eds. F. Nissl and A. Alzheimer, vol. 6, 245–432. Jena: Gustav Fischer [Figure 47, 50, 51, 52, 53].

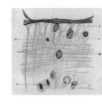

**FIGURE 269.**

Spatz, 1918. Normal histology of the spinal cord of the newborn rabbit, I.

Glia limitans externa. *a* = Rindenschicht; *b* = Grenzschicht (HELD); *c* = Radiärfasern; *F.x.* = Form *x*, kleines Gebilde,

vermutlich Teilstück eines karyorrhektisch veränderten Gliaelements. *M.* = Mitose im Stadium des Toctersterns; *Sp.* = Spirem. Nicht ganz ausgetragenes Kaninchen. MANNsches Gemisch. Spatz, H. (1918) Beiträge zur normalen Histologie des Rückenmarks des neugeborenen Kaninchens.
In *Histologische und histopathologische Arbeiten über die Grosshirnrinde*, eds. F. Nissl and A. Alzheimer, vol. 6, 477–604. Jena: Gustav Fischer [Figure 27].

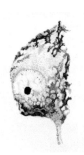

**FIGURE 270.**

Spatz, 1918. Normal histology of the spinal cord of the newborn rabbit, II.

Motorische Nervenzelle. 5 Tage altes Kaninchen. Vorderhorn. Thionin. Spatz, H. (1918) Beiträge zur normalen Histologie des Rückenmarks des neugeborenen Kaninchens. In *Histologische und histopathologische Arbeiten über die Grosshirnrinde*, eds. F. Nissl and A. Alzheimer, vol. 6, 477–604. Jena: Gustav Fischer [Figure 28].

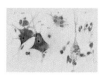

**FIGURE 271.**

Creutzfeldt, 1921. Pathological changes in the brain, I.

Alle Bilder sind nach Tionin- bzw. Toluidinblaupräparaten mit dem ABBEschen Zeichenapparat gezeichnet. Vergrößerung Zeiss-Ölimmersion 1/12, Kompensationsokular 4, nur Fig. 2 wurde mit Kompensationsokular 6 hergestellt. FIG. 1. Zeigt zwei Pyramidenzellen *(gaz)* der Lamin. pyramidal. aus der Übergangszone zu einem Herd. Die NISSL-Substanz ist größtenteils aufgelöst, nur am Rande liegen einige erhaltene Schollen oder Klumpen, die Zelleiber sind diffus dunkel. Fortsätze weithin sichtbar. Kerne diffus dunkel, ihr Gerüst verwaschen, die Grenze unscharf. An der linken Zelle Chromatinanlagerungen an der Kernwand. Bei *pglz* eine plasmareiche progressiv veränderte Gliazelle, bei *fglz* eine fortsatzreiche Gliazelle. Alle anderen Kerne sind Gliakerne. FIG. 3. Um die Ganglienzelle ist nur noch ein Rest des homogenisierten Plasmas sichtbar *(gaz)*. Ihre Form, einschließlich der Fortsätze, wird von Glia ersetzt. Dem Spitzenfortsatz entspricht ein stäbchenzellartiger Gliaplasmafortsatz. Die übrigen Gliazellen sind plasmareich. Bei *stz* eine gliogene Stäbchenzelle. FIG. 4. Ausgebildeter

Gliastern mit beginnenden regressiven Veränderungen an den Kernen. Creutzfeldt, H. G. (1921) *Über eine eigenartige herdförmige Erkrankung des Zentralnervensystems*. In Histologische und histopathologische Arbeiten über die Grosshirnrinde, eds. F. Nissl and A. Alzheimer, 1–48. Jena: Gustav Fischer [Figures 1, 3, 4].

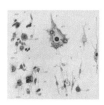

**FIGURE 272.**

Creutzfeldt, 1921. Pathological changes in the brain, II.

Alle Bilder sind nach Tionin- bzw. Toluidinblaupräparaten mit dem ABBEschen Zeichenapparat gezeichnet. Vergrößerung Zeiss-Ölimmersion 1/12, Kompensationsokular 4, nur Fig. 2 wurde mit Kompensationsokular 6 hergestellt. FIG. 2. Bei *gaz* sieht man den homogenisierten Plasmaleib, der von einem Gliasymplasma umschlossenen untergehenden Nervenzelle, deren dunkler pyknotischer Kern *n* mit zahlreichen basophilen Körnchen erfüllt ist und ein etwas helleres metachromatisches Kernkörperchen *(nc)* enthält. Die drei Gliakerne sind progressiv verändert. FIG. 5. Aus einem Herde: bei *pglz* plasmareiche Gliazellen, bei *eglz* mehr epitheloide Elemente. Bei *g* ein Gefäß mit Kernsprossen an einem Endothelkern. FIG. 6. Aus einem Herde: Plasmareiche, zum Teil 1-3 kernige Gliazellen mit zahlreichen Fortsätzen, bei *s* synzytialer Verband, der noch die Konturen der geschwundenen und ersetzten Ganglienzelle verrät. Bei *stz* losgelöste Stäbchenzelle. Bei *glr* ein Gliaring. FIG. 7. Stäbchenzellen in radiärer Anordnung mit senkrecht vom Zelleibe abgehenden Fortsätzen. In der Mitte eine Totenlade. Bei *glz* eine Gliazelle mit perinukleärer Plasmaansammlung und peripherer Vakuolisierung. FIG. 8a u. b. Zeigt Zellen aus einem Herde, die wahrscheinlich gliöse Elemente sind und lediglich die Form der ersetzten Ganglienzelle angenommen haben. Creutzfeldt, H. G. (1921) *Über eine eigenartige herdförmige Erkrankung des Zentralnervensystems*. In Histologische und histopathologische Arbeiten über die Grosshirnrinde, eds. F. Nissl and A. Alzheimer, 1–48. Jena: Gustav [Figures 2, 5–8].

**FIGURE 273.**

Creutzfeldt, 1921. Pathological changes in the brain, III.

FIG. 14–20 und 24, 25, 27 sind nach

HERXHEIMER-Präparaten gezeichnet und mit dem ABBEschen Zeichenapparat. Vergrößerung Zeiss homog. Immersion 1/12, und Kompensations-Okular 4. Fig. 21, 26, 28 nach ALZHEIMER- VI- Präparaten. Vergrößerung Zeiss homog. Immers. 1/12, Kompensations-Okular 6. Fig. 22 und 29, nach BIELSCHOWSKI-Präparat mit Kompensations Okular 6. Fig. 23, nach SNESSAREW-Präparat mit Kompensations-Okular 4. FIG. 21. Große Zelle der fünften Rindenschicht. Fuchsinophile Granula in der homogenisierten Innenzone. Nukleolus unverändert. Kern an den Rand gedrückt, Struktur erhalten. FIG. 22. BEETZsche Zellen. Diffuse Zellveränderung. Kern und Lipochrom peripher verlagert. Außenfibrillen gut imprägniert, Innenfibrillen lösen sich in der Zelle zu staubartiger Masse auf, die die Zellmitte erfüllt. *af*= Außenfibrillen; *if* = Innenfibrillen; *x* = zentrale Masse; *n*=Kern.; *ne* = Kernkörperchen; *lp* = Liprochrom; *plm* = Plasmabälkchen zwischem den Fettkörnern. FIG. 23. Fortsatzreiche, faserbildende Gliazelle aus einem Rindenherde. FIG. 24. Ganglienzelle aus dem Talamus. Verdrängung von Kern und Fett an den Zellrand. Zellinneres homogen, blaß. Bei *glz* Trabantzellkern. Nukleolus des Ganglienzellkerns zeigt Vakuole. FIG. 25. Kleinere fettarme Talamuszelle mit gleicher Veränderung wie *k*. Bei *glz* liegt fettbeladene Trabantzelle. FIG. 29. Zelle aus dem Talamus, die der in Taf. I, Fig. *9a* wiedergegebenen entspricht. Beachtenswert ist das Schwinden der intrazellulären Fibrillen und die Maschenbildung des Zellplasmas um die Fetteinlagerungen. FIG. 30. Talamuszelle mit Fetteinlagerung, die sich mit Eisenhämatoxylin zentral dunkel, peripher grau färbt. Creutzfeldt, H. G. (1921) *Über eine eigenartige herdförmige Erkrankung des Zentralnervensystems*. In Histologische und histopathologische Arbeiten über die Grosshirnrinde, eds. F. Nissl and A. Alzheimer, 1–48. Jena: Gustav Fischer [Figures 21–25, 29, 30].

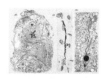

**FIGURE 274.**

Creutzfeldt, 1921. Pathological changes in the brain, IV.

FIG. 26. Diffuse Veränderung der Zellen der dritten Schicht. Fuchsinophile Granula zentral verändert und kleiner, bei der rechten Zelle osmophile Granula und Randansammlung der fuchsinophilen Granula, während die Zellmitte sie weniger enthält. FIG. 27. Windungsmark.

Fettbedeckter Achsenzylinder, von Gliakern begleitet. FIG. 28. Achsenzylinderschwellung und Achsenzylinderschlängelung. *axq* = geschwollener Kolben.  Creutzfeldt, H. G. (1921) *Über eine eigenartige herdförmige Erkrankung des Zentralnervensystems. In Histologische und histopathologische Arbeiten über die Grosshirnrinde,* eds. F. Nissl and A. Alzheimer, 1–48. Jena: Gustav Fischer [Figures 26–28].

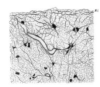

**FIGURE 275.**

Spielmeyer, 1922. Histopathology of the nervous system, I.

Abb. 86. Oberste Großhirnrindenschicht im Alzheimer-Mann-Präparat von einem etwa 50jährigen Menschen. Darstellung des Heldschen Gliaretikulums und seiner Versteifung durch Gliafasern. Insertion des Gliaretikulums und der Fasern an der Membrana limitans der Gefäße und der obersten Randzone meist deutlich. M.1 Membrana limitans superficialis mit darunter gelegenen Kammern.  Spielmeyer, W. (1922) *Histopathologie des Nervensystems.* Erster Band: Allgemeiner Teil. Berlin: J. Springer [Figure 86].

**FIGURE 276.**

Spielmeyer, 1922. Histopathology of the nervous system, II.

Abb. 116a [left], b [right]. Zwei Monstregliazellen. a. Gliazelle der Hirnrinde mit derben, Faserbündel führenden Plasmafortsätzen. b Zelle aus der tiefsten Rinde allseitig mit feineren ungemein zahlreichen, von Fasern versteiften Ausläufern. Weigerts Gliafärbung.  Spielmeyer, W. (1922) *Histopathologie des Nervensystems.* Erster Band: Allgemeiner Teil. J. Berlin: Springer [Figure 116].

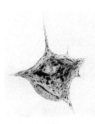

**FIGURE 277.**

Spielmeyer, 1922. Histopathology of the nervous sysrem, III.

Abb. 185. Vorderhornzelle im Lumbalmark eines Menschen, dem 1 ½Jahre zuvor ein Bein amputiert war. Große, anomal angeordnete Brocken im Innenteil der Zelle. Der Pigmenthaufen ist im wesentlichen noch an die Peripherie gedrängt geblieben.  Spielmeyer, W. (1922) *Histopathologie des*

*Nervensystems.* Erster Band: Allgemeiner Teil. Berlin: J. Springer [Figure 185].

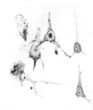

**FIGURE 278.**

Spielmeyer, 1922. Histopathology of the nervous system, IV.

Abb. 22a–f. Verschiedene pathologische Ganglienzellbilder bei Nisslfärbung. a, b: Akute Umwandlung des Granulabildes an Rindenzellen nach Status epilepticus. a Zerfall und Auflösung der Nisslsubstanz (sog. Chromolyse); die Auflösungsprodukte (Krümel) zum Teil noch entsprechend der normalen Anordnung. Die ungefärbten Bahnen leicht angefärbt. - b Weiter fortgeschrittene Umwandlung einer Ganglienzelle im gleichen Fall: leichte Schwellung und Abrundung des Zelleibs, körnige Auflösung der Granula. c, d. Schwellung, Verflüssigung und Imprägnation an zwei Ganglienzellen der Hirnrinde bei Kraepelins "Angstpsychose"; die Zellveränderung entspricht im wesentlichen dem Typus von Nissls "schwerer Ganglienzellerkrankung", zumal in der Zelle c, wo der Kern kleiner und dunkler geworden ist. Abschmelzungsvorgänge an der Zellperipherie und an den Fortsätzen. Von der Imprägnation ist, wie häufig, besonders die Basis betroffen. e, f. Weiter fortgeschrittenes Stadium des gleichen Prozesses (wie in Abb. c, d). Durch die Auflösung und Verflüssigung der Zelleibsubstanz sind Randpartien und Fortsätze der Zelle abgeschmolzen. Im Innern haben sich vakuoläre Räume und grobwabige Zerklüftungen ausgebildet. Injeder Zelle liegt ein Gliakern (mitKernwandhyperchromatose) in einem Hohlraum.  Spielmeyer, W. (1922) *Histopathologie des Nervensystems.* Erster Band: Allgemeiner Teil. Berlin: J. Springer [Figure 22].

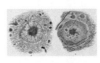

**FIGURE 279.**

Spielmeyer, 1922. Histopathology of the nervous system, V.

Abb. 201 a und b. Zwei senile Plaques. Bielschowskysche Silberimprägnation. In 201a gehen von dem amorphen Kerne Strahlen aus, welche wie Kristallnadeln einen hellen Hof durchsetzen und am Rande in einer schmalen, ringartigen Zone ansetzen. In 201b ist der Kern massiger, ebenfalls amorph, stellenweise etwas ausgezogen. In dem hellen Hof liegen Gliazellen und

dürftige Achsenzylinderauftreibungen. Die Außenzone besteht aus einem breiten dichten Wall.  Spielmeyer, W. (1922) *Histopathologie des Nervensystems.* Erster Band: Allgemeiner Teil. Berlin: J. Springer [Figure 201].

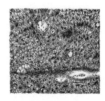

**FIGURE 280.**

Spielmeyer, 1922. Histopathology of the nervous system, VI.

Abb. 215. Anisomorphe Gliose in einem alten myelitischen Herd-Längsschnitt. Weigertsche Gliafaserfärbung.  Spielmeyer, W. (1922) *Histopathologie des Nervensystems.* Erster Band: Allgemeiner Teil. Berlin: J. Springer [Figure 215].

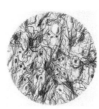

**FIGURE 281.**

Spielmeyer, 1922. Histopathology of the nervous system, VII.

Abb. 114. Fibrillisation sehr breiter, plasmatischer Verbände. Gliafaserpräparat.  Spielmeyer, W. (1922) *Histopathologie des Nervensystems.* Erster Band: Allgemeiner Teil. Berlin: J. Springer [Figure 114].

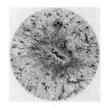

**FIGURE 282.**

Spielmeyer, 1922. Histopathology of the nervous system, VIII.

Abb. 250. Gliafasernarbe an Stelle einer alten Einschmelzung. Weigertsches Gliapräparat. Vorwiegend radiäre Anordnung der sich vielfach überkreuzenden Fasern gegen ein Gefäß. Im rechten oberen Teil des Bildes einige Monstregliazellen.  Spielmeyer, W. (1922) *Histopathologie des Nervensystems.* Erster Band: Allgemeiner Teil. Berlin: J. Springer [Figure 250].

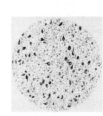

**FIGURE 283.**

Bozzi, 1929. Cortical histopathology.

Nucleo del III° paio. Riduzione numerica degli elementi cellulari. Cellule nervose povere di prolungamento con nucleo spesso lateralizzato. Metodo Nissl. Micr. Zeiss; oc. 15; obb, 2.  Bozzi, R. (1929) Contributo clinico ed anatomo-patologico allo studio dei tumori del lobo temporale. *Riv. Patol. Nerv. Ment.* 34, 429–523.

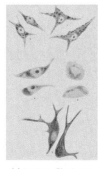

**FIGURE 284.**

Emma, 1929. Neurons of the substantia nigra.

FIG. 1 Cellule nervose della zona compatta della Nigra di nomo adulto: rapporti tra il pigmento melaniuico e le zolle di Niss1 (metodo di Niss1; oculare 8 C.; obbiettivo 1"/15 imm. omog.). Fig. 2 Cellule nervose della zona compatta della Nigra di feto al 9° mese (metodo di Nissl; oc. 8. C.; obb. 1"/15 imm. omog.). Fig. 3 Cellule nervose della zona compatta della Nigra di nomo adulto da sezioni di pezzi non fissatti senza alcuna colorazione (oculare 8 C.; obb. 1"/12 imm. omog.). Fig . 4 Cellule nervose della zona compatta della Nigra di nomo adulto: rapporti fra il pigmento melaninico e le sostanze grasse (Sudan III° ematossilina; oc. 8 C.; obb. 1"/12 imm. omog.). Fig. 5 Cellule nervose della zona compatta della Nigra: reticolo neurofibrillare e snoi rapporti con il pigmento melanico (metodo di Bielschowsky; oc. 8 C.; obb. 1"/15 imm. omog.). Emma, M. (1929) Contributo alla conoscenza della fine struttura della regione della substantia nigra. *Riv. Patol. Nerv. Ment.* 34, 579–615 [Figures 1–5].

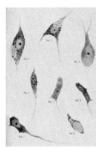

**FIGURE 285.**

Berlucchi, 1931. Histological changes of the corpus striatum, I.

Figure ricavate dai preparati col metodo del Nissl. Ingrandimento 820. Fig. 12–17. Piccole cellula nervose dello Striato del caso 25 con dissoluzione del protoplasma e pseudoneuronofagia. Fig. 17. Grossa cellula nervosa dollo Striato del caso 6. Sostanza cromofila piuttosto' scarsa disposta a zolle regolari. Fig. 18. Grossa cellula nervosa dello Striato del caso 34. Zolle cromofile regolari come nella cellula precedente. Presenza di pigmento. Fig. 20. Grossa cellula nervosa dello Striato del caso 25. Le zolle cromofile sono completamente

scomparse; il protoplasma ha assunto un aspetto alveolare. Il nucleo è intensamente colorato tanto che a mala pena si distingue il nucleolo. Fig. 21. Grossa cellula nervosa dello Striato del caso 8. Il protoplasma ha aspetto omogeneo pallido. Il nucleo è intensamente colorato. Berlucchi, C. (1931) Modificazioni del quadro istologico del Corpo Striato in soggetti morti di malattie varie. *Riv. Patol. Nerv. Ment.* 38, 152–378 [Plate 18, Figures 17, 18, 20, 21].

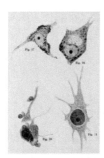

**FIGURE 286.**

Berlucchi, 1931. Histological changes of the corpus striatum, II.

Figure ricavate da preparati col metodo del Nissl. Ingrandimento 820. Fig. 1–2. Cellula nervose del Pallido del caso 39. Sostanza cromatica regolarmente distribuita in zolle. Fig. 3. Cellula nervosa del Pallido del caso 33. Protoplasma colorato in modo pallido ed omogeneo. Fig. 4–5. Cellule nervose del Pallido del caso 21. Raggrinzamento. Scomparsa delle zolle cromofile. Aspetto areolare del protoplasma. Limiti mal definiti del protoplasma. Fig. 6. Cellula nervosa del Pallido del caso 3. Le stesse alterazioni del caso precedente ma più gravi. Fig. 7. Cellula nervosa del Pallido del caso 17. Protoplasma diffusamente colorato col Nissl in modo uniforme ed intenso. Fig. 8. Cellula nervosa del Pallido caso 52. Enorme aumento del Pigmento. Nucleo senza membrana, mal delimitato. Berlucchi, C. (1931) Modificazioni del quadro istologico del Corpo Striato in soggetti morti di malattie varie. *Riv. Patol. Nerv. Ment.* 38, 152–378 [Plate 19, Figures 1–8].

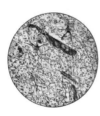

**FIGURE 287.**

Zanetti, 1931. Cortical histopathology.

Dis. da prep. Cajal-Bielschowsky. Reticulo fibrillare nevroglico e metamorfosi ameboide. Immers. 1/15 color.

Nat. Zanetti, G. (1931) Sulla struttura ed istogenesi della gomma cerebrale. *Riv. Patol. Nerv. Ment.* 37, 147–265 [Figure 26].

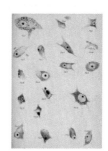

**FIGURE 288.**

Tronconi, 1932. Histology and histopathology of the dentate nucleus.

Fig. N. 1 – Cellula nervosa di struttura normale. Colorazione col metodo di Niss : X 950. Fig. N. 3-4-6-7 - Cellule nervose come si riscontrano sovente nella maggior parte dei casi. Tigrolisi, lieve eccentricità del nucleo; in complesso non segni di grave alterazione cellulare. Metodo di Nissl : X 650. Fig. N. 2 - Due cellule nervose piccole con segni di evidenti alterazioni sia a carico della struttura protoplasmatica sia del nucleo. Metodo di Nissl : X 650. Fig. N. 5 - Cellula nervosa con tigrolisi, eccentricità del nucleo ed evidente spostamento periferico del nucleolo. Metodo di Nissl : X 650. Fig. N. 8-9-10-11-14 - Altri tipi di cellule nervose nelle quali si osservano caratteri patologici (incipiente o completa tigrolisi, una struttura spongiosa del protoplasma, nucleo più o meno centrale ecc.). Si trovano in numerosi casi. Metodo di Bielschowsky-Plien: X 650. Fig. 12 - Cellula nervosa con eccentricità e scomparsa del nucleo che è distinguibile soltanto per la presenza del nucleolo. Metodo di Bielschowsky-Plien: X 650. Fig. N. 13-15 - Cellule nervose con evidente eccentricità del nucleo che fa ernia al di fuori del pirenoforo. Metodo di Bielschowsky-Plien: X 650. Fig. N. 16 - Cellula nervosa con limiti protoplasmatici indistinti; nucleo ridotto ad un piccolo spazio chiaro con nucleolo ipercromatico. Metodo di Bielschowsky-Plien: X 650. Fig. N. 17-18 – Cellule nervose con nucleo caratterizzato da aspetto granuloso, mammellonato. Evidenti alterazioni nella struttura protoplasmatica. Metodo di Bielschowsky-Plien: X 650 . Fig. N. 19 Cellula nervosa alterata nella forma. Addensameuto gliale perineuronico. Metodo di Bielschowsky-Plien: X 650. Tronconi, V. (1932) Osservazioni sulla fine struttura normale e patologica del Nucleo Dentato umano. *Riv. Patol. Nerv. Ment.* 40, 132–240 [Plate 1].